Manual of Anesthesia

Manual of Anesthesia

Second Edition

John C. Snow, M.D.
Professor of Anesthesiology,
Boston University School of Medicine;
University Hospital, Boston

Little, Brown and Company
Boston

Copyright © 1982 by John C. Snow

Second Edition

Published September 1982
Second Printing December 1982

Previous edition copyright © 1977 by
Little, Brown and Company (Inc.)

All rights reserved. No part of this book may be reproduced in any form or by any electronic or mechanical means, including information storage and retrieval systems, without permission in writing from the publisher, except by a reviewer who may quote brief passages in a review.

Library of Congress Catalog Card No.
82-82799

ISBN 0-316-80222-0

Printed in the United States of America

HAL

To Anne

Preface

The purpose of this edition, like that of its predecessor, is to present step by step the methods of anesthesia, together with management of specific anesthesia situations, and to provide a number of references for further study.

The **Manual of Anesthesia** has been written for clinical anesthesiologists, resident anesthesiologists, nurse-anesthetists, and medical and dental students. They will find herein the essentials of the practice of anesthesia in the operating room, the recovery room, the delivery room, the intensive care unit, and the emergency room.

For this second edition the format is unchanged, but the text has been revised and some of it has been rewritten. There have been added two new chapters: Blood Gases: Acid-Base Balance and Oxygen Transfer; and Invasive Hemodynamic Monitoring—including sections on arterial cannulation, central venous pressure monitoring, and pulmonary artery pressure monitoring (Swan-Ganz catheterization).

The second edition contains the latest information on malignant hyperthermia, diabetes, glycopyrrolate, pyridostigmine, nitroprusside, nitroglycerine, etidocaine, isoflurane, Norton's endotracheal tube, the fiberoptic laryngoscope and bronchoscope, and vitrectomy. In addition, a bibliography for further study has been added at the end of each of the 44 chapters.

In the practice of anesthesia, it is difficult to demonstrate that one technique is better than another. With experience, particular methods will come to be preferred by individual anesthesiologists and nurse-anesthetists. For this reason, although more than one technique is described for some of the procedures discussed here, most often no preference is stated.

I wish to express my deepest appreciation for reviewing parts of the manuscript to Drs. Donald Booth, Patrick J. Breen, George Chasapakis, Dusan B. Dobnik, Albert J. Finck, Alan W. Grogono, Istrati Kupeli, Demetrios G. Lappas, Howard M. Leibowitz, Simmons Lessell, John I. Loewenstein, Marlene R. Meyer, Martin L. Norton, Melvin M. Pick, Stanley M. Shapshay, and M. Stuart Strong.

For their fine chapters, I also owe many thanks to the contributing authors: Drs. George Chasapakis, Dusan B. Dobnik, Alan W. Grogono, Benjamin J. Kripke, Istrati Kupeli, Demetrios G. Lappas, Marlene R. Meyer, Martin L. Norton, and Melvin M. Pick.

I thank Mrs. Madeline Typadis for her help in correcting the manuscript and galley and page proofs.

I also extend my thanks to the members of the staff of the Medical Division of Little, Brown and Company and acknowledge their interest, advice, and guidance in the publication of the second edition of the *Manual of Anesthesia*.

J. C. S.

Contents

Contributing Authors

George Chasapakis, M.D., D.A. (London)	Director, Department of Anesthesiology and Intensive Care Unit, Municipal Hospital of Athens, Athens, Greece
Dusan B. Dobnik, M.D.	Associate Professor of Anesthesiology, Boston University School of Medicine; Associate Anesthesiologist, University Hospital, Boston
Alan W. Grogono, M.D., F.F.A.R.C.S.	Professor and Chairman, Department of Anesthesiology, Tulane Medical Center, New Orleans, Louisiana
Benjamin J. Kripke, M.D.	Professor of Anesthesiology, U.C.L.A. School of Medicine, Los Angeles; Chairman, Department of Anesthesiology, San Bernardino County Medical Center, San Bernardino, California
Istrati Kupeli, M.D.	Clinical Assistant in Anesthesia, Harvard Medical School; Associate in Anesthesia, Department of Surgery, New England Deaconess Hospital, The Faulkner Hospital, Boston
Demetrios G. Lappas, M.D.	Associate Professor of Anesthesia, Harvard Medical School; Associate Anesthetist, Massachusetts General Hospital, Boston
Marlene R. Meyer, M.D., J.D.	Instructor in Anesthesia, Harvard Medical School; Assistant Anesthetist, Massachusetts General Hospital, Boston
Martin L. Norton, M.D., J.D.	Professor of Anesthesiology, University of Michigan Hospital, Ann Arbor, Michigan
Melvin M. Pick, M.D.	Assistant Professor of Anesthesiology, University of Colorado Medical Center, Denver, Colorado; Chief, Anesthesiology, Anesthesia Department, St. Francis Hospital, Colorado Springs, Colorado

General Considerations

Notice The indications and dosages of all drugs in this manual have been recommended in the medical literature and conform to the practices of the general medical community. The medications described do not necessarily have specific approval by the Food and Drug Administration for use in the diseases and dosages for which they are recommended. The package insert for each drug should be consulted for use and dosage as approved by the FDA. Because standards for usage change, it is advisable to keep abreast of revised recommendations, particularly those concerning new drugs.

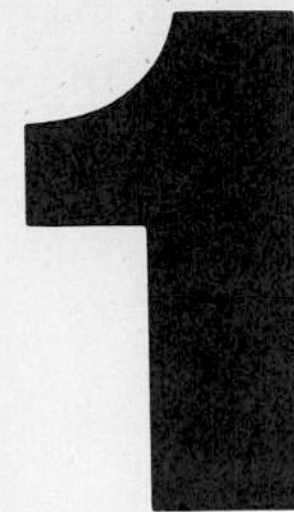

Preanesthetic Preparation of the Patient

I. The preanesthetic visit and examination

A. The preanesthetic visit and examination are an essential part of each patient's preparation and assessment prior to surgery. Customarily, this visit is made on the day before the operation. At this visit, information that is of importance to both the patient and the anesthesiologist is exchanged.

1. **A properly done visit** and examination is equivalent to pentobarbital 100 mg in its calming effect and is superior to the drug in terms of decreasing the patient's anxiety and providing emotional support.
2. **For elective operations,** admission to the hospital usually takes place 1 day before surgery. This permits time for a complete examination. If a patient has severe cardiac or pulmonary restrictions, more than 1 day may be required.
3. **An ambulatory program** may be allowed for admission early on the morning of surgery, provided the medical workup has been done within 2 days before or in the early morning prior to the operation. The **Joint Commission for Accreditation of Hospitals** requires that a patient's laboratory values be determined within 48 hr before surgery.
4. **The interview** should be carried out in such a way that meaningful information on the patient's status and experience can be gained by the anesthesiologist.

B. The preoperative visit and examination enable the anesthesiologist **to study the patient and his records,** to inspect the teeth, and to evaluate the patient's physical status, appearance, weight, and general condition.

1. **The patient's record** includes the history, preoperative physical examination findings, and essential laboratory data, including a complete blood count, urinalysis, electrolytes, and chest x-ray.
2. **An ECG** is recommended on all patients who are 35 years old or older and on younger ones as indicated.
3. On completion of study of the patient's records, the anesthesiologist proceeds to **examine the patient.**
   a. If the patient is a **minor,** the presence of the mother or father is a great help.
   b. **The questionnaire** includes previous experience with surgery and anesthesia, history of allergies to drugs, hay fever, bronchial asthma, diabetes, hypertension, blood dyscrasias, psychotic states, heart disease, chronic lung disease, or history of anesthetic problems in blood relatives.
   c. **The patient is questioned regarding his personal and social habits.**
   d. The patient is asked about the current use of such **medications** as insulin, oral antiglycemic agents, corticosteroids, nitroglycerine, anticoagulants, digitalis, narcotics, sedatives, amphetamines, or other psychotropic agents.

e. If a decision has been made to use **regional anesthesia,** the area selected for nerve block, spinal, epidural, or caudal anesthesia is examined, and a neurologic examination is done. If the patient is taking anticoagulants, regional anesthesia is contraindicated.

II. Other essential steps

A. During the preanesthetic visit, the anesthesiologist examines the patient's **teeth** and discusses the likelihood of damage during laryngoscopy and endotracheal anesthesia, especially if the teeth are loose or capped.

B. **Dentures** and removable bridges are removed and kept in the patient's room.

C. Patients scheduled for surgery must take **nothing by mouth** after midnight.

D. On completion of the examination, the anesthesiologist requests the patient to sign the **informed consent to anesthesia** form. If the patient is a **minor,** it is signed by a parent or a legal guardian.

E. **Finally,** the anesthesiologist writes the anesthesia summary on the patient's record, classifies the patient's physical status, orders the preanesthesia medication, and requests that the patient's records accompany the patient to the operating room.

F. **If a consultant is required,** the patient is referred to an internist or pediatrician. A consultant's advice is not binding, especially when it may deal with matters out of his area of specialization, such as anesthetic drugs or techniques. The role of the consultant is to ensure design of a program that will lead to an optimal preoperative status for the patient.

III. Drug interactions

A. **Smoking** one to two packs of cigarettes daily may be regarded as an indication of the presence of **chronic bronchitis.** Smoking should be decreased or stopped for 2 weeks prior to surgery to diminish coughing and secretions of the tracheobronchial tree.

B. Corticosteroids

1. The systemic administration of small amounts of corticosteroids is not without risk. **Therapeutic amounts of corticosteroids** result in functional depression and microscopic signs of atrophy of the **adrenal cortex.**
2. **In response to stress,** as with anesthesia and surgery, such a patient's adrenals may not secrete sufficient amounts of steroids required to meet the demand.
3. **The main manifestation of adrenocortical insufficiency** is hypotension.
4. If steroids have been administered during the previous 3 months for more than 1 week, **cortisone 100 mg** is administered IM in the evening and in the morning before surgery. In addition, 100 mg of hydrocortisone is diluted in 1000 ml of 5% D/W and is administered IV by a slow drip during the intraoperative and postoperative periods for at least 8–10 hr. Additional cortisone is administered during the following 2–3 postoperative days.

C. Antihypertensive agents

1. **The reserpine group of drugs** has been considered responsible for some cases of cardiovascular collapse encountered during the operative and postoperative periods.
2. Studies show that anesthetic drugs may be given safely to patients being maintained on **antihypertensive agents** and that an operation on such a patient need not be delayed.

3. **The fundamental cardiovascular defect** of these patients presents a greater-than-normal anesthetic hazard that demands preoperative medical evaluation and careful administration of the anesthetics.

D. Antibiotics

1. The administration of some antibiotics is followed by **respiratory insufficiency.** Their action has been described as intrinsically curare-like or synergistic to curare and certain anesthetics.

2. Studies and clinical experience have shown that **neuromuscular block** has been followed in patients receiving antibiotics such as neomycin, streptomycin, kanamycin, polymyxin B, bacitracin, viomycin, gentamicin, and colistin.

3. Some of these antibiotics are given **PO for intestinal antisepsis** before abdominal surgery, but there is no absorption from the intestines. However, if these antibiotics are administered by **injection, muscular paralysis and apnea** may result. Thus it is important that provisions be made for support of the patient's respiration during the postanesthesia period.

E. Levodopa and parkinsonism. Levodopa (Larodopa, Dopar) is administered for treatment of Parkinson's disease. It relieves the rigidity, tremor, and diminished mobility, but under anesthesia it may produce orthostatic hypotension and arrhythmias. In surgical patients under therapy with levodopa, treatment must be continued until the night before the operation and resumed as soon as possible postoperatively.

F. Monoamine oxidase inhibitors

1. Monoamine oxidase inhibitors are administered for the **treatment of mental disorders** associated with anxiety or depression.

2. The administration of monoamine oxidase inhibitors results in **increased production of norepinephrine, dopamine, and 5-hydroxytryptamine** with very dangerous and sometimes fatal reactions. These reactions may occur particularly in patients either receiving **sympathomimetic drugs** or meperidine, or ingesting foods and beverages with a high amine (tyramine) content (Chianti wine, ripe cheese, pickled herring).

3. **Monoamine oxidase inhibitors with vasopressors,** such as ephedrine, dopamine, and the amphetamines, may cause **forceful heartbeat, severe headache, and hypertension.** Some of these episodes have progressed to nausea, vomiting, stiff neck, and death due to intracranial hemorrhage.

4. When an attack of hypertension develops, **therapy** includes phentolamine (Regitine), trimethaphan (Arfonad), or nitroprusside (Nipride).

5. The monoamine oxidase inhibitors that may cause these reactions include amitriptyline (Elavil), tranylcypromine (Parnate), phenelzine (Nardil), and pargyline (Eutonyl).

G. Propranolol. The beta-adrenergic blocking drug propranolol (Inderal) is employed in the therapy of severe cardiac arrhythmias and to decrease the effort of the myocardium in angina pectoris. Propranolol is usually discontinued 12 hr prior to general anesthesia.

IV. Pulmonary function testing

A. A patient in the **acute phase of a respiratory infection** should not undergo surgery. At least a week must pass after complete recovery before surgery is rescheduled. General or spinal anesthesia is excluded in such patients for the following reasons:

1. **Trauma to an inflamed mucosal surface** may be caused by airway devices, and it is possible that sepsis will be introduced to the lower airway.

2. There is potential for occasional central nervous action from nasopharyngeal viruses.

B. Extreme cases of **respiratory insufficiency** are usually recognized, and preparations are made for postoperative support. However, many surgical patients have **borderline** respiratory insufficiency. These cases would include patients with obesity, spinal arthritis, obstructive lung disease, or a neuromuscular disorder.

1. Patients in these groups may lapse into **respiratory failure** when subjected to surgery involving the abdominal wall or intraperitoneal or intrathoracic organs.

2. The well-known decrease in the mechanical activity of breathing associated with incisions in these areas may leave a patient unable to cope with secretions and with an inappropriate sigh volume, leading to atelectasis and eventual pneumonia.

3. **Pulmonary function testing** of the vital capacity and timed vital capacity is an excellent screen for determining those patients at risk. Pulmonary function tests are ordered preoperatively in patients with the following histories:

   a. Smoking more than one pack of cigarettes per day.

   b. Chronic cough, whether or not productive.

   c. Obesity.

   d. Bronchial asthma.

   e. Bronchitis or emphysema.

   f. Neurologic or muscular disease.

   g. Arthritis or skeletal deformities involving the ribs or thoracic vertebrae.

   h. All patients undergoing thoracic or abdominal surgery; this includes procedures that involve the abdominal wall musculature, as in ventral or inguinal herniorrhaphy.

V. Anemia

A. The guideline that elective surgery should not be performed if the **hemoglobin** concentration is less than 10 gm/100 ml is no longer followed. Wide experience with little occurrence of morbidity in the care of patients with **chronic renal disease** whose hemoglobin bordered on 5–6 gm/100 ml has influenced this less dogmatic stance. However, **unexplained anemia** should stimulate efforts by the physician to better understand the patient before elective surgery.

B. The taking of the history may suffice to rule out the possibility of a **bleeding disorder.** Questions should be directed toward past experience with bleeding associated with tooth extractions, the catamenia, or trauma from play. It is well known that simple tests, such as bleeding or clotting times, are not reliable. If a positive history for a bleeding disorder is obtained, referral for a complete hematologic study prior to surgery is mandatory.

C. Normal circulating blood volume is more important than the red blood cell count in producing a stable circulating response to anesthesia or surgery.

1. The presence of a **normal hemoglobin or hematocrit** does not rule out a dangerously low blood volume, nor does the presence of anemia indicate that the blood volume is low.

2. **A simple method** that yields reliable numbers for most elective situations utilizes an indicator technique of radioactive iodinated serum albumin and a semiautomatic radioactivity counter and calculator. Valuable information is gained when blood volume determinations are made in patients with the following histories:

a. Chronic or acute hemorrhage.

b. Recent weight loss.

c. Anemia.

d. Prior to major traumatic surgery, such as abdominal-perineal resection, aortic aneurysmectomy, pancreatectomy, or total hip replacement.

3. **If more than a 20% reduction** is found, circulatory instability will be noted on induction of anesthesia, whether general or spinal. Such deviations should be treated prior to anesthesia so that all the signs of transfusion reaction can be noted.

VI. Patients who have recently eaten

A. No patient who has ingested food or drink within 6 hr of surgery is acceptable for anesthesia for **elective surgery.** This is a minimal time period; considerations of pain, other medications, marked anxiety, and the fat content of the last meal all influence gastric emptying time adversely and might justify prolongation beyond 6 hr.

B. **In an emergency situation,** it is necessary to go ahead rapidly if there are bona fide life-, limb-, or organ-threatening circumstances, even if the patient is not properly prepared. Of course, the anesthesiologist's fear in such a situation is that pulmonary aspiration may occur, with its more-than-theoretical potential for causing disability and even death. This potential for harm must be weighed against the gravity of the surgical emergency. If the surgeon decides that surgery is justifiable at that time, a note by him to this effect in the patient's chart will sanction the anesthesiologist's presence and action in behalf of the patient.

C. Acceptance of a patient for anesthesia, general or local, involves **medicolegal considerations and responsibilities.** If advice with regard to deferring a case is not heeded, the anesthesiologist will continue to assist and support the patient, with the clear understanding that no depressants nor analgesics will be used in conjunction with local anesthesia.

VII. **Emergencies.** There are a few acute emergency situations that demand immediate surgical intervention without regard to the patient's situation. Among these are airway obstruction, uncontrolled hemorrhage, rapidly increasing intracranial pressure, ruptured aortic aneurysm, and cardiac tamponade.

VIII. **Physical status.** The classification of physical status adopted by the American Society of Anesthesiologists is as follows:

Class 1: A normal, healthy person.

Class 2: A patient with a mild systemic disease.

Class 3: A patient with a severe systemic disease that limits activity but is not incapacitating.

Class 4: A patient with an incapacitating systemic disease that is a constant threat to life.

Class 5: A moribund patient who is not expected to survive 24 hr with or without surgery.

Emergency (E): A patient in one of the preceding classes who is undergoing surgery as an emergency. The letter E is written next to the numerical classification.

Bibliography

Cullen, B. F., and Miller, M. G. Drug interactions and anesthesia. A review. *Anesth. Analg.* (Cleve.) 58:413, 1979.

Dornette, W. H. L. Informed consent and anesthesia. *Anesth. Analg.* (Cleve.) 53:832, 1974.

Kaplan, J. A., and Dunbar, R. W. Propranolol and surgical anesthesia. *Anesth. Analg.* (Cleve.) 55:1, 1976.

Lankton, J. W., Batcheder, B. M., and Ominsky, A. J. Emotional response to a detailed risk disclosure for anesthesia, a prospective, randomized study. *Anesthesiology* 46:294, 1977.

Lappas, D. G., Powell, M. W. J., and Daggett, W. M. Cardiac dysfunction in the perioperative period. Pathophysiology, diagnosis, and treatment. *Anesthesiology* 47:117, 1977.

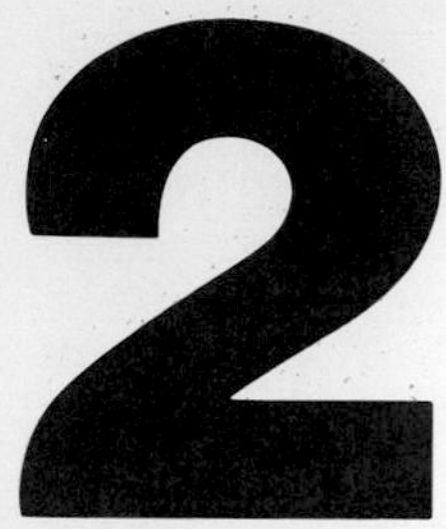

Choice of Anesthesia

I. **General comments.** In a general hospital, about 70–75% of surgery is performed under general anesthesia, and the remainder is performed under regional or local anesthesia. Operations about the head, neck, chest, and abdomen are best performed under general endotracheal anesthesia, since with this method the airway is free and under control at all times. However, the final decision concerning the type of anesthesia to be employed rests with the anesthesiologist in consultation with the surgeon.

II. **Factors in selecting the type of anesthesia**

A. **Age**

1. **In infants and children,** general anesthesia is the method of choice.

2. **In adults,** short and superficial procedures call for local anesthesia.

B. **Physical status of the patient**

1. **Preoperative disease.** Some anesthetic drugs are poorly accepted by patients with certain diseases, such as muscle relaxants in a patient who has had poliomyelitis with involvement of the chest muscles or in a patient with myasthenia gravis. Spinal anesthesia is contraindicated in a patient with diabetic neuropathy or central nervous system syphilis. Regional or spinal anesthesia is contraindicated in a patient on anticoagulant therapy.

2. **Severe impairment of the vital functions,** particularly reduction of the pulmonary or cardiovascular reserve, dictates use of regional or local anesthesia.

3. **Emotional, mentally ill, uncooperative, senile, or disoriented patients** are candidates for general anesthesia.

4. **In an obese patient** with a short, thick neck, airway obstruction easily develops soon after induction of general anesthesia. Regional or spinal anesthesia may be a better selection. If general anesthesia is indicated, it must be endotracheal anesthesia.

C. **Type of surgery.** Lengthy operations require general anesthesia. In addition, procedures performed in prone, lateral, or other awkward positions require general endotracheal anesthesia to secure satisfactory control of ventilation.

D. **The skill and requirements of the surgeon.** The presence of electrocautery, the need for muscle relaxation in abdominal operations, the use of epinephrine solution during ear, oral, or plastic surgery, and the skill of the surgeon are important factors in selecting the anesthetic agents and techniques.

E. **The skill and preference of the anesthesiologist.** An anesthesiologist who is experienced in a variety of anesthetic methods and drugs may apply the experience to solving the problem of choice of anesthesia. In some situations one technique and drug may be preferable to another in the hands of a particular anesthesiologist. Following the study of all the factors, indications, and contraindications, the final selection of techniques and agents is often a matter of personal experience and preference.

F. **The patient's wishes.** A few patients insist on general anesthesia in spite of the surgeon's assurance that the operation can be performed under regional or local anesthesia. The patient's wishes are respected only if his condition permits it and the success of surgery will not be jeopardized.

G. **Presence of fire and explosion dangers.** Use of nonflammable and nonexplosive anesthetics is mandatory when there is risk of fire or explosion hazards.

H. **Teaching purposes.** In teaching institutions the operations last longer, and general anesthesia is the choice, particularly for lengthy procedures. In these operative situations, the instructor and resident physicians are more relaxed and can speak freely, without the need to choose their words carefully to avoid alarming the patient. If regional or local anesthesia is selected, however, the patient is well sedated.

Bibliography

Bamford, C., Sibley, W., and Laguna, J. Anesthesia in multiple sclerosis. *Can. J. Neurol. Sci.* 5:41, 1978.

Foex, P. Preoperative assessment of patients with cardiac disease. *Br. J. Anaesth.* 50:15, 1978.

Hannallah, R., and Rosales, J. K. Acute epiglottitis: Current management and review. *Can. Anaesth. Soc. J.* 25:84, 1978.

Mustajoki, P., and Heinonen, J. General anesthesia in "inducible" porphyrias. *Anesthesiology* 53:15, 1980.

Tinker, J. H., Noback, C. R., Vlietstra, R. E., et al. Management of patients with heart disease for noncardiac surgery. *J.A.M.A.* 246:1348, 1981.

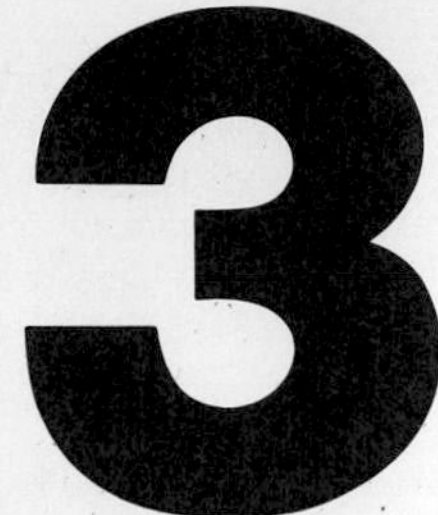

Preanesthesia Medication

I. General comments

A. Purposes of preanesthetic medication

1. Psychic sedation to allay apprehension.
2. Amnesia.
3. Analgesia.
4. Smoother, easier induction of anesthesia.
5. Reduction in the amount of drug needed for local, regional, or general anesthesia.
6. Decreased undesirable reflexes.
7. Diminished flow of secretions in the upper respiratory tract.
8. Inhibition of nausea and vomiting.

B. Criteria for prescribing preanesthesia medication

1. **The preoperative anesthetic agents,** usually prescribed in combination, include sedatives, tranquilizers, phenothiazines, narcotics, and belladonna alkaloids. These agents may be given intravenously in the operating room just before the induction of anesthesia.
2. **Drugs are administered** according to the patient's age, sex, weight, and general physical and mental condition, as well as the type of operation to be performed. All drugs used in premedication are given IM; oral administration is not recommended, since absorption is slow and not dependable.
3. **The metabolism of drugs** may be delayed during anesthesia and surgery. Their action may be prolonged for 4–6 hr during the recovery period.
4. **Patients who are acutely or chronically ill,** those who have heart disease, those who are elderly, anemic, or febrile; or patients with hypothyroidism or esophageal stenosis require considerably smaller amounts of drugs than others, since they already exhibit a degree of psychic or physical depression. Conversely, patients who are emotionally unstable, apprehensive, or addicted to drugs may require heavy premedication.
5. **In the presence of pain,** analgesics are always indicated; barbiturates are contraindicated.
6. Barbiturates are contraindicated in the presence of an **acute intermittent porphyria.** This rare metabolic disease is exacerbated by the administration of barbiturates, causing episodes of acute abdominal pain, paralysis, psychiatric manifestations, and the passage of reddish urine; a fatal outcome is possible.
7. For patients with a history of **bronchial asthma** or allergies, hydroxyzine (Vistaril), with or without diphenhydramine (Benadryl), is preferred to pentobarbital (Nembutal).

8. Patients who have been receiving **corticosteroids** for more than a week during the preceding 3 months are given 100 mg of cortisone IM in the evening and again in the morning prior to surgery. In addition, 100 mg of hydrocortisone diluted in 1000 ml of 5% D/W or lactated Ringer's solution is infused IV by a very slow drip during the intraoperative and postoperative periods for 8–10 hr. Additional hydrocortisone is given for the following 2–3 postoperative days.
9. **Chronic alcohol abuse** increases the patient's tolerance for barbiturates and general anesthetic agents. Postoperative seizures may be prevented by administering 200 mg of phenytoin sodium (Dilantin) IM preoperatively and 100 mg tid for 2–3 days postoperatively. Delirium tremens, or the onset of withdrawal symptoms, may be prevented by IV injection of alcohol during the postoperative period, along with liberal use of chlordiazepoxide (Librium) or diazepam (Valium).
10. The belladonna drugs are not contraindicated in patients with a history of **glaucoma.**
11. If surgery is delayed for 1–2 hr or lasts for more than 3 hr, **atropine** may be repeated, since there is no risk of toxic reactions to the repeated injections.

II. Modes of administration. For adults and children in reasonably good health, the following preanesthetic drugs are recommended for IM administration:

A. For local or regional anesthesia in adults

1. Nothing by mouth after midnight.
2. Pentobarbital, 100 mg PO at bedtime.
3. Pentobarbital, 100 mg IM 2 hr preoperatively.
4. Diazepam (Valium), 10 mg PO, or meperidine (Demerol), 75 mg, or morphine, 10 mg, IM 1 hr preoperatively.

Or

1. Nothing by mouth after midnight.
2. Pentobarbital, 100 mg PO at bedtime.
3. Innovar, 1–2 ml IM 1 hr preoperatively.

B. For general anesthesia in adults

1. Nothing by mouth after midnight.
2. Pentobarbital, 100 mg PO at bedtime.
3. Pentobarbital, 100 mg IM 2 hr preoperatively.
4. Atropine, 0.5 mg SQ 1 hr preoperatively.

Or

1. Nothing by mouth after midnight.
2. Pentobarbital, 100 mg PO at bedtime.
3. Innovar, 1–2 ml IM 1 hr preoperatively.
4. Atropine, 0.5 mg SQ 1 hr preoperatively.

C. For general anesthesia in children

1. **A hypnotic,** with or without morphine, is ordered both for amnesia and to reduce fear and excitement. Atropine is also given to inhibit secretions and vagal tone. The combination of a barbiturate and a belladonna derivative is satisfactory.
2. **The dosages of preanesthetic agents** are calculated according to the patient's age, weight, and general condition (Table 3-1). Pentobarbital or sec-

Table 3-1. Premedication for Children

Age	Weight		Pentobarbital or Secobarbital	Morphine	Atropine or Scopolamine
Newborn	7 lb	3.5 kg	—	—	0.1 mg
6 months	16 lb	7.5 kg	—	—	0.1 mg
1 year	22 lb	10 kg	35 mg	1 mg	0.2 mg
2 years	26.5 lb	12 kg	50 mg	1.2 mg	0.3 mg
4 years	33 lb	15 kg	65 mg	1.5 mg	0.3 mg
6 years	44 lb	20 kg	75 mg	2 mg	0.4 mg
8 years	55 lb	25 kg	90 mg	2.5 mg	0.4 mg
10 years	66 lb	30 kg	100 mg	3 mg	0.4 mg
12 years	88 lb	40 kg	100 mg	4 mg	0.4 mg

obarbital (Seconal) is prescribed for the mother if she stays with the child overnight. The following schedule is recommended for general anesthesia in children:

a. Nothing by mouth after midnight.

b. Pentobarbital, ______ mg IM 2 hr preoperatively (see Table 3-1).

c. Atropine, ______ mg SQ 1 hr preoperatively (see Table 3-1).

III. Sedatives

A. Pentobarbital and secobarbital

1. These barbiturates are administered before surgery, most often to **relieve anxiety and tension.** They have a short hypnotic effect and a pronounced sedative action. Barbiturates have no analgesic effect in the doses prescribed for premedication.

2. Pentobarbital (Nembutal) and secobarbital (Seconal) have minimal depressant effects on ventilation and circulation; their main effect is **cerebral cortical depression.** On the average, patients receiving these drugs awaken more easily from general anesthesia than if a narcotic had been administered, but the incidence of emergence excitement tends to be higher, because barbiturates lack analgesic action.

3. No teratogenic effects on the **embryo** have been observed.

4. These barbiturates are detoxified mainly in the **liver;** for this reason, barbiturates are useful in patients with impaired kidney function. While they may relieve that part of pain associated with apprehension, they also may cause delirium in the presence of pain and may be habit-forming.

5. **These barbiturates may be prescribed PO or IM** for adults in doses of 100 mg (1.5 mg/kg) and for children in doses of 3–4 mg/kg. Sedation occurs in 60 min, reaches its maximum peak effect in 1–1½ hr, and lasts 3–4 hr. The IM injection is preferable, but there is pain at the site of injection when barbiturates are administered SQ because of the solvent propylene glycol.

B. Phenobarbital

1. Phenobarbital is excreted through the **kidney,** so it is the indicated barbiturate in patients with impaired liver function.

2. In adults, the sedative dose of phenobarbital is 15–30 mg, and the hypnotic dose is 100 mg. It may be administered PO or IM.

C. Chloral hydrate

1. **This safe, well-tolerated drug** is one of the oldest and best hypnotics. It very seldom causes excitement or delirium except in the presence of pain. It is a perfect alternative to secobarbital or pentobarbital, particularly for elderly patients.

2. Chloral hydrate is hydroscopic and causes gastric irritation associated with nausea and emesis. It is tolerated best if prescribed in capsules (Noctec or Somnos).

3. In adults the dose is 0.5–1 gm PO. Sedation occurs within 30 min; sleep occurs within the hour and lasts 5–6 hr. There are no unpleasant aftereffects.

D. Diazepam

1. **Diazepam produces a satisfactory sedative and amnesic** effect with minimal action on circulation. However, as the dose is increased, increased depression of respiration occurs. Diazepam is indicated to prevent or treat **convulsions,** and it is the drug of choice prior to cardioversion of arrhythmias and cardiac catheterization. IV injection causes pain at the injection site, and the possibility of phlebitis exists. When diazepam is administered prophylactically to animals, an increase in the lethal dosage of the local anesthetic agents is observed.

2. Diazepam is frequently ordered to premedicate surgical patients. The dosage is 5–10 mg 1 hr before the induction of anesthesia. It is administered PO with 30 ml of water. The absorption is better by the gastrointestinal route than by IM injection.

E. Hydroxyzine

1. **Hydroxyzine (Vistaril) has sedative, antihistaminic, antiemetic, and bronchodilating properties.** It is classified as a psychotherapeutic antihistamine. Because it is a central nervous system depressant, it is used clinically as a calming drug to relieve anxiety and tension.

2. **No toxic effects of hydroxyzine on the liver** or blood-forming organs have been reported, and there are no adverse effects on ventilation, blood pressure, or heart rate. However, hydroxyzine may increase the effects of the other central nervous system depressants, narcotics, and barbiturates.

3. Hydroxyzine is an **effective premedicant** that is tolerated by all age groups, particularly in patients with a history of bronchial asthma. The dosage is 50–100 mg IM in adults and 1 mg/kg IM in children. Deep IM administration via the Z method is advised.

F. Droperidol-fentanyl (Innovar)

1. Innovar is a 50:1 mixture of droperidol and fentanyl (the latter is a narcotic analgesic). The two drugs are formulated in solution, of which 1 ml contains 2.5 mg of droperidol and 0.05 mg of fentanyl. Innovar is injected IM or IV. The effects of Innovar can be described best as a combination of those produced by droperidol and fentanyl (see **G** and sec. **IV.A**).

2. **As premedication,** the dosage is 1–2 ml IM 1 hr preoperatively.

G. Droperidol

1. The main effects of droperidol (Inapsine) appear to be **tranquillity** and peripheral vasodilation. When infused intravenously, droperidol produces sleepiness and mental detachment, which may last for several hours. It decreases blood pressure very little, controls emesis, and decreases the increased blood pressure caused by injection of epinephrine and norepinephrine.

2. In large doses, this drug may produce **uncoordinated muscular movements** that simulate extrapyramidal effects (akathisia, dystonia, and oculogyric crises). These may be controlled or reversed with antiparkinsonism drugs.

3. **As premedication,** the dosage for adults is 2.5–5 mg (1–2 ml) IM 1 hr preoperatively. This tranquilizing agent takes effect 5–10 min following IV or IM injection, and the effects are detectable 6–12 hr after a single dose.

IV. Narcotic analgesics

A. Fentanyl

1. Fentanyl (Sublimaze) is a powerful **narcotic analgesic.** It produces depression of ventilation and transient rigidity of the somatic musculature. Fentanyl does not release histamine. It may cause euphoria and miosis and, very rarely, hypotension. It has a strong cholinergic action that is mediated through the vagus nerve; this effect may be blocked by atropine.

2. **Ventilatory depression** appears to be more rapid following the injection of fentanyl than after other potent narcotics. However, this action is of short duration and is reversed by the injection of a narcotic antagonist, such as naloxone. Too-rapid injection of fentanyl may result in rigidity of muscles, particularly the muscles of the thorax, abdomen, and extremities.

3. **During surgery,** the use of muscle relaxants reverses any muscular rigidity that may be produced by fentanyl.

4. **As premedication,** the dosage is 0.05–0.1 mg (1–2 ml) IM 1 hr preoperatively. The peak effect is reached within 3–5 min following IV administration, and the analgesic effect lasts 50–60 min. The analgesic action of fentanyl rarely continues much into the postoperative period. Following IM injection, the onset of effect takes place within 7–8 min, and the duration of action is 1–2 hr.

B. Morphine

1. Morphine is the **standard analgesic narcotic drug** for the relief of severe pain. It depresses the central nervous system, including the respiration and cough reflex centers. In addition, it decreases gastrointestinal motility, causing constipation; it produces biliary spasm; it constricts the bronchi; and it lowers the metabolic rate. Morphine has sedative and strong analgesic properties.

2. Morphine is **contraindicated** for intraocular surgery because it frequently causes emesis. It is also contraindicated in acute alcoholism, bronchial asthma, intracranial injury, ureteral obstruction, and respiratory obstruction.

3. The **adult dose** is 10–15 mg, injected IM or SQ. The effects last 6–10 hr. The **dose in children** is 0.1 mg/kg. Morphine 1.5–3 mg IV is a satisfactory analgesic and sedative drug in the postanesthesia recovery room.

4. It should be kept in mind when using morphine that excessive depression of the **cough reflex** during the postoperative course may result in the accumulation of pulmonary secretions and thus may cause atelectasis, particularly in patients with chronic pulmonary diseases.

C. Meperidine

1. Meperidine (Demerol) has **analgesic, sedative, and spasmolytic** properties. In conjunction with barbiturates, it induces amnesia. This drug also produces dryness of the mouth, sweating, flushing of the face, minimal respiratory depression, euphoria, dizziness, and emesis. **More severe reactions** include fainting, great weakness, profuse perspiration, and marked dizziness. Meperidine also greatly decreases corneal sensitivity.

2. Meperidine is **contraindicated** in patients with atrial flutter or intracranial lesions that cause increased intracranial pressure.

3. The **adult dose** of meperidine is 50–100 mg, and in **children** it is 1–2 mg/kg, injected IM or SQ at 3-hr or 4-hr intervals. The effects last 3–4 hr. When meperidine is injected IM, the analgesic action occurs within 15 min, and the peak effect is apparent in 45–60 min. When it is infused IV, the analgesic effect becomes evident immediately, and the full effect is reached in 15 min.

D. **Other synthetic narcotic analgesics** are alphaprodine (Nisentil) 20–40 mg IM, oxymorphone (Numorphan) 0.5–1.5 mg IM, anileridine (Leritine) 25–50 mg IM, and pentazocine (Talwin) 30–50 mg IM.

E. **Undesirable side effects**

1. Narcotic analgesic agents may produce the following side effects: **respiratory depression,** circulatory depression, pupillary constriction, psychomimetic effects, **emesis,** and **physical dependence.** Peristalsis is decreased, causing constipation. The smooth muscles in the biliary tract, ureter, and bronchioles are constricted, and the release of histamine results in bronchoconstriction.

2. **Patients with bronchial asthma,** kyphoscoliosis, pulmonary emphysema, or cor pulmonale react poorly to narcotics.

3. Because of placental transfer, there is a respiratory depression in the **fetus** when a narcotic is given to the mother.

4. **Undesirable effects** are much more common with narcotics than with nonbarbiturate sedatives, barbiturates, and some of the tranquilizers.

5. **Narcotics may be habit-forming** and are subject to the U.S.A. Controlled Substance Act of 1970.

F. **Narcotic antagonist**

1. **Naloxone** (Narcan) is a satisfactory narcotic antagonist of the respiratory depression induced by narcotics.

2. The **adult dose** is 0.2–0.4 mg (0.5–1.0 ml) IV.

3. Naloxone reverses the analgesic effects of the narcotics.

V. Tranquilizers: Phenothiazines

A. Phenothiazines are prescribed for preanesthetic medication because of their sedative, antiemetic, antihistaminic, and temperature-regulating effects.

B. The phenothiazines vary in degree of **side effects,** which include **extrapyramidal excitation,** agranulocytosis, photosensitivity, jaundice, and pigmentary retinopathy. **Hypotension and postanesthetic lethargy** may appear in the postoperative recovery period. Depression of respiration is increased and prolonged when narcotics are given in association with phenothiazines. Slough or gangrene has been observed following the IV injection of phenothiazines; this complication can be prevented by diluting the IV solution.

C. **Contraindications.** Phenothiazines increase cortical motor activity in patients with epileptiform electroencephalographic patterns. Therefore this group of drugs must be avoided in patients with a history of convulsions, especially those associated with epilepsy.

D. These drugs may be administered PO, IM, or IV. The **single IM dose** for an adult is as follows:
Chlorpromazine (Thorazine) 15–25 mg.
Promazine (Sparine) 25–50 mg.
Triflupromazine (Vesprin) 20–40 mg.
Prochlorperazine (Compazine) 5–10 mg.
Promethazine (Phenergan) 25–50 mg.

VI. Belladonna compounds (atropine and scopolamine)

A. Atropine

1. **Atropine decreases secretions** and is the drug of choice to reduce bronchial and cardiac effects of parasympathetic origin. **It increases the heart rate** by blocking the vagus nerve. Atropine also **stimulates the cortex.** It relaxes the smooth muscles in various organs and is indicated for the relief of gastrointestinal spasm and in treatment of parkinsonism. Atropine does not prevent the appearance of laryngospasm associated with general anesthetics.

2. Atropine is superior to scopolamine as a **vagolytic** agent. This vagolytic effect is important, especially in the presence of vagotonic agents, such as halothane (Fluothane) and succinylcholine. Atropine can prevent severe bradycardia and asystole. **Bradycardia** and **hypotension** resulting from reflex stimulation may occur during intrathoracic, abdominal, neck, or eye surgery. IV-injected atropine may restore heart rate and blood pressure to normal.

3. Atropine and scopolamine are **bronchodilators** and are indicated in relieving bronchospasm.

4. Patients who are **allergic** to atropine may be given scopolamine and the antiallergic drug diphenhydramine (Benadryl).

5. When drops of atropine solution are **applied topically,** the pupil is dilated and the ciliary muscle used for accommodation is paralyzed. However, **systemic** use of atropine as a preoperative medication has minimal effect on the smooth muscle of the iris. The recommended parenteral dose of **atropine for premedication does not increase intraocular pressure** and is not contraindicated in patients with **glaucoma.** If an increased intraocular pressure occurs in a patient with **narrow-angle glaucoma,** topically applied **pilocarpine** will counteract this effect.

6. **Blacks** are prescribed higher doses of atropine or scopolamine because they have increased production of secretions within the respiratory tract.

B. Scopolamine

1. Scopolamine is an effective drug for **psychic sedation** and **amnesia.** The **drying effect** is superior to that of atropine, but it is less effective than atropine in preventing reflex bradycardia during general anesthesia, particularly in children.

2. **Rarely,** excitement, restlessness, disorientation, and **prolonged postoperative emergence** are seen. These occurrences may be treated effectively with **physostigmine (Antilirium)** 1–3 mg IV.

3. A child awakens faster in the postanesthesia recovery room if he is premedicated with atropine than with scopolamine.

C. Atropine and scopolamine

1. Atropine or scopolamine can be injected SQ, IM, or IV. The **adult dose** is 0.5 mg SQ (for **children,** 0.1–0.4 mg).

2. **The onset of action** occurs within 10–15 min, and the effects last for 90 min. A larger dosage of atropine (1–2 mg) is necessary for a major blockade of the vagus nerve prior to use of **neostigmine (Prostigmin)** or for treatment of **organophosphate poisoning.**

D. Side effects of atropine and scopolamine

1. Following therapeutic doses, there is drying of the mouth and blurring of vision.

2. Patients receiving belladonna derivatives may complain of uncomfortable

Table 3-2. Effects of Atropine and Scopolamine on Secretions, Cardiac Vagus Nerve, Eye, and Central Nervous System

Drug	Effect on Secretions	Effect on Cardiac Vagus Nerve	Effect on Eye	Effect on CNS
Atropine	Effective	Effective	Mydriasis	Stimulates
Scopolamine	Effective	Less than atropine	Less than atropine	Depresses cortex

dryness of the mouth. Therefore it is preferable that atropine or scopolamine be omitted in patients scheduled for surgery to be performed under **local or regional anesthesia.**

3. Atropine or scopolamine is administered with caution to patients with **fever** and **cardiac abnormalities,** especially atrial fibrillation.
4. The reduced tone of the urinary bladder may lead to **urinary retention,** particularly in the presence of prostatic hypertrophy.
5. A **blotchy rash** may be seen in children, but this is insignificant.
6. **Heat retention** with increased temperature may appear in children, especially in the hot summer months or when they are ill or dehydrated. In these conditions, decreased doses of belladonna compounds are infused IV prior to induction of anesthesia.
7. A toxic dose may produce restlessness, giddiness, hallucinations, and confusion. **Treatment** includes 1–3 mg of physostigmine IV.

E. **Summary.** See Table 3-2.

F. **Glycopyrrolate**

1. Glycopyrrolate (Robinul) is a synthetic anticholinergic drug and antagonizes the **muscarinic effects** such as bradycardia, bronchospasm, bronchorrhea, and intestinal hypermotility.
2. It can be injected **in place of atropine** in the reversal of nondepolarizing muscle blockade with neostigmine or pyridostigmine. The dose is half that of atropine.
3. The **tachycardia** produced by glucopyrrolate is less than with atropine, but the protection against vagal-induced bradycardia is greater.
4. Glycopyrrolate does not cross the blood-brain barrier, and thus it does not have mind-confusing and central stimulating properties.
5. **Peak effects** occur in 45 min. The vagal blocking effects persist for 2–3 hr, and the antisialagogue action remains up to 7 hr. With IV administration, the effect is present within 1 min.
6. It is injected SQ, IM, or IV. The **dose** is 0.1–0.2 mg.

Bibliography

Conner, J. T., Bellville, J. W., Wender, R., et al. Morphine, scopolamine and atropine as intravenous surgical premedicants. *Anesth. Analg.* (Cleve.) 56:606, 1977.

Forrest, W. H., Brown, C. R., and Brown, B. W. Subjective responses to six common preoperative medications. *Anesthesiology* 47:241, 1977.

Gal, T. J., and Suratt, P. M. Atropine and glycopyrrolate effects on lung mechanics in normal man. *Anesth. Analg.* (Cleve.) 60:85, 1981.

McCubbin, T. D., Brown, J. H., Dewar, K. M. S., et al. Glycopyrrolate as a premedicant. Comparison with atropine. *Br. J. Anaesth.* 51:885, 1979.

Rieser, J. C., and Snow, J. C. Atropine and glaucoma. *Anesth. Analg.* (Cleve.) 55:460, 1976.

Shutt, L. E., and Bowes, J. B. Atropine and hyoscine. *Anaesthesia* 34:476, 1979.

Tornetta, F. J. A comparison of droperidol, diazepam, and hydroxyzine as premedication. *Anesth. Analg.* (Cleve.) 56:496, 1977.

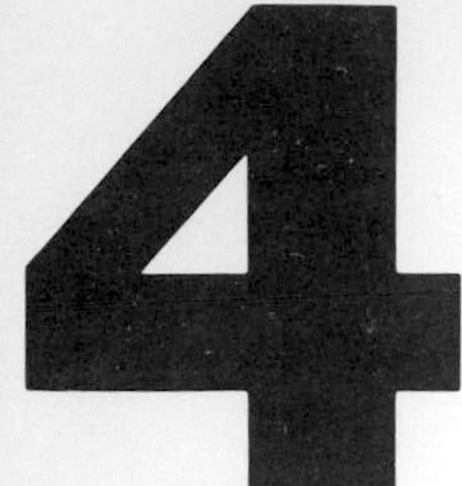

Medicolegal Aspects of Anesthesia

I. Background and present trends

A. The number of legal actions against physicians is increasing every year. According to the American Medical Association, one out of four physicians currently practicing in the United States will be sued for malpractice before the end of his career.

B. In recent years, anesthesiology has become one of the most litigious areas of medicine.

II. Precautions against malpractice claims and their consequences

A. Today, every anesthesiologist should be aware of the possibility of malpractice suits and of the need for protection against them. The main purpose of malpractice insurance is to provide recompense for the patient while at the same time assuring the physician of legal representation. Secondarily, it provides a source of funds that will prevent depletion of the physician's personal and family resources.

B. Discuss complications with the patient and family and the referring and/or operating physician. State the facts only and not opinions as to propriety of action. **Communication** is the best malpractice defense when coupled with good medical practices.

C. The plaintiffs' main complaints in suits against anesthesiologists indicate the following areas for caution:

1. Overdosage of anesthetic drugs.
2. Injury from the mask, mouth gag, improper position on the operating table, or struggling.
3. Damage to eyes or skin.
4. Damage to teeth.
5. Spinal anesthesia administered without the patient's consent.
6. Injury from improperly conducted spinal anesthesia.
7. Fire, explosion, and burns from electrocautery (improper grounding).
8. Injury in the postanesthesia recovery room.
9. Death of the patient as a result of anesthetic mismanagement.

D. Recommended precautions to prevent malpractice claims

1. Public criticism of the work of other physicians should be avoided, although proper peer review is indicated.
2. Complete medical records must be kept.
3. It should be remembered that promising the patient too much or guaranteeing results sets up a basis for complaints.

4. Equipment must be examined regularly, and every possible safety installation must be used.

5. Preoperative consultation by the anesthesiologist with the patient will reduce the possibility of misunderstanding concerning the administration of anesthesia.

6. The anesthesiologist must have adequate malpractice insurance coverage to protect the patient's rights and to avoid personal financial catastrophe in professional liability judgments.

III. The informed consent doctrine

A. General considerations

1. A **mentally competent adult has the right to decide** what will be done with his body. Any intentional touching of a person without the person's consent constitutes a battery.

2. The anesthesiologist who administers anesthetic agents without **the patient's written informed consent** risks a charge of battery for which he is liable in damages, except in the following circumstances:

   a. **Emergencies** (for saving life, limb, or a vital organ).

   b. **Legally designated minors** (for treatment related to drug addiction, pregnancy, venereal disease).

   c. Patients under the **influence of drugs or alcohol** to the point of mental incompetence (this is a gray area in law, and consent of the next of kin or guardian should be obtained).

3. It is very important that the **written informed consent be properly executed** during the preoperative visit and before the preanesthesia medication is given.

4. **A consent to surgery** does not necessarily imply consent to the use of anesthetics; a written informed consent for each must be obtained. The anesthesiologist and the surgeon may be jointly responsible for each other's omissions and acts.

5. **The doctrine of informed consent** holds a physician liable for any unfortunate result of therapy if the patient is not made fully aware of the nature, extent, and risks of the operation. Except in an acute emergency, the patient must be given a nontechnical explanation of the planned treatment, its associated hazards, complications, and chances of success or failure, and this must be done without causing undue apprehension. The patient should also be informed about alternatives to the planned surgical and anesthetic procedures and the possible consequences of those alternatives. When it is possible, the patient must be given a choice.

B. Minors or mentally incompetent persons

1. If a patient is either a **minor or mentally incompetent,** the written informed consent must be received from a **parent** or **guardian.** No anesthetic drugs can be administered to a child until informed consent is obtained by a parent or guardian. If the parents are divorced, consent should be obtained from the parent who has custody of the minor.

2. In case of an **emergency**, if a parent or guardian cannot be found, the physician must do for the child or mentally incompetent person what the situation requires. The question of the existence of an emergency is decided by the physician who has responsibility for the minor (this is a joint responsibility of the surgeon and the anesthesiologist as well as the referring physician).

IV. General considerations

A. All patients, especially children, must at all times wear **identification bracelets or name tags** bearing the hospital's unit number.

B. Negligence is defined as a breach of a duty owed by one person to another in which injury to the latter results. The plaintiff-patient, to obtain a verdict and judgment against an anesthesiologist, must plead and prove that the physician failed to exercise the degree of care ordinarily exercised by the reasonable and prudent physician in similar circumstances. When there are claims based on negligence and maltreatment, adequate compensation is legally available and morally sanctioned. It is desirable to reach a satisfactory settlement and, if possible, to avoid trial.

C. *Res ipsa loquitur*

1. In certain limited factual circumstances, the plaintiff will plead *res ipsa loquitur*, which means "the act speaks for itself." It is implied that the planned instrumentality (procedure) or method, if used with care, would not, under normal circumstances, cause such damage. The instrumentality must be under the control of the physician-defendant.

2. If the plaintiff is not in a position to obtain expert medical testimony, the court may invoke the doctrine of *res ipsa loquitur*.

D. Interns, residents, and fellows may be held liable for negligence, along with the supervising anesthesiologist, the surgeon, and the hospital's director. They must also carry malpractice insurance.

E. The nurse-anesthetist and anesthesiologist's assistants are also open to court action for negligence connected with their acts during the administration of anesthetics. Supervising anesthesiologists or surgeons are held responsible for their acts under the doctrine of *respondeat superior*, by which principals are responsible for the acts of their agents. This does not relieve the nurse-anesthetist or anesthesia assistant from liability.

F. Records. The case history, preoperative anesthesia conference with the patient, physical examination findings, and laboratory workup should all be entered in the patient's record before any anesthetic is administered. In addition to the preanesthesia history and examination, detailed records of the actual anesthetic procedure and the postanesthesia visit must be kept. If a patient's record must be changed postoperatively, a note to this effect should be made, so that any subsequently recorded information or change is very clearly an addition. **The records of the hospital** and/or physician are always demanded in a medicolegal case, and their degree of thoroughness and accuracy can be vital to the outcome of the suit.

G. Jehovah's Witnesses

1. Jehovah's Witnesses' interpretation of the Scriptures has caused them to believe that blood is sacred, and that therefore they must "abstain from blood." In addition, the Bible says that blood removed from a body must be disposed of. This rules out all blood and blood products transfusions for Jehovah's Witnesses.

2. Jehovah's Witnesses may refuse transfusion of blood or blood products components. In an elective operation, the mentally normal adult patient has a lawful right to demand that he not be given blood or blood components. In turn, the anesthesiologist or surgeon may elect to refuse to undertake the care and treatment of the patient.

3. A more difficult situation exists in an emergency, when the patient or the person legally responsible for him demands that no blood or blood components be transfused. In such a case, an appeal to a court for an emergency writ must be made.

4. If a blood transfusion for a minor child has been refused, the courts have seen fit to declare the child a ward of the court and to appoint a guardian authorized to consent to the blood transfusion. In one case, a federal court in the District of Columbia ordered a blood transfusion for a child despite the re-

fusal of the parents, who were Jehovah's Witness. In another case, the court declared that parents may make martyrs of themselves but that they cannot make martyrs of their children before they reach the age of legal discretion, at which time they may make their own choices.

V. Conclusion

A. As a general rule, the best way for an anesthesiologist to avoid legal hazards and prevent litigation of all types is to know his patient and to watch him with special attention. This is very important, particularly during the postoperative period. The anesthesiologist can do much to prevent complications or accidents, or, if they happen, can help to control them and to explain their cause to the patient or the parents. This attention and care may prevent the prejudicial feelings that stand behind many lawsuits and thus prevent the suits themselves.

B. If a potentially litigious complication occurs, the anesthesiologist must notify the insurance carrier agents and provide them with a detailed and accurate report within the time limit specified in the policy (usually 72 hr).

Bibliography

Curran, W. J. Malpractice insurance. *N. Engl. J. Med.* 292:1223, 1975.

Dornette, W. H. L. The medical malpractice problem and some possible solutions. *Anesthesiology* 44:230, 1976.

Gray, T. C., and Shelley, F. C. A medicolegal view. *Br. J. Anaesth.* 50:721, 1978.

Louiselle, D. W., and Williams, H. B. *Medical Malpractice.* New York: Matthew Bender, 1981.

Norton, M. L. When does an experimental/innovative procedure become an accepted procedure? *Pharos* 34(4):161, 1975.

Norton, M. L. Medicolegal Aspects of Anesthesia. In J. C. Snow, *Anesthesia in Otolaryngology and Ophthalmology.* New York: Appleton-Century-Crofts, 1982.

Rosoff, A. J. *Informed Consent: A Guide for Health Care Providers.* Rockville, Md.: Aspen Systems Corp., 1981.

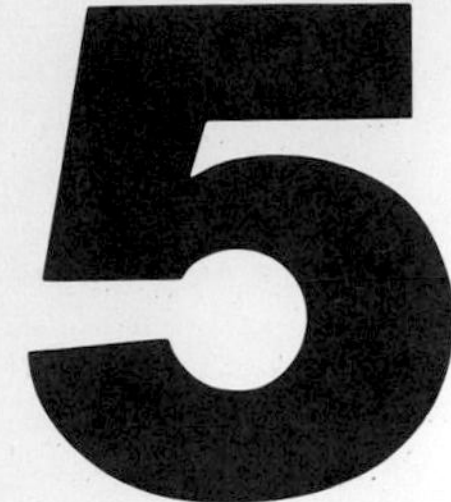

Cleaning and Sterilization of the Anesthesia Equipment

I. General Comments

A. Cross-infection from antibiotic-resistant pathogens poses a serious threat to every patient in the hospital. About 15% of hospital patients acquire an infection in this manner. The majority of these nosocomial infections are caused by gram-negative bacilli, and this type of gram-negative bacteremia occurs with a frequency of 1 per 100 admissions in the hospital and a 30% fatality rate.

B. Within 2 days, one-third of **intravenous catheters** become colonized with bacteria. Bacteremia occurs in 1% of patients who have an intravenous catheter in place longer than 48 hr. The hazard of sepsis increases to 5% as the length of time the catheter remains in place increases. In spite of advances in chemotherapy and antibiotic therapy and the development of more aseptic patient-care methods, infections continue.

C. The infectiousness of a disease is equal to the **virulence** of the pathogenic germs plus the **total dosage** of pathogens minus the **resistance** of the patient. An effective approach to fighting infection in the hospital is to decrease the number of bacteria below the level necessary to produce infection.

D. Sources of infection

1. Patients, personnel, anesthesia equipment, air conditioning equipment, cleaning techniques, and intravenous fluid therapy equipment.
2. Inhalation therapy equipment, nebulizers, humidifiers, resuscitation equipment, and ventilators used for intermittent positive-pressure breathing.
   a. **An anesthesiologist and nurse-anesthetist** have many contacts with ill people in the hospital, especially within the operating room, delivery room, recovery room, and intensive care unit. They must share in the responsibility for decreasing and controlling cross-infection. They cannot control the virulence of the pathogenic bacteria or the resistance of a patient, but they can control the total amount of pathogens.
   b. **It has been clearly demonstrated** in both the operating room and in the laboratory that all parts of anesthesia breathing equipment can become contaminated and cause cross-infection. It is well known that mechanical ventilators and humidifiers used in inhalation therapy can be responsible for cross-infection. The means are available to eliminate this hazard.

II. Techniques of cleaning and sterilization

A. Solutions for preparing the skin for needle puncture

1. Ethyl or isopropyl alcohol 70%.
2. Tincture of benzalkonium (Zephiran) 1:1000 in 70% alcohol.
3. Iodine 2% in 70% alcohol.

B. Sterilization for anesthesia and inhalation therapy equipment

1. Heat sterilization

a. **Moist heat.** High-pressure steam sterilization (autoclaving) is the most dependable, effective, and efficient means of destroying pathogenic bacteria. It is applicable to sterilization of the equipment used in hospitals that is not damaged by heat and moisture. The principle involved is thermal denaturation of proteins of pathogenic organisms: **Moisture** increases cellular permeability, and **heat** coagulates protein.

b. **Dry heat,** 160°C for 1 hr, is useful for powders, oils, greases, and glass syringes.

2. Chemical sterilization

a. General considerations

(1) The techniques of sterilization that utilize **heat** and **steam** are damaging to the rubber and plastic equipment used in anesthesia, in the postanesthesia recovery room, and in inhalation therapy.

(2) **Cold chemical techniques** with antiseptic solutions and disinfectants are time-consuming and are not reliable. Tubercle bacilli, viruses, and spores are very resistant to chemical drugs, and *Pseudomonas aeruginosa* is resistant to the quaternary ammonium compounds. A great number of chemicals act only at the exposed surfaces, and some will react with metals. Others will remain on the surfaces, producing irritation. Satisfactory control of this problem is a very difficult task, because the pathogens are not killed, and they will not grow until the chemical drug is neutralized.

(3) Injuries to the patient occurring during anesthesia that can cause him to take legal action include **dermatitis** and **facial burns** from rubber treated with antiseptics.

b. Ethylene oxide sterilization

(1) Sterilization of the anesthesia and inhalation therapy equipment with ethylene oxide is reliable and has the following **advantages:**

(a) It is safe for the anesthesia equipment that would be damaged by high heat and moisture.

(b) Sterility is obtained by destruction of all microbes and spores. The bactericidal effect, which is tested by biologic and chemical controls, is increased by physical techniques that consist of both **vacuum pressure** to aid penetration and **heat.**

(c) Ethylene oxide destroys all pathogenic bacteria at room temperature.

(d) Ethylene oxide is noncorrosive and nondestructive.

(e) It readily penetrates rubber, paper, plastic material, cellophane, and cardboard.

(f) It can be removed by aeration and has low toxicity for humans.

(g) The **tubercle bacillus** is killed by ethylene oxide, which destroys all vegetating bacteria and fungi, has strong sporicidal action, and kills at least the larger viruses. Its effect on the virus causing **human hepatitis** is unknown.

(h) The **main advantage** of ethylene oxide is its ability to sterilize heat-sensitive and moisture-sensitive anesthesia equipment that cannot be sterilized by dry heat or steam under pressure.

(2) Disadvantages

(a) At room temperature, ethylene oxide is a colorless gas, but it can easily become liquid because of its boiling point, 10.6°C (51°F). If the liquid is kept in ordinary containers, it presents a safety risk because **the vapor is flammable** in a concentration between 3% and 80% by volume. But if it is diluted with carbon dioxide or Freons, the substance will not produce a flammable mixture in air.

(b) Sterilization with ethylene oxide is **slow** and is done in airtight cabinets. It is **expensive**, and dilution with Freons or carbon dioxide is necessary. Aeration must be sufficient for rubber and plastic goods, which absorb ethylene oxide very quickly. An aeration period of 5–7 days at ambient temperature or aeration at 50°C (122°F) for 6–8 hr in a specially designed vacuum aerator with bacteria filters is usually satisfactory for all materials.

(c) Ethylene oxide inhalation irritates the tracheobronchial tree and may cause headache and vomiting.

(d) If the liquid compound is in contact with the skin for some time, blisters may result. Very rare complications, such as facial burns from face masks and tracheal inflammation following intubation, have been reported.

(e) Due to the vacuum pressure process, ethylene oxide sterilization is contraindicated for articles with closed spaces that the vacuum could injure.

III. Disposable anesthesia and respiratory care equipment

A. A satisfactory alternative to the cleaning and sterilizing of articles and supplies used in anesthesia, in the postanesthesia recovery room, in the delivery room, in inhalation therapy, and in the intensive care unit is the use of **disposable items,** which can be economically replaced rather than resterilized.

B. The use of single-use, **sterile, disposable pieces of equipment** solves many of the problems presented by both sterilizing anesthesia equipment and nosocomial cross-infections. The use for each patient of sterile disposable equipment, such as syringes, needles, endotracheal tubes, oropharyngeal airways, suction catheters, Y-pieces, connectors, masks, corrugated-rubber breathing hoses, breathing bags, and complete anesthetic circle absorbers help to prevent infections, especially in the presence of tuberculosis or other infections caused by virulent microbes and viruses.

IV. Summary

A. Pathogenic microbes in equipment constitute one of the main factors contributing to the spread of **hospital cross-infections.** Bacteria, spores, and viruses can remain for long periods of time in the moist, dark interior of corrugated-rubber breathing hoses.

B. **The anesthesiologist and nurse-anesthetist** must share the responsibility for preventing and controlling nosocomial infections by (1) using detergents or soap containing bacteriostatic agents to suppress the pathogenic microorganisms on their hands before starting to administer an anesthetic and (2) meticulous cleaning and sterilizing of the anesthesia and respiratory care equipment for every patient.

C. All anesthesia and inhalation therapy articles may be cleaned with a detergent and sterilized with **steam** if the articles and supplies can withstand heat at 121°C (250°F) under 15 psi pressure for 30 min.

D. Sterilization with **ethylene oxide gas** is an excellent special method for sterilizing equipment that would be damaged by heat or by exposure to strong liquid disinfectants. Ethylene oxide is the agent of choice in sterilizing heat-sensitive and moisture-sensitive articles and supplies used in anesthesia, in the recovery room, and in inhalation therapy.

E. A very satisfactory alternative to the sterilization of anesthesia and respiratory care equipment is the use of **single-use disposable items.**

Bibliography

Albrecht, W. H., and Dryden, G. E. Five-year experience with the development of an individually clean anesthesia system. *Anesth. Analg.* (Cleve.) 53:24, 1974.

Berry, F. A. Comparison of bacteremia occurring with nasotracheal and orotracheal intubation. *Anesth. Analg.* (Cleve.) 52:873, 1973.

Burton, R., and Eliason, K. The sterilization of anesthesia equipment by ethylene oxide. *Anesth. Analg.* (Cleve.) 49:957, 1970.

Dryden, G. E. Anesthesia equipment sterility. *Anesth. Analg.* (Cleve.) 52:167, 1973.

Dryden, G. E. Uncleaned anesthesia equipment. *J.A.M.A.* 233:1298, 1975.

Dryden, G. E., and Brickler, J. Stopcock contamination. *Anesth. Analg.* (Cleve.) 58:141, 1979.

Rendell-Baker, L., and Roberts, R. B. Safe use of ethylene oxide sterilization in hospitals. *Anesth. Analg.* (Cleve.) 49:919, 1970.

Roberts, R. B. The eradication of cross-infection from anesthetic equipment. *Anesth. Analg.* (Cleve.) 49:63, 1970.

Snow, J. C., Mangiaracine, A. B., and Anderson, M. L. Sterilization of anesthesia equipment with ethylene oxide. *N. Engl. J. Med.* 266:443, 1962.

Stetson, J. B., Whitbourne, J. E., and Eastman, C. Ethylene oxide degassing of rubber and plastic materials. *Anesthesiology* 44:174, 1976.

Thomas, E. T. The sterilization dilemma: Where will it end? Clinical aspects. *Anesth. Analg.* (Cleve.) 47:657, 1968.

Thomas, E. T., and Levy, A. A. Dissipation of ethylene oxide from anesthetic equipment. Use of a mechanical aerator. *Anesthesiology* 32:261, 1970.

Walter, C. W. Cross-infection and the anesthesiologist. *Anesth. Analg.* (Cleve.) 53:631, 1974.

White, C. W. Ethylene oxide sterilization of anesthesia apparatus. *Anesthesiology* 33:120, 1970.

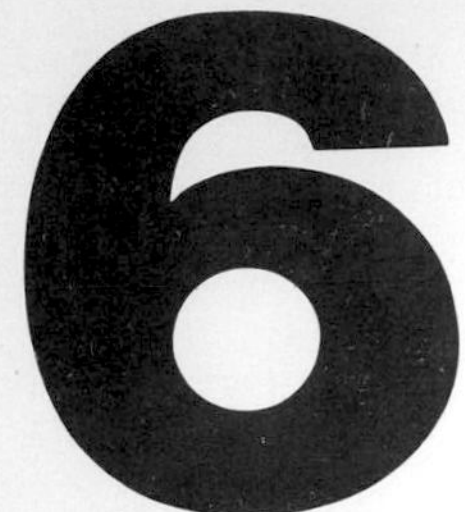

Monitoring During Anesthesia and Postanesthesia Period

I. Definition and general comments

A. A **monitor** is defined as one who reminds and warns. **Monitoring instruments** record respiration, pulse, blood pressure, central venous pressure, blood gases, temperature, and electrical activity of the heart and brain. These devices should function as assistants and not as substitutes for constant personal contact with the patient. As adjuvants, they provide very useful information; as substitutes, they are dangerous because they tend to encourage detachment of the anesthesiologist from the patient. **Monitors** should not replace sound clinical judgment and observation.

B. During a 10-yr period (1955–1964), **115,000 anesthetics,** including general, spinal, and regional anesthesia, were administered by a group of anesthesiologists in Springfield, Massachusetts. Of this total, 1000 patients died in the hospital, 180 of them within 24 hr following surgery. Anesthesia contributed to or was responsible for 65 (6.5%) of all surgical deaths. The chief mistake of the anesthesiologists involved was **improper administration of anesthetics;** a secondary error was poor management in the immediate postanesthesia period. It was concluded that the error in almost all cases was the **lack of proper monitoring** of the patient. This was especially apparent in those deaths that occurred in patients who had been in good health.

II. Monitoring devices.

The proper and safe practice of anesthesiology requires adequate monitoring. To assist the anesthesiologist in observation and evaluation of the patient's condition during the preoperative, intraoperative, and postoperative periods, the following instruments and monitoring systems are used:

A. Stethoscope

1. Monitors by auscultation, directly or electronically, heart rate, heart rhythm, and breath sounds.
2. May be taped to the precordium and used throughout surgery, particularly during head and neck procedures. Following endotracheal intubation, the **precordial stethoscope** is usually replaced by an **esophageal stethoscope.**
3. May be connected to an individual **earpiece** for continuous monitoring by the anesthesiologist or nurse-anesthetist with maximal comfort.

B. The Doppler monitor sends out high-frequency sound waves that are reflected by the tissues involved. The distinction in frequency between emitted and reflected waves due to blood circulation or arterial pulsation may be translated to an audible note. The Doppler monitor is useful for measuring blood pressure, particularly in infants.

C. The pulsometer determines **capillary flow.** This device registers **cardiac rate** and **rhythm.** A photoelectric cell, placed on the earlobe or finger, views the capillary bed. The differential absorption of light during the systolic and diastolic congestion of the capillary field triggers a visible or audible signal. This signal is absent when the peripheral pulse is weak or nonpalpable due to intense vasoconstriction, or during peripheral circulatory failure.

D. **The sphygmomanometer** is used for the **indirect** determination of the arterial systolic and diastolic blood pressure. The monitoring of **systolic** and **diastolic** pressure indicates the vitality of the heart, its functional efficiency as a pump, and the status of the circulation. Arterial blood flow is occluded in the extremity by external pressure. When the external pressure is reduced, the flow is reestablished by the appearance of Korotkoff's sounds. These sounds are produced by changes in the rate of blood flow through partially constricted tubes.

1. The sphygmomanometer includes a manometer (aneroid or mercury), cuff, and stethoscope.
2. The blood pressure **cuff** is wide enough to cover two-thirds of the length of the upper arm. When it is narrower, the readings are high; when it is wider, the readings are low. The center of the rubber inflatable bag is placed over the brachial artery, with the lower border just above the cubital fossa.
3. **Palpation method.** The cuff pressure is increased to about 30 torr above the point at which the radial pulse is not palpable. The pressure is then decreased at a rate of 2–3 torr per heartbeat. The cuff pressure is read as **systolic pressure** when the radial pulse first reappears regularly. The systolic pressure taken by the palpation technique is usually 10 torr lower than by the auscultation method.
4. **Auscultation method.** The cuff is inflated until the radial pulse is not palpated and then is decompressed at a rate of 2–3 torr per heartbeat. Turbulence is created as blood begins to circulate through the compressed artery. This is transmitted as sounds or vibrations, which can be detected by placing the stethoscope over the brachial artery. The **systolic pressure** is determined when the first sound is heard. The **diastolic pressure** is determined at the point when there is a sudden decrease of sound. In the presence of **venous stasis,** the readings may show low systolic and high diastolic pressure.
5. The pressure may be taken by watching the **oscillations** of the needle of the aneroid manometer.

E. **Electrocardiogram**

1. **Electrocardiography monitors the electrical activity of the heart.** It is of great help in recognizing arrhythmias, conduction defects, myocardial ischemia, and myocardial infarction and in estimating the effects of anesthetics, cardiac drugs (digitalis and quinidine), and electrolytes (potassium and calcium). An ECG should be taken preoperatively on all patients who are 35 years old or older and on younger ones as indicated.
2. **The electrocardioscope** is an electrocardiographic monitoring instrument that displays visually, on a cathode ray tube, the various electrical potentials associated with the myocardial contraction. It differs from the electrocardiograph in that there is no written record.
3. **During a 3-yr period (1958–1960)** there were 16 deaths from cardiac arrest in 20,000 operations in a hospital in Chicago, Illinois. In the following few years, electrocardioscopic monitoring of heart rate and rhythm and observing for signs such as hypotension, tachycardia, bradycardia, cyanosis, arrhythmias, and unexplained changes in the level of anesthesia or in ventilation decreased the incidence to 1 death in 20,000 surgical procedures.
4. **Advantages of the electrocardioscope**
    a. The electrocardioscope provides a continuous **visual display** of the ECG, allowing immediate recognition and differential diagnosis of arrhythmias.
    b. Tachycardia, bradycardia, extrasystoles, and other arrhythmias are **recognized immediately** and with precision.

c. S–T segment depression and an **inverted T wave** indicate that the coronary artery perfusion is not adequate and that oxygenation of the myocardium is not efficient.

d. **A permanent ECG tracing** can be obtained.

e. In the presence of a **cardiac arrest,** the diagnosis and differential diagnosis between ventricular asystole and ventricular fibrillation can be obtained in a few seconds.

f. The monitor sounds an **audible note** and displays a **visual signal** with each QRS complex that represents ventricular contraction.

5. **Limitations of the electrocardioscope**

a. The electrocardioscope corresponds approximately to that of **standard leads I and II.**

b. **It does not foretell heart failure,** but it may give warning signals.

c. **It does not record hemodynamic events,** such as the efficiency or force of contraction of the myocardium.

d. **The tracing portrays only the electrical activity of the heart** and provides no indication of the strength of myocardial contraction.

e. **Artifacts** must be differentiated from changes originating in the myocardium. The electrocardioscope records the electrical activity of the heart, but it cannot separate cardiac potentials from those originating elsewhere and conducted into the device.

F. Direct measurement of arterial pressure

1. Measurement of arterial pressure is best done by **percutaneous** or **cutdown** positioning of a plastic catheter into the **radial artery** after checking for adequacy of distal perfusion.

2. **To ascertain patency of the ulnar artery,** the hand is blanched through compression of the radial and ulnar arteries and the flush on release of the ulnar artery is observed while the radial artery remains closed **(Allen's test).**

3. In patients in whom **ulnar arterial pulsations are absent** and satisfactory collateral circulation cannot be demonstrated, the brachial or femoral artery must be selected.

4. **The arterial catheter,** filled with heparinized solution, is connected to a strain-gauge transducer, which allows changes in pressure by displacing a diaphragm, in turn changing the electrical resistance of a wire. Change in resistance is picked up through a Wheatstone bridge circuit, amplified, and displayed on a cathode ray tube or other appropriate recorder.

5. **Indications**

a. Critically ill patients.

b. Shock.

c. Major traumatic surgery.

d. Cardiopulmonary bypass.

e. Hypothermic or hypotensive anesthetic techniques.

6. **Advantages.** Reveals actual intraarterial or intracardiac blood pressure and moment-to-moment variations in pressure.

G. Direct arterial cannulation for PO_2, PCO_2, and pH determinations

1. Direct arterial catheterization is necessary for the proper care of **critically ill patients.** Blood received allows analysis for PO_2, PCO_2, pH, and bicarbonate.

Thus diagnosis and therapy of cardiopulmonary inadequacy can be done on a rational basis.

2. Arterial blood samples are of **great value in determining** (a) acid-base status, (b) efficiency of oxygenation of the patient, and (c) adequacy of ventilation.

H. Monitoring central venous pressure

1. Central venous pressure (CVP) reflects the **right heart competence.** It measures the pressure exerted by the blood returning to the right side of the heart and the ability of the right side of the heart to manage this return effectively.

2. It serves to distinguish between hemorrhage and congestive heart failure. **Hemorrhage** is associated with a fall in venous pressure, even before the arterial pressure is decreased. In the **failing heart,** the venous pressure is increased.

3. **A rough estimation of the CVP** can be made by (a) watching the degree of distention of the **neck veins** and (b) lowering or raising an **upper extremity** while observing the degree of distention of the **cubital or hand veins** and the level at which they collapse when referred to the heart.

4. **More accurate determinations** of the CVP can be obtained by a catheter introduced through the median cubital vein or the external jugular vein and threaded to the superior vena cava. The catheterization of the femoral, subclavian, or internal jugular vein is hazardous and must be done by an experienced physician. Normal CVP range is 3–10 cm H_2O (2–7 torr) (1 cm H_2O $\div$ 1.36 = torr).

5. **To adjust zero level** of monitoring equipment (water manometer or transducer) to the position of the right atrium, various techniques are used.

   a. For accurate readings, the **zero point** of the manometer scale should be at the level of the right atrium.

   b. Two practical reference points are the midaxillary line or the midpoint of the anterior-posterior diameter of the thorax at the level of the fourth intercostal space.

6. **Indications**

   a. **Elderly patients** undergoing extensive surgical operations.

   b. Patients in whom a **large blood or fluid exchange** is expected, to prevent overhydration or overtransfusion.

   c. In patients known to have **cardiac disease.**

   d. **Major traumatic surgery.**

   e. Anticipation of **major blood loss** during surgery.

   f. In patients with **uncertain preoperative volume status** (immediate preoperative fluid, weight, or blood loss).

   g. Facilitation of postoperative care in **critically ill patients.**

   h. **Craniotomy** or **cervical laminectomy,** when either is done in the upright position to treat potential **air embolism.**

   i. **Multiple transfusions.**

   j. **Open heart surgery.**

   k. During and following removal of a **pheochromocytoma.**

I. Measurement of pulmonary artery and wedge pressures

1. The Swan-Ganz catheter is advanced into the right atrium by various routes, and then the small balloon located at the catheter's tip is inflated and carried

by the circulating blood through the heart and into the pulmonary artery. These various routes are:

a. Through the median cubital vein by needle or cutdown.

b. Through the subclavian vein.

c. Through the internal jugular vein.

2. **Pulmonary artery diastolic pressure** and **wedge pressure** correspond more closely to left atrial pressure than does CVP. Hence they reflect incipient left heart failure more promptly.

J. **Measuring urine output.** Collection and determination of urine flow by **indwelling catheter** is a simple, useful method for testing hydration of the body. Increased urine output per hour approaching normal (40–60 ml/hr) indicates satisfactory fluid replacement. The normal kidney will excrete any excess fluid to restore a normal water balance.

K. **Monitoring cardiac output.** During anesthesia, determination of cardiac output is used very rarely, since there are some difficulties with the present techniques. However, in special operations the measurement of cardiac output is necessary. Techniques used are:

1. **The Fick principle.** Central venous blood samples are taken from a catheter inserted through a cubital fossa vein to the right ventricle or pulmonary artery. Blood from the radial or femoral artery is obtained. Oxygen consumption is estimated, and measurements are computed by:

$$\text{Cardiac output (ml/min)} = \frac{\text{Total body } O_2 \text{ consumption (ml/min)}}{\text{Arteriovenous } O_2 \text{ difference (ml/100 ml)}} \times 100$$

2. **Dye dilution technique.** Through a catheter, dye is injected into the pulmonary artery, and blood specimens are obtained from a peripheral artery and examined by a photoelectric technique. Successive estimations are plotted on a graph, and the area under the curve is computed by:

$$\text{Cardiac output (ml/min)} = \frac{\text{mass of dye injected}}{\text{area under curve}} \times 60$$

3. **Thermodilution technique.** A known quantity of a cold solution is administered into the right atrium or superior vena cava through the **Swan-Ganz catheter,** and the resultant change in blood temperature is detected by the thermistor in the pulmonary artery.

a. Cardiac output is inversely proportional to the integral temperature change.

b. This method provides good correlation with the dye dilution technique and direct Fick method.

4. **Noninvasive techniques**

a. Impedance measurement system, which uses the changes in conductivity of high-frequency currents through the extremities produced by the pulsatile blood flow.

b. Echocardiogram.

c. The Doppler method is not yet available, but extensive research on this method is in progress.

L. **Blood loss and blood volume measurements**

1. The methods of **estimation of blood loss** are:

a. Intraoperative weighing of sponges and towels.

b. Volumetric measurement of blood loss.

c. Monitoring central venous pressure.

d. Repeated blood volume estimations.

e. Serial microhematocrits.

2. The simplest, most often used method is to **weigh all sponges, packs, and towels** as they are removed from the surgical area, as well as **blood** found and estimated in **suction bottles, drapes, and on the floor.** The quantities of irrigation solutions must be known and taken into account.

3. **Blood volume measurements**

a. **In special procedures** the estimation of blood volume before surgery is useful. It is based on the **principle of dilution.** A known amount of tracer material is injected intravenously and is allowed to mix with the circulating blood. Then blood is removed and examined. The quantity of tracer introduced is compared with the concentration of the tracer in the blood specimen to determine the dilution proportion.

b. **Radioactive iodinated human serum albumin** is incorporated into albumin, and **radioactive chromium** is incorporated into red cells. With these detectable nontoxic materials, the blood volume can be determined up to 10 times daily, because the total quantity of radiation in 20 measurements does not exceed the dose delivered in taking an x-ray chest film. The **Volemetron computer** is a semiautomatic instrument for blood volume estimations that yields a whole-blood volume or plasma volume, depending on the specimen.

c. A normal blood volume estimation can be obtained from a **nomogram** showing height and weight. If weight and height are in reasonable proportion, a rough estimation can be made by assuming blood volume to be **7% of body weight** in kilograms.

d. A normal patient **without anesthesia** may lose 30% of his blood before showing signs of decompensation. **Under anesthesia** a 20% loss in adults (15% loss in children) is the point at which decompensation may begin.

e. Due to technical difficulties and apparent imprecision of direct means to estimate blood volume, **indirect methods** are used. These include:

(1) Intraarterial blood pressure monitoring and (occasionally) pulmonary artery catheterization.

(2) Central venous pressure monitoring.

(3) Determination of urine output.

M. **Monitoring tidal volume and minute volume of respiration**

1. **Tidal volume (V_T)** is the quantity of air breathed in and out with each ordinary respiratory effort (V_T = 450 ml).

2. **Anatomic dead space (V_D)** includes the airway passages extending from the nose and mouth down to the alveoli (150 ml). This space is about 2 ml/per kilogram of body weight; the space of the alveoli is not included.

3. **Effective tidal volume** is the air that actually reaches the alveoli. It is found by subtracting the anatomic dead space (V_D) of the lungs from the tidal volume (V_T).

4. Effective V_T, multiplied by the number of respirations per minute, gives the **alveolar minute ventilation ($\dot{V}_A$).**

5. **Tidal volume (V_T)** can be quantitatively estimated by using different spirometers (mechanical or electronic). The spirometer should be located on the expiratory limb of the anesthesia circle and close to the endotracheal

tube or face mask, so that the results will not be influenced by fresh gas flows. The **Wright spirometer** measures tidal volume, minute volume, and vital capacity in a spontaneously breathing and a manually ventilated patient. Gas passes through 10 tangential slots in a cylindrical stator ring to turn a flat two-bladed rotor. Gas volumes are displayed on a calibrated meter.

N. Gas chromatography

1. **Gas chromatography** is used for quantitative analysis of anesthetic compounds in respired mixtures and blood.
2. The essential elements in gas chromatography are the **column,** the **carrier gas,** and the **detector.**
3. The basic principle of this method is that the gas or gases are selectively absorbed by an inert material **(stationary phase).** The **moving phase** is gaseous.
4. The absorption varies, so that when a mixture is passed through a long analyzing **column** containing the absorbant, the gas with the least attraction for the compound will reach the end first.
5. **Helium,** a nonabsorbable gas, is used as a **carrier.**
6. **The detector** is the part of the machine that actually estimates the amount of the agent to be analyzed.

O. Neuromuscular block monitoring. During general anesthesia and the postoperative period, the anesthesiologist and nurse-anesthetist must know the **degree of the effects** of the neuromuscular blocking agents. This can be done several ways:

1. **Clinically,** by observing any movements of the patient, the surgical working conditions, the degree of relaxation of the abdominal wall, and the chest and lung compliance.
2. **With a peripheral nerve stimulator.** Following placement of skin or needle electrodes in the area of a peripheral nerve, usually in the forearm (ulnar nerve), an evoked response of the muscle can be observed on application of a stimulus. Either single or tetanic stimuli can be administered.
3. By observing and recognizing that each group of the neuromuscular blocking drugs yields a **characteristic depression of the evoked response.** By maintaining a response barely perceptible by the fourth and fifth fingers when the stimulus is applied to the ulnar nerve at the wrist, excellent muscle relaxation during surgery can be obtained. In addition, the peripheral nerve stimulator gives accurate guidance as to the need for reversal drugs, thus preventing both postoperative respiratory depression and atelectasis.

P. Electroencephalogram

1. An EEG reveals the **electrical activity of the brain,** which can be picked up by scalp electrodes, amplified, and recorded.
2. Electroencephalographic monitors are used to observe the **surgical patient.** During general anesthesia, the EEG represents the degree of cortical depression associated with anesthesia or the effects of accompanying adverse circumstances, such as hypoxia or hypercapnia.
3. **The value of the EEG** has been downgraded during the last 10 years, because it was recognized that many extraanesthetic factors can influence the EEG pattern. The EEG is seldom used today to evaluate depth of anesthesia. However, it is useful to monitor cerebral hypoxia in special conditions, such as during extracorporeal circulation, during surgery on the carotid artery, and in any form of anesthesia or surgery in which marked physiologic trespass is contemplated.

Q. Temperature monitoring

1. A continuous temperature indicator with a **rectal, esophageal,** or **tympanic membrane** probe is very useful for detecting hypothermia or malignant hyperthermia. It is recommended especially in children, in young adults, in patients with fever, and in procedures involving induced hypothermia.
2. **Rectal temperature** is peripheral and only poorly and inconsistently reflects the central body core temperature changes. The position of the probe is far from either the main output channels of the heart or the central nervous system, where the thermoregulatory centers are located.
3. Most commonly used in the operating room is **esophageal** thermometry. The position for measurement is the lower mediastinum below the pulmonary veins, between the heart and descending aorta. In this site, the temperature-monitoring instrument should clearly follow changes in the temperature of the blood in the central circulation.
   a. Insertion of an esophageal probe may be difficult, and it may become displaced during intubation, extubation, and surgical manipulations.
   b. Epistaxis may follow placement or removal of the probe, particularly in patients on anticoagulants or with histories of hypertension or blood dyscrasias.
4. **Tympanic membrane temperature** reflects accurately the temperature of blood flowing through the brain.
   a. Measurements obtained at the tympanic membrane parallel those in a properly positioned esophageal probe and reflect subtle changes in temperature.
   b. The tympanic membrane is considered safe, reliable, and clinically very useful for monitoring body temperature.

R. Fetal monitoring is important to the obstetrician and anesthesiologist for the early diagnosis of **fetal distress.** The **fetal heart rate** is obtained directly from electrocardiographic electrodes attached to the fetus or indirectly by ultrasonic detection of fetal heart motion. **Fetal distress** is detected by studying the relationship of uterine contractions and fetal heart rate changes. Uterine contractions are detected by (1) a pressure transducer connected to an intrauterine catheter, (2) use of the tokodynamometer, or (3) electromyography of the uterus.

S. Monitoring pressures in the breathing circuit is important during controlled respiration. A pressure-sensing device, preset to a certain pressure range, emits audible and visual signals, alerting the anesthesiologist or nurse-anesthetist to the presence of difficulties requiring evaluation and correction.

T. The oxygen gas analyzer is a device for measuring the oxygen content of the gaseous mixture in the circuit of the anesthesia machine.

Bibliography

Buchbinder, N., and Ganz, W. Hemodynamic monitoring. Invasive techniques. *Anesthesiology* 45:146, 1976.

Hall, G. M. Body temperature and anesthesia. *Br. J. Anaesth.* 50:39, 1978.

Herbert, M. Assessment of performance in studies of anesthetic agents. *Br. J. Anaesth.* 50:33, 1978.

Holdcroft, A., and Hall, G. M. Heat loss during anesthesia. *Br. J. Anaesth.* 50:157, 1978.

Lowenstein, E., and Teplick, R. To (PA) catheterize or not to (PA) catheterize. That is the question. *Anesthesiology* 53:361, 1980.

Lowry, R. L., Lichti, E. L., and Eggers, G. W. N. The Doppler, an aid in monitoring blood pressure during anesthesia. *Anesth. Analg.* (Cleve.) 52:531, 1973.

Mangano, D. T. Monitoring pulmonary arterial pressure in coronary-artery disease. *Anesthesiology* 53:364, 1980.

Mazel, M. S., Bolton, H. E., Tapia, F. A., et al. Prevention of cardiac arrest during surgery. *Dis. Chest* 45:639, 1964.

Memery, H. N. Anesthesia mortality in private practice. A ten-year study. *J.A.M.A.* 194:1185, 1965.

Saidman, L. J., and Smith, N. T. *Monitoring in Anesthesia.* New York: Wiley, 1978.

Snow, J. C., and Dobnik, D. B. Central venous pressure monitoring. A simple device to determine zero level. *Anesthesiology* 43:678, 1975.

Vaughan R. W., and Wise, L. Postoperative arterial blood gas measurements in obese patients: Effect of position on gas exchange. *Ann. Surg.* 182:705, 1975.

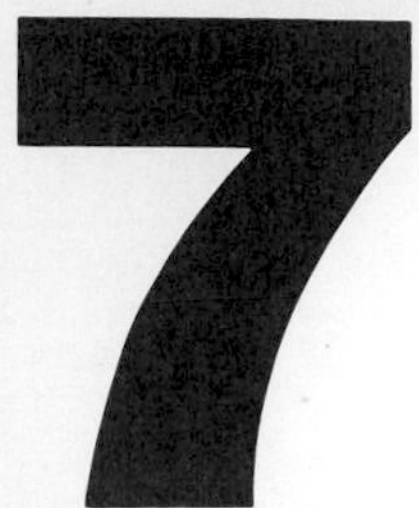

Electrocardiography

Electrocardiography is the graphic representation of the **electrical currents** associated with the **contraction of the heart** muscle. The basic function of the electrocardiographic monitor is to amplify the small voltage formed by the depolarization of the heart so that it can be presented on the screen for visual monitoring or so that a graphic record can be made.

I. **Conducting mechanism of the heart. In the normal heart,** the electrical impulse is formed in the **sinoatrial (SA) node,** which is the physiologic **pacemaker** of the heart. The SA node is located at the junction of the right atrium and superior vena cava. The impulse spreads to the atria and, at the junction between atria and ventricles, it stimulates the **atrioventricular (AV) node.** Then the impulse travels rapidly through the bundle of His, the right and left bundle branches, Purkinje's fibers, and the ventricles.

II. **The normal electrocardiogram**

A. **An ECG reveals** (1) the condition of the cardiac conducting system, (2) the heart rate and rhythm, and (3) the area and extension of a cardiac injury. This graphic tracing **does not reflect** mechanical factors, such as the efficiency or force of cardiac systole; thus a normal ECG can be obtained when there is no measurable blood pressure.

1. **In the normal ECG,** the **P wave** indicates the results of the electrical activity during the atrial depolarization that initiates atrial contractions. The **P–R interval** represents the time it takes the impulse to spread from the SA node to the ventricles. The **normal P–R interval** is 0.12–0.20 sec.

2. **The QRS complex** is due to the depolarization of the ventricles, which triggers their contraction. It indicates the time it takes for ventricular depolarization. The QRS complex is 0.06–0.10 sec.

3. **The T wave** occurs at the end of ventricular systole. It is followed by an isoelectric line or by a U wave during diastole.

4. **The P, QRS, and T waves represent** the rhythmic electric depolarization or repolarization of the myocardium that precedes or follows the contraction.

B. **The recording paper** has horizontal and vertical lines.

1. **The horizontal lines** indicate **voltage** and are 1 mm apart **(1 mm represents 0.1 mV).**

2. **The vertical lines** indicate time and are separated from one another by an interval of 0.04 sec. **The heavy vertical lines** represent 0.2 sec (5 × 0.04) intervals, and **five large squares** represent 1 sec (5 × 0.2).

3. **Heart rate per minute** is determined by **counting the numbers of QRS complexes** that occur in 3 sec (15 large squares) from left to right and multiplying by 20. At the upper border of the strip there is a mark for every 15 large squares, representing 3 sec (15 × 0.2).

III. ECG leads

A. **The standard leads (I, II, III)** are bipolar indirect leads. They record the difference, between two points on the body, in electrical events formed by the cardiac action. The electrodes are attached on the right arm, left arm, and left leg. The right leg is used for grounding and does not have any relation to the graphic records of the ECG. The **terminals are placed** as follows:

Lead I. Right arm, left arm.

Lead II. Right arm, left leg.

Lead III. Left arm, left leg.

B. **The unipolar extremity leads** indicate the electrical potentials at one point. The electrodes of three limbs are attached together to form one electrode, called the **central terminal lead.** The differences of the electrical potentials are recorded between the central terminal and each of the three extremities. Lead aVR is positioned at the right arm; lead aVL, at the left arm; and lead aVF, at the left foot.

C. **The precordial leads** are unipolar leads that indicate the variation of electrical potentials at a given cardiac anatomic site. The central terminal lead is used, and the exploring electrode is positioned on the chest and in six different locations, V1 to V6.

IV. ECG during anesthesia

A. During anesthesia, **the ECG is a very useful method** for evaluating and monitoring the cardiac electrical activity, which cannot be done by any other technique. The ECG is essential to recognizing cardiac arrhythmias, conduction defects, myocardial hypoxia, and myocardial infarction and in estimating the cardiac effects of anesthetics, cardiac drugs (digitalis and quinidine), and electrolytes (potassium and calcium).

B. An ECG **should be taken preoperatively** on all patients who are 35 years old or older and on younger patients as indicated.

V. Electrocardioscopy in the operating room and recovery room

A. **The electrocardioscope,** or oscilloscope, is an electrocardiographic monitoring instrument that displays on a cathode ray tube the different electrical potentials deriving from the cardiac contractions. It differs from the electrocardiograph by not recording a written tracing, although it can be connected to a direct electrocardiographic writer.

1. **A vacuum tube is utilized.** The discharge of electrons by the cathode is passed through the anode and forms a beam, which is projected on the screen in a horizontal sweep.

2. The electrocardioscope includes an electronic device that produces an **audible signal** and a **blinking light** with each cardiac systole. This method allows a constant, inexpensive monitoring of the heart rate and rhythm.

3. Electrocardiographic changes accompany the decrease of body temperature during **deliberate hypothermia.** Heart rate is decreased, the QRS complex widens, the S–T segment is elevated, the T wave changes in configuration, and atrial fibrillation is frequently observed. These changes disappear when the patient is rewarmed.

B. **The electrocardioscope** is the most useful electronic apparatus in the operating room, delivery room, recovery room, and intensive care unit. Dependence on the palpating finger and precordial or esophageal stethoscope is **not satisfactory** for detection of arrhythmias.

1. **In the operating room,** the electrodes are often attached so as to measure from the right shoulder to the cardiac apex, with the electrode on the side at the costal margin.

2. Most anesthesiologists prefer to observe **lead II,** because the transmission of the electrical impulses from the atrium to the ventricles is more obvious there.

VI. Advantages and limitations of the electrocardioscope.
See Chapter 6.

VII. Arrhythmias during anesthesia and surgery

A. Cardiac arrhythmias

1. **The incidence** of arrhythmias during administration of anesthetic agents is 15–30%.
2. **Precipitating factors** are:
   - a. Anesthetic drugs.
   - b. Intubation.
   - c. Anoxia.
   - d. Duration of surgery.
3. **Complications** due to dangerous arrhythmias are:
   - a. Ischemia of the brain, heart, or kidney.
   - b. Congestive heart failure and pulmonary edema.
   - c. Intrathoracic thrombosis with subsequent embolism.
   - d. Myocardial infarction.
   - e. Ventricular fibrillation (cardiac arrest).

B. Sinus rhythm and sinus arrhythmia

1. **Sinus rhythm** is a normal cardiac rhythm that originates in the SA node.
2. **Sinus arrhythmia** is a normal sinus rhythm with periodic variations in cardiac contraction during the respiratory cycle, since heart rate increases during inhalation and decreases on exhalation. It is caused by changes in vagal tone. This arrhythmia is common in children and young adults and has no clinical significance. It can be prevented or abolished by administration of **atropine.**

C. Sinus tachycardia

1. **The heart rate** is 100–160 beats/min. This rate is considered a sign of a normal sinus mechanism.
2. Sinus tachycardia can be produced by emotional stress, exercise, fever, anemia, hemorrhage, hypoxia, hypotension, hyperthyroidism, heart failure, epinephrine, or atropine.
3. It may occur in light planes of anesthesia with painful stimuli.
4. If allowed to persist or if the rate is very rapid (over 160), it may lead to congestive heart failure in compromised hearts, especially in children.
5. **Therapy** is directed at the underlying cause. Sinus tachycardia usually is not primarily treated. Digitalis is used only for heart failure.

D. Sinus bradycardia

1. The ECG shows a **normal sinus rhythm** with a rate of 40–60 beats/min and without a blocking of the conducting system of the heart.
2. **Hypotension** will result if the cardiac output is decreased.
3. Sinus bradycardia may be observed:
   - a. In athletes and elderly patients.

b. In patients with a history of myxedema, obstructive jaundice, or increased intracranial pressure.

c. During external pressure on the carotid sinus, eye muscle surgery, or vagal stimulation.

d. During (1) anesthesia with halothane, narcotics, or IV injection of succinylcholine and (2) administration of digitalis or quinidine.

4. **Therapy.** Usually, increased vagal tone is the cause, and **atropine** is the preferred drug for treatment. Also used are isoproterenol and cardiac pacing. No treatment is necessary if the cardiac rate is above 40 beats/min and there is no evidence of decreased cardiac output and blood pressure.

E. Premature atrial contractions

1. **Premature atrial contractions** may arise from any site on the atrial muscle, and they are difficult to detect on the electrocardioscope. However, they can be suspected when the periods between the QRS complexes become irregular.

2. **Premature atrial contractions may be observed** in patients with:

   a. Normal and abnormal hearts.

   b. History of heavy intake of alcohol, tobacco, or coffee.

   c. Digitalis toxicity.

   d. All forms of anesthesia.

   e. Myocardial ischemia or infarct and chronic lung disease.

3. **Diagnosis** can be made by ECG and careful palpation of the radial pulse; there is no compensatory pause as in premature ventricular contractions.

4. Whenever possible, **therapy** is directed at the cause. Sedation and quinidine are also used.

F. Paroxysmal atrial tachycardia

1. Paroxysmal atrial tachycardia is a **rapid succession of abnormal P waves** and usually occurs in paroxysmal attacks. The atrial rate is regular, **150–250 beats/min** with a 1:1 ventricular response. It may be observed in **normal** and **abnormal hearts.**

2. Paroxysmal atrial tachycardia usually **responds to vagal stimulation** (carotid massage or Valsalva's maneuver) as well as to sedation, vasopressors, digitalis, propranolol, or atrial pacing. The **paroxysms** of atrial tachycardia **usually stop suddenly.**

G. Atrial flutter

1. **The atrial rate** is 250–350 beats/min. The **ventricles respond slowly** in a ratio of 2:1, 3:1, or 4:1. The ECG shows P waves replaced by regular flutter waves. The baseline has a **sawtooth appearance.**

2. Atrial flutter is **due to** organic cardiac diseases. **Digitalis** is used to control the heart rate and may convert it to sinus rhythm in 50% of the cases. **DC countershock** with low energy is always successful in converting atrial flutter to sinus rhythm.

H. Atrial fibrillation

1. **The P waves are not visible,** and the occurrence of **QRS complexes** is irregular. The true P waves are **replaced** by irregularly shaped **F waves,** at a rate of **400–600 beats/min.**

2. This arrhythmia **occurs often** in rheumatic mitral valve disease, coronary artery disease, and hyperthyroidism.

3. **Clinical diagnosis** is made from:

a. The pulse deficit between the apex and radial pulse.

b. The complete irregular pulse.

4. Symptoms are present when the ventricular rate is more than 120 beats/min, and the results are **diminished diastolic filling time** and subsequent **decreased cardiac output.** This drop in organ perfusion pressure **may lead** to congestive heart failure, syncope, and hepatic and renal insufficiency.

5. Atrial stasis and thrombosis are frequently associated with atrial fibrillation, and about 30% of these patients may experience **emboli** (brain, kidney, extremities, and spleen).

6. Therapy. Digitalis is given to slow the heart rate. Digoxin must be given IV if sudden, rapid atrial fibrillation occurs during surgery. **DC countershock** is indicated if atrial fibrillation persists. **Quinidine** or **procainamide** are often given before and/or after cardioversion to maintain sinus rhythm.

I. Heart blocks. The excitation waves of the heart are **decreased** or **interrupted** in a portion of the conduction pathways.

1. AV block is associated with **organic cardiac disease.** There is a delay or failure of the passage of impulses through the conducting pathways of the AV node and the bundle of His.

2. An ECG is essential for diagnosis of an AV block.

3. Drugs that prolong the AV conduction time include digitalis, potassium, and procainamide. The sympathomimetic drug **isoproterenol** has good effects, particularly if the pulse rate is less than 40 beats/min. **Atropine** has minimal effect on AV block.

4. Implantation of a pacemaker is indicated in all patients with symptomatic heart block.

5. Temporary myocardial pacing wires before surgery may be indicated.

6. On all patients who have **conduction abnormalities,** temporary myocardial **pacing wires** are placed at the time of **open heart surgery.**

7. The three degrees of AV block are:

a. First-degree. The AV conduction time is prolonged. The P–R interval is more than the normal 0.2 sec.

b. Second-degree. Only one impulse every second or third atrial impulse is passed to the ventricles (2:1 or 3:1 block).

(1) Wenckebach's phenomenon is a form of second-degree block; there is a progressive **increase of the P–R interval** until one P wave is not transmitted to the lower chamber of the heart (dropped beat).

(2) Patients with a second-degree block as the result of a **myocardial infarction** must be **monitored constantly,** since complete heart block (third-degree) with cardiac standstill may suddenly develop in these patients.

c. Third-degree (complete heart block). All **atrial impulses fail to be transmitted** to the ventricles. There is a nonspecific form of **AV dissociation** in which the atria and ventricles contract independently. The regular **P waves** and **QRS complexes** are totally unrelated to each other, the **P–R interval** varies, and the **ventricular rate** is about 30 beats/min. In **Adams-Stokes syndrome,** there are episodes of giddiness, syncope, temporary loss of consciousness, and convulsions as the result of the complete heart block.

8. Bundle branch block (BBB). There is damage in one of the branches of the **bundle of His.** The **impulses arise** at the SA node and pass the AV node and bundle of His, but they can be **delayed** or **blocked** after the bifurcation of the bundle of His, either in the left or right bundle. BBB is divided into right (RBBB) and left (LBBB) block. The **rhythm** is regular, the **QRS complex** is wide and notched, and the **T wave** is directed in the opposite direction to the main deflection.

a. **RBBB may be found** in normal hearts but is usually associated with congenital defects, coronary artery disease, and hypertensive and valvular heart disease.

b. **LBBB is seen** more often in coronary artery disease, hypertensive heart disease, and aortic stenosis.

J. Wolff-Parkinson-White (preexcitation) syndrome

1. Wolff-Parkinson-White syndrome is characterized by a **short P–R interval** and a **prolonged QRS time.** This is a form of accelerated AV conduction as a **result** of the existence of congenital short-circuit muscle pathways. This syndrome may occur in **healthy individuals** and is **not** indicative of organic cardiac disease.

2. There is a 40% **incidence of episodes** of paroxysmal tachycardia, atrial fibrillation, and atrial flutter in affected patients, as well as a possibility of **sudden death** from a ventricular arrhythmia.

3. **Therapy** includes digitalis, quinidine, propranolol, and atrial pacing.

K. Premature ventricular contractions

1. Premature ventricular contractions (PVCs) are **produced** by an ectopic focus in any part of the **ventricular myocardium,** and they are more common than all the other arrhythmias. The **premature QRS complex** is broad, large, and coarsely notched, with **the T wave** pointing in the opposite direction from the **QRS deflection.** The PVCs are **followed** by a compensatory pause.

2. Occasionally, PVCs occur regularly with every second contraction (bigeminy) or every third contraction (trigeminy). These contractions may be due to **actual heart disease** or may be present in normal hearts as the result of medications, metabolic abnormalities, or unknown causes. If they appear during **anesthesia,** the cause may be inadequate oxygenation or deep anesthesia.

3. **Multifocal PVCs** may lead to **ventricular fibrillation.**

4. **Therapy** consists of **hyperventilating** the lungs with oxygen and decreasing the amounts of the anesthetic agents. If **PVCs persist,** the drug of choice is an IV injection of **lidocaine,** 1–3 mg/kg. Preference for this agent is based on clinical evidence showing that lidocaine is effective and has minimal effect on blood pressure and on the cardiac contractile force. The **duration of the antiarrhythmic effect** following lidocaine is brief (10–20 min), but this should be adequate time to discover and correct the underlying abnormality responsible for the arrhythmia. **Also useful** are procainamide, phenytoin sodium, and quinidine.

L. Ventricular tachycardia

1. The contractions occur in succession at a rate of **150–250 beats/min.** The **impulses arise** from an irritable ectopic focus located in one of the lower chambers of the heart.

2. **The ECG shows bizarre and irregular QRS complexes.** The **S–T segment** is covered by the next **QRS complex.** The **P waves** are difficult to recognize.

3. Ventricular tachycardia is a **very serious arrhythmia** because the increased irritability suggests severe ischemia of the myocardium, digitalis toxicity, electrolyte disturbances, anoxia, heart block during Adams-Stokes attacks, or overdosage of catecholamines, and it can lead to **ventricular fibrillation.**

Table 7-1. Treatment of Cardiac Arrhythmias

Arrhythmia	Therapy	Remarks
Sinus tachycardia	Correct underlying condition	Digitalis only for heart failure
Sinus bradycardia	Atropine, isoproterenol, cardiac pacing	
Atrial premature contractions	Correct underlying condition, sedation, quinidine	
Paroxysmal atrial tachycardia	Sedation, vagal stimulation, digitalis, propranolol, atrial pacing	
Atrial flutter	Digitalis, DC countershock	
Atrial fibrillation	Digitalis, DC countershock	Administer quinidine or procainamide before and after elective cardioversion
Complete heart block	Isoproterenol, cardiac pacing	Prepare for insertion of a permanent pacemaker
Wolff-Parkinson-White syndrome	Digitalis, quinidine, propranolol, atrial pacing	
Premature ventricular contractions	Lidocaine, treatment of digitalis toxicity, procainamide, phenytoin sodium, quinidine	Multifocal PVCs may lead to ventricular fibrillation
Ventricular tachycardia	Sedation, lidocaine, procainamide, DC countershock, phenytoin sodium	May lead to ventricular fibrillation
Ventricular fibrillation (cardiac arrest)	DC countershock, artificial ventilation and artificial circulation, sodium bicarbonate, epinephrine, etc.	

4. **Diagnosis is made by a clinician** from the presence of a fast, thready pulse, distant cardiac sounds, low BP, and a narrow pulse pressure (the difference between systolic and diastolic pressures) in patients with a history of cardiac disease.
5. **Therapy**
   a. **Lidocaine** (IV bolus of 50–100 mg, which may be repeated once) is tried first, and if it fails, **DC countershock** is tried. Procainamide or quinidine is used to prevent recurrence of this arrhythmia.
   b. **In the operating room,** hyperventilation with oxygen and lidocaine are a great help.
   c. **Vagal stimulation** does not lower the cardiac rate as it does in sinus tachycardia. **Digitalis** is **not** indicated, because it may precipitate ventricular fibrillation.

M. Ventricular fibrillation (cardiac arrest)

1. This is the **gravest of all arrhythmias** and is characterized by **irregular and uncoordinated** movements of the ventricles. The **impulses travel** in a disorganized fashion throughout the ventricles. The **contractions are not effective,** and **cardiovascular failure** and **death** result.

2. Ventricular fibrillation is **difficult to differentiate clincially** from ventricular asystole.
3. **Diagnosis** is made by **ECG** or **by inspection** during open chest surgery. The **ECG shows a few deflections** similar to PVCs; the deflections become smaller and erratic in shape and frequency. Ventricular fibrillation is **followed by** ventricular asystole with no recorded electrical ventricular activity.
4. **Therapy**
   a. Immediate external electrical defibrillation with DC countershock with 200–400 watt-sec.
   b. External cardiac compression.
   c. Hyperventilation with oxygen.
   d. Sodium bicarbonate.
   e. Epinephrine.
5. **Cardiac arrest** and **cardiopulmonary resuscitative measures** are discussed in Chapter 8.

N. **Treatment** of specific arrhythmias is outlined in Table 7-1.

Bibliography

Crehan, J. P., and Nicholson, M. J. A cardiac monitor-pacemaker. Its role in clinical anesthesia. *J.A.M.A.* 185:604, 1963.

Katz, R. L., and Bigger, J. T. Cardiac arrhythmias during anesthesia and operation. *Anesthesiology* 33:193, 1970.

Mazzia, V. D. B., Ellis, C. H., Siegel, H., and Hershey, S. G. The electrocardiograph as a monitor of cardiac function in the operating room. *J.A.M.A.* 198:103, 1966.

Snow, J. C. Monitoring with an electrocardioscope during anesthesia and surgery. *Anesth. Analg.* (Cleve.) 47:144, 1968.

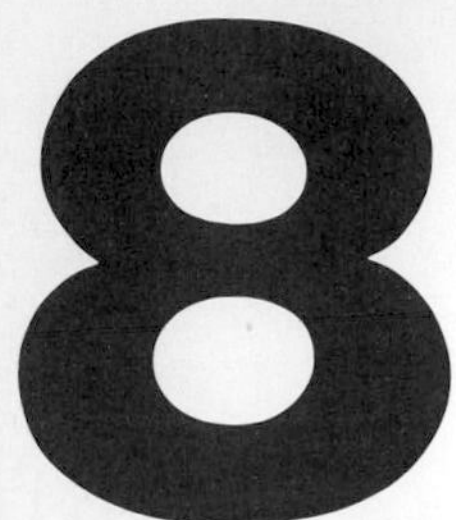

Cardiac Arrest and Cardiopulmonary Resuscitation

Cardiopulmonary arrest is the **sudden, unexpected cessation of respiration and functional circulation.** During respiratory and cardiac arrest, cardiopulmonary resuscitation (CPR) may be successful if performed before biological death of vital tissue develops.

Survival of the patient depends on (1) the degree of preexisting hypoxia of the cells and (2) whether circulatory or respiratory arrest occurs first. The **brain** depends totally on oxygen and is the organ least able to withstand hypoxia; in case of **circulatory arrest,** the pupils dilate in 45 sec and respiration stops within 1 min due to medullary depression. In the adult, the brain may be damaged within 4–6 min. However, if **respiratory arrest** occurs first, the circulation may continue for 5 min, with decreasing effectiveness, and damage to the brain may not become irreversible for 3–6 min.

I. Cardiac arrest

A. Cardiac asystole. There is total absence of electrical activity; **the ECG tracing** shows only a **straight line.** IV administration of a **positive inotropic agent** is of vital importance in such a case.

B. Ventricular fibrillation accounts for 75% of cardiac arrests in intensive care units and is the next most common form of cardiac arrest after myocardial infarction. The **ECG tracing** shows **wavy, irregular, and chaotic activity.** Electrical **defibrillation** is required to reestablish spontaneous and effective cardiac electrical activity. The precordial thump is considered to be effective usually only in the initial stages of fibrillation, when a small amount of energy may be sufficient to produce defibrillation.

C. Electromechanical dissociation may be caused by **anesthetics, hypoxia,** or **arrhythmia.** Regular electrical activity may be seen with a recognizable electrocardiographic complex, but there is **inadequate cardiac output,** as evidenced by the absence of a palpable pulse.

D. Artificial respiration and **external cardiac compression** must be begun; at the same time, efforts must be made to correct the inciting or underlying disease process.

II. Etiology

A. The etiologic factors of cardiac arrest are many and complex. In all patients, the treatment is directed toward correcting **hypoxia.** In some cases, e.g., electrocution, coronary occlusion, or overdose of isoproterenol, arrhythmia and fibrillation occur first, then hypoxia.

B. Causes of respiratory failure

1. **Airway obstruction** by vomitus, foreign body, blood, secretions, solid material, mucous plugs, laryngeal or bronchial spasm, or tumor.
2. **CNS depression** caused by stroke, head trauma, hypercapnia, barbiturates, narcotics, tranquilizers, or anesthetics.

3. **Neuromuscular failure** secondary to poliomyelitis, muscular dystrophy, myasthenia, or muscle relaxant drugs.

C. **Primary causes of cardiac or respiratory arrest**
   1. Flail chest.
   2. Pneumothorax.
   3. Massive atelectasis.
   4. Acute pulmonary embolism.
   5. Congestive heart failure.
   6. Overwhelming pneumonia.
   7. Gram-negative septicemia.
   8. Lung burns.
   9. Carbon monoxide poisoning.
   10. Massive blood loss.

D. **Causes of cardiac arrest**
   1. **Low cardiac output** as a result of cardiac tamponade or blood loss.
   2. **Hypercapnia** secondary to obesity, chronic lung disease, or incorrect anesthetic methods.
   3. **Hyperkalemia** following rapid transfusion of cold blood or excessive potassium replacement therapy.
   4. **Hypoxia and vagal stimulation** associated with drowning, intubation, aspiration, cor pulmonale, or traction on abdominal viscera.
   5. **Stimulation of the heart** by an intracardiac catheter or electrode.
   6. **Coronary occlusion** by embolus, thrombus, ligature, or replacement of coronary blood flow by contrast medium.
   7. **Overdosage** of cardiac glycosides, catecholamines, or anesthetic drugs.
   8. Hypothermia.
   9. Hyperthermia.
   10. Acidosis.
   11. Electrocution.

E. **Cardiac arrest may occur** as a result of anesthetics and other complicating factors during:
   1. Induction of anesthesia.
   2. Surgery.
   3. Postanesthesia recovery period.

F. Cardiac arrest is **more frequent:**
   1. In **geriatric** or **pediatric** patients.
   2. In patients with a history of **arrhythmias, heart block,** digitalis toxicity, myocarditis, myocardial infarction, congestive heart failure, electrolyte imbalance, or dehydration.
   3. In **massive hemorrhage.**
   4. During or following **heart surgery.**

III. **Prevention.** The majority of the situations that tend to promote cardiopulmonary arrest are preventable. Points of importance are:

A. **Identification of high-risk patients** by careful attention to a previous history of heart, lung, or kidney diseases; diabetes; drug allergy or addiction; and blood dyscrasias. Patients on digitalis, diuretics, steroids, or anticoagulants must be handled with special care.

B. **Collecting adequate information** and correcting serious omissions. Special attention should be given to the following:

1. Maintenance of **adequate blood volume.**
2. Proper choice of **preanesthetic medication.**
3. **Vagal stimulation** by intubation or other maneuvers should be done during induction of anesthesia following hyperoxygenation.
4. **Blood loss** during surgery must be checked and replaced properly.
5. **Arterial blood gases,** pH, and electrolytes must be monitored continuously.
6. **Respiratory insufficiency** should be watched for and anticipated during recovery. Postoperatively, respiration is frequently depressed, and additional oxygen or assistance with a respirator may be necessary. While a patient may be well ventilated during surgery, during recovery the patient may develop a progressive hypoxia and hypercapnia, possibly leading an irritable myocardium into ventricular fibrillation.

C. **Avoid hazardous maneuvers. Suctioning of the trachea** in a hypoxic patient is often the stimulus for arrest.

D. **Induction of anesthesia** must always be done very carefully, particularly in high-risk patients, with the following precautions:

1. Continuous ECG monitoring.
2. Use of chest or esophageal stethoscope.
3. Availability of a DC defibrillator.
4. Ready availability of all drugs for therapy of cardiopulmonary arrest.

IV. Diagnosis

A. **Early symptoms and signs** of hypoxia and/or heart failure, including:

1. **CNS.** Restlessness, anxiety, and disorientation. A cooperative patient who becomes difficult to manage in the recovery room is more likely to be hypoxemic than psychotic.
2. **Respiratory.** Dyspnea, tachypnea, gasping, laryngeal stridor, pallor, and cyanosis.
3. **Cardiovascular.** Cyanosis, venous distention, irregular pulse, hypotension, and profuse diaphoresis.

B. **Late symptoms and signs** of cardiopulmonary arrest, including:

1. **Absence** of carotid or femoral pulse. The radial pulse is not dependable.
2. **Heart sounds** are not obtainable.
3. **Respiratory standstill** or gasping respirations. Circulatory arrest is followed within 45–60 sec by respiratory arrest.
4. **Pupillary dilation** occurs within 45 sec following cardiac arrest. This indicates beginning damage to the anoxic brain.
5. **Absence of bleeding** and dark-colored blood in the surgical field.
6. **Flaccidity.**

7. **Convulsions** or loss of consciousness. If convulsion occurs, the brain is not yet anoxic.

8. The **ECG** shows cardiac asystole or ventricular fibrillation.

V. Therapy

A. The initial goal of therapy is oxygenation of the brain. The second goal is **restoration of circulation.** In addition, **the underlying condition** must be corrected.

1. Cardiopulmonary resuscitation **is not indicated for all** patients. Natural death in the aged or in the terminal stages of a chronic illness should not be reversed in this manner.

2. Cardiopulmonary resuscitation should be performed in cases of **reversible unexpected death** that occur as a result of myocardial infarction, general and local anesthetic drugs, electric shock, adverse reaction to drugs, cardiac catheterization, or suffocation.

B. Emergency cardiopulmonary resuscitation includes the following **ABCD** steps, which should always be started as quickly as possible.

1. **A, airway.**

2. **B, breathing.**

3. **C, circulation.**

4. **D, drugs and definitive therapy.**

5. In a witnessed cardiac arrest (when treatment can be initiated within 1 min of the onset of arrest), the **ABCD** sequence should include use of a **precordial thump.**

C. Pulmonary resuscitation

1. **Airway (A).** Time is the critical factor. Establishment of an **airway** as soon as possible is vital in a successful resuscitation. Artificial **ventilation** and artificial circulation must be initiated within 2–4 min.

   a. **Immediate opening of the airway.** This can be done easily and quickly by tilting the patient's head backward as far as possible. Many times this maneuver is all that is required for breathing to resume spontaneously. To carry out the **head tilt,** the patient must be lying on the back. The operator places one hand beneath the victim's neck and the other hand on the victim's forehead. Then the neck is raised by the operator with one hand (neck lift), and the head is tilted backward by the pressure with the other hand on the forehead. This effort flexes the neck, extends the head, and raises the tongue away from the back of the throat. Thus anatomic obstruction of the airway, created by the tongue dropping against the back of the throat, is relieved (chin lift).

   b. **The head-tilt technique** is satisfactory in most victims. If head tilt is not successful in opening the airway satisfactorily, additional forward displacement of the lower jaw, **jaw thrust,** may be necessary.

   c. This can be done by a **triple airway maneuver:** (1) the physician places the fingers behind the angles of the patient's jaw and forcefully displaces the mandible forward, (2) tilts the head backward, and (3) uses the thumbs to retract the lower lip to allow the patient to breathe through the mouth and nose.

2. **Breathing (B).** If the patient does not promptly resume spontaneous breathing after the airway is opened, **artificial ventilation** must be started immediately by **mouth-to-mouth,** mouth-to-nose, or mouth-to-mask breathing. There is enough oxygen (16%) in expired air to ensure oxygenation of a

patient's circulating blood. By doubling normal tidal volume, the rescuer increases the expired oxygen to 18%.

a. **A self-filling, nonrebreathing bag** and **well-fitting** anesthesia **mask** with oxygen supplied from a cylinder of compressed oxygen may be used as soon as they are available. Room air may be used if oxygen is not available.

b. **Endotracheal intubation** must be carried out at the earliest possible moment, but not before ventilation is produced for a few minutes by another method.

c. **An emergency tracheotomy** is indicated when an adequate airway cannot otherwise be effective. Alternative methods to tracheotomy are: (1) cricothyreotomy, (2) transtracheal catheter ventilation, and (3) esophageal obturator airway.

d. In a patient with a **laryngectomy,** direct **mouth-to-stoma** artificial respiration must be carried out. The head-tilt and jaw-thrust maneuvers are unnecessary for mouth-to-stoma resuscitation.

e. During artificial ventilation, the following adverse effects may take place:

(1) **Inflation** of the patient's **stomach** with air, followed by regurgitation and/or transmission of **infection** to the operator. These may occur when there is no endotracheal tube in place.

(2) **Rupture** of the patient's lungs.

(3) Aspiration of gastric contents.

3. **Pulmonary ventilation** is not adequate during external cardiac compression, so artificial ventilation must be carried out concurrently by any means available.

D. Artificial circulation–external cardiac compression

1. **Circulation (C).** In a case of sudden, unexpected cardiac arrest, all the ABCs of basic life support must be applied in rapid succession. This includes artificial ventilation and artificial circulation–external cardiac compression.

2. **Artificial circulation** can be carried out by **external cardiac compression,** which must be started at once. The exact instant of cardiac arrest is seldom known, and anoxia may cause irreversible damage to the brain after 4 min. After that interval, if resuscitation is successful, the patient will probably remain decerebrate.

3. Proper application of external cardiac compression requires that the patient be in a **horizontal position** and on a **firm surface.**

4. Application of pressure must be restricted to the **lower half of the sternum,** but not over the xiphoid process, to obtain maximum compression of the heart and to minimize the dangers of fractured ribs and damage to the liver.

5. **The heel only of one hand** is placed in the center of the chest **over the lower half of the sternum,** and the heel of the **other hand** is placed **on top of the heel of the first hand.** It is very important that the fingers be kept elevated at all times and not allowed to touch the chest wall. If pressure is incorrectly applied directly over the xiphoid, it may drive this bony process into the **liver,** which can result in a **fatal rupture** of this vascular organ.

6. Adequate force must be exerted **vertically downward** to move the lower sternum 4–5 cm toward the vertebral column, forcing blood into the pulmonary and systemic arteries. This requires 35–45 kg of pressure on the chest of an adult.

7. Following sternal compression, the sternum is released, and one cycle is repeated. When the pressure is released, the chest expands and the heart fills with oxygenated blood, which is circulated through the tissues with the next compression of the heart. **For one worker alone,** the compression and relaxation cycle of external chest compression should be repeated at a rate of 80 per minute; 15 compressions alternate with 2 quick lung inflations. **If there are two rescuers,** it should be repeated at a rate of 60 per minute for compressions, which is a **5:1 ratio,** with no interruption in compressions for ventilation. If the patient's trachea has been intubated, the compression rate can be 80 per minute.

8. Under optimum conditions, external heart compression produces only **30–40% of the normal amount of blood flow.**

9. **For infants and young children,** less pressure is required. Pressure with the fingertips alone on the middle third of the sternum is recommended for infants. For children up to 9–10 years of age, the use of one hand is considered adequate. The compression rate should be 100 per minute with ventilation every five compressions. There should be a ratio of 5:1 whether there are one or two rescuers.

E. Drug therapy

1. **Intracardiac** or **IV-**injected positive inotropic and vasoactive agents are of great help in stimulating heart contraction and in increasing perfusion pressure during external cardiac compression.

   a. The intracardiac route may be used when there has been a delay in starting an IV infusion.

   b. Intracardiac injections necessitate interruption of cardiac compression and ventilation, and there is the additional risk of laceration of a coronary artery, pneumothorax, or cardiac tamponade. Also, intramyocardial injection may precipitate intractable fibrillation.

2. The drugs that may be used under any condition of cardiac arrest are **sodium bicarbonate** and **epinephrine.**

3. **Ventricular fibrillation**

   a. The specific therapy includes **epinephrine** (to convert a fine fibrillation to a coarse fibrillation, to improve the perfusion pressure, and to increase myocardial contractility).

   b. **Sodium bicarbonate** (to facilitate the fibrillation, to enhance the effects of epinephrine, and to treat metabolic acidosis).

   c. **Electrical defibrillation.**

   d. **If the preceding therapeutic measures are not successful,** make sure that ventilation and external cardiac compression are being performed as optimally as possible, and repeat the epinephrine and sodium bicarbonate. If defibrillation is still unsuccessful, add **lidocaine** (1 mg/kg IV bolus) and repeat the above regimen. **If still unsuccessful,** substitute **procainamide** (1 mg/kg IV bolus) for lidocaine and repeat defibrillation.

   e. If still unsuccessful, add **propranolol** (0.5–1 mg IV) and repeat defibrillation.

   f. The principal indication for **isoproterenol** (2–20 micrograms/min drip rate, not bolus) is immediate control of hemodynamically significant bradycardia to get the heart started again and/or to boost the rate to about 60 beats/min.

F. Establishment of an IV route must be achieved as soon as possible by (1) **percutaneous peripheral puncture,** (2) **cutdown** over the greater saphenous vein at the ankle or another vein, or (3) percutaneous puncture of the **subclavian, external jugular,** femoral, or internal jugular vein.

G. **Correction of metabolic acidosis**

1. **Profound metabolic acidosis** occurs within a few minutes in the presence of cardiovascular collapse, and it persists in spite of efforts at cardiopulmonary resuscitation, which perfuses tissues but at a reduced rate.
2. **Sodium bicarbonate** should be infused promptly. The IV dose is 1 mEq/kg. Repeat after 10 min. Then give 0.5 mEq/kg every 10 min until arterial blood gases and pH are known.
3. Blood pH and base deficit are useful guides in the maintenance of acid-base balance.
4. A normal pH renders the heart more responsive to circulating and injected catecholamines and defibrillation.

H. **Therapy in asystole**

1. ECG shows a straight line.
2. Tilt the head to open the airway, and palpate the carotid pulse.
3. If the carotid pulse is absent at any time in any witnessed arrest, it is reasonable to apply a precordial thump with the knowledge that this is usually successful only in fibrillation, not in asystole.
4. If the victim is not breathing, give four quick, full lung inflations.
5. If pulse and breathing are not immediately restored, begin one-rescuer or two-rescuer cardiopulmonary resuscitation.
6. **Epinephrine** (0.5 mg) is injected IV, and the injection is repeated every 5 min.
7. **Sodium bicarbonate** is given by IV bolus only (see **G.2**).
8. **Isoproterenol,** 2–20 micrograms/min (drip rate, not bolus).
9. **Calcium chloride,** 5 ml of a 10% solution, administered slowly IV.
10. Prompt insertion of an **endocardial electrode,** by the transvenous or direct transthoracic route, with **artificial pacing** may be required.

I. **Therapy in electromechanical dissociation.** In electromechanical dissociation, the **ECG** shows a rhythmic electrical activity of the heart but no peripheral pulse or blood pressure. The therapy is the same as for asystole.

J. **Therapy in ventricular fibrillation** (see **E.3**). The **ECG** shows wavy, irregular, and chaotic activity.

1. Tilt the head to open the airway and palpate the carotid pulse. If the pulse is absent, give a precordial thump.
2. The administration of epinephrine and sodium bicarbonate is followed by **DC countershock.** Use maximum energy, 400 watt-sec.
3. Continued **external cardiac compression** and artificial **ventilation** are necessary.
4. If **defibrillation** with DC countershock **is not successful, give:**
   a. **Epinephrine,** 0.5 mg.
   b. **Sodium bicarbonate.**
   c. **Lidocaine,** 1 mg/kg IV bolus.
   d. **Repeat DC countershock.** If still not successful: First, substitute procainamide (1 mg/kg IV bolus) for lidocaine or bretylium (Darenthin) (5

mg/kg IV bolus); second, try propranolol (0.5–1 mg IV bolus), but extreme caution must be exercised when using it.

VI. Complications include rib fractures, fracture of the sternum, costochondral separation, pneumothorax, hemothorax, lung contusions, laceration of the liver, and fat emboli. A check for these conditions must be done in the postoperative period. Also check for intrathoracic and intraabdominal bleeding.

VII. Indications for open chest cardiac massage. Thoracotomy and direct cardiac massage are necessary in the following: (a) penetrating chest wounds, (b) tension pneumothorax, (c) cardiac tamponade, and (d) chest deformities, e.g., barrel chest and kyphoscoliosis.

VIII. Termination of effort. Resuscitation is considered **unsuccessful** if signs of **death of the heart and brain** are present after 1 hr of continuous cardiopulmonary resuscitative effort.

A. Signs of cardiac death

1. Absence of cardiac electrical activity.
2. Slurring and widening of the QRS complexes.
3. Persistent fibrillation with slowing and loss of amplitude.

B. Signs of central nervous system death

1. Unresponsiveness.
2. No movements.
3. No breathing.
4. Absence of reflexes.
5. Fixed and dilated pupils unresponsive to a direct light.
6. An isoelectric EEG.

Summary of Cardiopulmonary Resuscitation

1. Establish the **diagnosis:** apnea, absence of pulse, collapse, absence of heart sounds, absence of responsiveness, and ashen gray color.
2. **Summon help.** Note the time. **Time is critical;** you only have 4–6 min to reestablish ventilation and circulation.
3. **Thump the patient's chest** once sharply (only in witnessed arrest).
4. Check for absence of breathing first. Displace the patient's **mandible forward,** clear the airway manually only if obviously necessary, and give four rapid respirations by whatever means are available.
5. Place support under the patient's back and start mouth-to-mouth **breathing** (or use any other means available) and **external cardiac compression** in a 5:1 ratio (only in the two-rescuer sequence; otherwise the ratio is 15:2), depressing the lower sternum 4–5 cm.
6. **Insert an endotracheal tube** and ventilate with 100% oxygen.
7. Start **IV** infusion by needle or cutdown. Administer epinephrine and **sodium bicarbonate** (1 mEq/kg IV), and repeat bicarbonate injections 0.5 mEq/kg every 10 min until arterial blood gases and pH results are known.
8. Monitor ECG. If **ventricular fibrillation** is present following oxygenation, closed chest compression, and administration of epinephrine and sodium bicarbonate, defibrillate with **external DC countershock, 400 watt-sec,** placing one electrode to the right of the upper sternum below the clavicle and the

other electrode to the left of the apex or left nipple. If defibrillation is not effective, repeat countershock.

9. **Inject epinephrine.** If defibrillation is not successful, repeat external DC countershock.
10. Following restoration of heart function, inject **lidocaine** IV for excessive ventricular irritability.
11. **If asystole** is present, heart function may resume following myocardial oxygenation by ventilation and external cardiac compression.
12. **If asystole persists,** inject epinephrine and sodium bicarbonate IV. In addition, use calcium chloride and isoproterenol as indicated.
13. **If electromechanical dissociation** is present, take the therapeutic steps as in asystole.
14. **Corticosteroids** may be useful to decrease **cerebral edema.**
15. **Postcardiac arrest therapy.** This includes corticosteroids, diuretics, hypothermia, and hyperventilation. Monitor arterial blood gases, BP, ECG, CVP, urine, electrolytes, and chest x-ray.
16. **Essential drugs during cardiopulmonary resuscitation**
    Sodium bicarbonate
    Epinephrine
    Atropine
    Lidocaine
    Morphine
    Calcium chloride
    (Oxygen is also considered an essential drug)
17. **Useful drugs during cardiopulmonary resuscitation**
    Vasoactive drugs (levarterenol, metaraminol)
    Isoproterenol
    Propranolol
    Corticosteroids
    Procainamide

Bibliography

Bishop, R., and Weisfeldt, M. L. Sodium bicarbonate during cardiac arrest. Effect on arterial pH, Pco, and osmolality. *J.A.M.A.* 235:506, 1976.

Carveth, S. W., Burnap, T. K., Bechtel, J., et al. Training in advanced life support. *J.A.M.A.* 235:2311, 1976.

Chandra, N., Rudikoff, M. T., and Weisfeldt, M. L. Simultaneous chest compression and ventilation at high airway pressure during cardiopulmonary resuscitation. *Lancet* 1:175, 1980.

Donegan, J. H. New concepts in cardiopulmonary resuscitation. *Anesth. Analg.* (Cleve.) 60:101, 1981.

Eisenberg, M. S., Bergner, L., and Hallstrom, A. Cardiac resuscitation in the community. Importance of rapid provision and implications for program planning. *J.A.M.A.* 241:1905, 1979.

Gascho, J. A., Crampton, R. S., Cherwek, M. L., et al. Determinants of ventricular defibrillation in adults. *Circulation* 60:231, 1979.

Gascho, J. A., Crampton, R. S., and Sipes, J. N. Energy levels and patient weight in ventricular defibrillation. *J.A.M.A.* 242:1380, 1979.

Goldberg, A. H. Cardiopulmonary arrest. *N. Engl. J. Med.* 290:381, 1974.

Guildner, C. W. Resuscitation—opening the airway. A comparative study of techniques for opening an airway obstructed by the tongue. *JACEP* 5:588, 1976.

Lown, B., Crampton, R. S., DeSilva, R. A., et al. The energy for ventricular defibrillation—too little or too much? *N. Engl. J. Med.* 298:1252, 1978.

Luce, J. M., Cary, J. M., Ross, B. K., et al. New developments in cardiopulmonary resuscitation. *J.A.M.A.* 244:1366, 1980.

National Conference Steering Committee, American Heart Association and National Academy of Sciences–National Research Council. Standards for cardiopulmonary resuscitation (CPR) and emergency cardiac care (ECC). *J.A.M.A.* 227:833, 1974.

Rogers, M. C., Weisfeldt, M. L., and Traystan, R. J. Cerebral blood flow during cardiopulmonary resuscitation. *Anesth. Analg.* (Cleve.) 60:73, 1981.

Rudikoff, M. T., Maughan, W. L., Effron, M., et al. Mechanisms of blood flow during cardiopulmonary resuscitation. *Circulation* 61:345, 1980.

Snow, J. C. Treatment in cardiopulmonary resuscitation. *Acta Anaesth. Hellenica* 7:54, 1973.

Standards and guidelines for cardiopulmonary resuscitation (CPR) and emergency cardiac care (ECC). *J.A.M.A.* 244:453, 1980.

Taylor, G. J., Tucker, W. M., Green, H. L., et al. Importance of prolonged compression during cardiopulmonary resuscitation in man. *N. Engl. J. Med.* 296:1515, 1977.

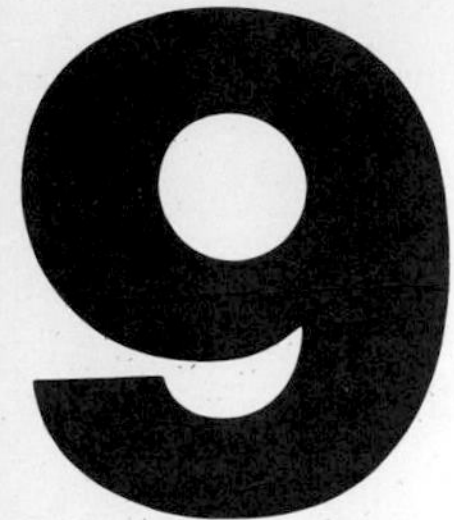

The Anesthesia Machine

The anesthesia machine is an apparatus for the administration of inhalation anesthetic agents.

I. **Components of the anesthesia machine** include sources of compressed oxygen and anesthetic gases, reducing valves, flowmeters, vaporizers, carbon dioxide absorption system, inspiratory and expiratory valves, escape valve, reservoir bag, and breathing tubes and face masks (Fig. 9-1).

A. **Gas sources**

1. **Oxygen** and **anesthetic gases** are supplied in cylinders as gases or liquids under pressure.
2. Anesthesia machines have two **yokes** for oxygen and two yokes for nitrous oxide. In many hospitals these gases are also supplied by high-pressure pipes from a remote central supply to the anesthesia machine.
3. Anesthesia machines are equipped with:
    a. A **pin index system**, designed to prevent accidental attachment of a cylinder to the wrong yoke. On the intended cylinder, the pins on the yoke match the holes on the valve seat.
    b. **Pressure gauges**, showing the pressure of the gas in the cylinder.
    c. A **fail-safe system** or **warning devices** to alert the anesthesiologist in case of failure of the oxygen supply. These systems regulate the flow of nitrous oxide in proportion to oxygen pressure, thus avoiding hypoxic mixtures. The newest machines also have a special valve to permit room air intake when **both nitrous oxide and oxygen** are shut off. Thus the patient will breathe room air containing approximately 20% oxygen concentration, rather than inhaling against a vacuum.
4. The cylinders are identified by their **labels** and by the **color** of their exteriors (see Table 9-1).
5. **In cylinders containing liquefied compressed gas** (nitrous oxide, cyclopropane, or carbon dioxide), the pressure within the cylinder is determined only by the gas pressure of the liquid. It is **not related** to the quantity of liquid that remains in the cylinder. At a given temperature, the pressure in a cylinder with a liquefied compressed gas will remain constant until all the liquid has been removed, at which time the pressure falls and **is related** to the rate at which the leftover gas is removed. As long as liquid remains in the cylinder, the amount can be determined only by weight.
6. **In cylinders containing nonliquefied compressed gas** (oxygen, helium, or oxygen mixtures), the pressure in the cylinder is related to both temperature and the amount of the gas within the cylinder. The cylinder content is measured by pressure; at a given temperature, the pressure will decrease proportionately as the cylinder contents are removed (e.g., when the pressure is decreased to half the given pressure, the cylinder will be half full).

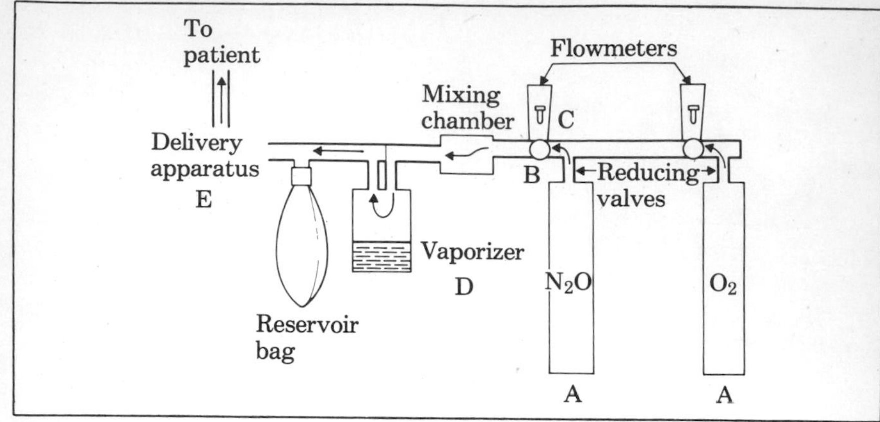

Fig. 9-1. The basic components of the anesthesia machine.

7. **Regulations** for production, packaging, handling, transportation, and storage of gases are set by (1) the Interstate Commerce Commission, (2) the Compressed Gas Association, and (3) the National Fire Protection Association.

B. **Reducing valves** or **pressure regulators** permit fine control of gas **flows** by lowering tank pressure to a less dangerous pressure. A pressure of 2000 psi in a full oxygen cylinder is reduced to 50 psi. **No grease** should ever be applied to a yoke, pressure gauge, or reducing valve because of the risk of combustion and explosion.

C. **Flowmeters**

1. Flowmeters are devices to **measure the volumes of gases** under pressure as they flow from cylinders.

2. They are calibrated, tapered glass tubes in which **bobbins float** in the flow of gas. Most common are **rotameter** flowmeters.

3. The flow rate of gas through the meter is regulated by an adjustable **needle valve.** As the orifice becomes wider, the flow rate of gas increases and the

Table 9-1. Color Coding of Gas Cylinders

Compressed Gases	Color	Physical State in Cylinder
Cyclopropane (C_3H_6)	Orange (silver WHO)	Liquid
Ethylene (C_2H_4)	Red (violet WHO)	Liquid
Nitrous oxide (N_2O)	Blue	Liquid
Helium (He)	Brown	Gas
Oxygen (O_2)	Green (white WHO)	Gas
Carbon dioxide (CO_2)	Gray	Liquid
Carbon dioxide–oxygen	Gray-green (gray-white WHO)	Gas
Helium–oxygen	Brown-green (brown-white WHO)	Gas

WHO = World Health Organization.

bobbin rises in the tube, coming to rest when the force of gravity is balanced by the upward stream of the gas. Gas flow rates are read directly from the calibrated tube.

4. Each flowmeter is **calibrated** specifically for the gas that it is to measure.
5. The gases are measured according to the **metric system,** in liters or fractions of a liter per minute.
6. **The flowmeters are gauged** for use at atmospheric pressure (760 torr) and room temperature (25° C). They become inaccurate at high altitudes or in hyperbaric chambers.
7. After the gas passes through the flowmeter, it goes into the **common mixing chamber,** where oxygen and anesthetic gases are mixed before delivery to the patient.

D. Vaporizers

1. A vaporizer is used **to vaporize** low-boiling-point, volatile, liquid anesthetic agents. There are many vaporizers: Copper Kettle, Vernitrol, Fluotec, Pentec, Fluomatic, Pentomatic, Drager, and others. Each is manufactured for use with a particular anesthetic.
2. These vaporizers are gauged so that, for a given flow, a known concentration of vapor is delivered.
3. **In the Copper Kettle vaporizer** (a heavy copper container), small bubbles of oxygen are passed through the anesthetic liquid. This oxygen, with the anesthetic vapor, is then joined with other gases in the common mixing chamber. The high heat conductivity of copper allows heat to be transmitted rapidly from the room and the metal parts of the anesthesia machine to the liquid, thus maintaining the volatile anesthetic at a relatively constant temperature.
4. **The Fluotec vaporizer** is a precision-control, temperature-compensated device. It delivers halothane vapor in a concentration range of 0.1–4%. A flow of oxygen, with or without nitrous oxide, passes through the vaporizer, with a flow rate of 2–10 L/min. A metallic valve expands and contracts according to the variations of the temperature of the anesthetic liquid, allowing a proportionately increased or decreased quantity of vapor to go through the vaporizer.

E. Carbon dioxide absorption system

1. **In the closed system** (with complete rebreathing of anesthetic mixtures) and in the **semiclosed system** (with partial rebreathing), there is the hazard of accumulation of carbon dioxide.
2. To overcome this danger, a carbon dioxide absorption system is used with **alkalies.**
3. A transparent **canister** containing a strong alkali is incorporated into the anesthesia circle system. During exhalation, the carbon dioxide is absorbed by the alkalies. In the semiclosed system, part of the carbon dioxide is returned to the patient and rebreathed.
4. **The transparent canisters** have the advantage of being easily inspected visually. The large canisters have a longer life before exhaustion, since they contain more absorbant.
5. **The alkalies** used are **soda lime,** a mixture of sodium and calcium hydroxides, and **barium hydroxide lime (Baralyme),** a mixture of barium and calcium hydroxides. Soda lime and barium hydroxide lime are efficient in removing the carbon dioxide from the anesthesia circuit.
6. **Soda lime for anesthesia** is white and contains **sodium hydroxide** 5%, **potassium hydroxide** 1%, and **calcium hydroxide** 94%. Small amounts of

silicates are added to prevent dust formation. For effective absorption, **moisture** is added to the granules (14–19%) (water is needed for the neutralization reaction). The **granules** are graded with a screen into sizes 4-mesh to 8-mesh, the mesh of a screen being determined by the number of holes per inch of screen. A 4-mesh screen has four quarter-inch-square openings per inch. The **size and shape of the granules** are very important, because effective absorption depends on the size of the surface presented to the gases.

a. During absorption, the **carbon dioxide** is converted chemically, the gas first going into solution and forming **carbonic acid,** which then reacts with the hydroxide to form **sodium carbonate,** at the same time regenerating the water used earlier. The sodium carbonate then reacts with the hydrate lime and forms **calcium carbonate,** regenerating caustic soda and caustic potash.

b. The **reaction of absorption and neutralization** of carbon dioxide with soda lime may be expressed by the following equations:

(1) $CO_2 + H_2O \rightleftharpoons H_2CO_3$

(2) $2\ H_2CO_3 + 2\ Na^+ + 2OH^- + 2\ K + 2\ OH^- \rightarrow 2\ Na^+ + CO_3^= + 2\ K^+ + CO_3^= + 4\ H_2O$

(3) $Ca(OH)_2 + H_2O \rightleftharpoons Ca^{++} + 2\ OH^- + H_2O$

(4) $2\ Ca^{++} + 4\ OH^- + 2\ Na^+ + CO_3^= + 2\ K^+ + CO_3^= \rightleftharpoons 2\ CaCO_3 + 2\ Na^+ + 2\ OH^- + 2\ K^+ + 2\ OH^-$

7. Barium hydroxide lime is pink and is as efficient as soda lime. It contains **barium hydroxide** 20% and **calcium hydroxide** 80%. The barium hydroxide is a chemical hydrate with eight molecules of water, which function as the bonding substance for the granule, so no inert material is needed. In addition, carbon dioxide is dissolved with this water. The **granules** are mesh size 4 to 8.

a. The procedure utilized to **manufacture** barium hydroxide lime absorbent granules combines barium hydroxide octahydrate, calcium hydroxide, which is a minimally active base addition (potassium hydroxide), and a wetting agent in a dustless noncaking granular form.

b. In the presence of gaseous **carbon dioxide**, the **barium hydroxide octahydrate** reacts chemically to form **barium carbonate** and simultaneously liberates sufficient **water** from the crystal structure to wet the admixed calcium hydroxide and propagate the continuing absorption of carbon dioxide by the moistened calcium hydroxide.

c. The following equations illustrate the chemical reactions that take place in barium hydroxide lime:

(1) $Ba(OH)_2 \cdot 8\ H_2O + CO_2 \rightarrow BaCO_3 + 9\ H_2O$

(2) $9\ H_2O + 9\ CO_2 \rightarrow 9\ H_2CO_3$

(3) $9\ H_2CO_3 + 9\ Ca(OH)_2 \rightarrow 9\ CaCO_3 + 18\ H_2O$

(4) $2\ KOH + H_2CO_3 \rightarrow K_2CO_3 + 2\ H_2O$

(5) $Ca(OH)_2 + K_2CO_3 \rightarrow CaCO_3 + 2\ KOH$

8. Indicators

a. Chemical dyes are incorporated into the soda lime and barium hydroxide lime granules; these dyes change color when exposed to different acids or alkalies. Thus **color indication** is, for the anesthesiologist, an adjunct guide to carbon dioxide absorption.

b. In all acid-base indicators, the color change is fully reversible.

c. Presence of an indicator does not affect absorption.

d. Soda lime

(1) To signal the progressive exhaustion of soda lime, a colorless, sensitive acid-base, **ethyl violet indicator,** is added.

(2) The soda lime changes from **white** to **purple** as absorption proceeds, full exhaustion being indicated by deep purple color.

(3) **Ethyl violet** is an especially effective indicator for use with soda lime because the critical pH is 10.3. As the strong caustic NaOH is consumed and replaced by the weak base $CaCO_3$, the color changes parallel the falling pH in the canister.

e. Baralyme.

(1) The indicator color change in barium hydroxide lime absorbent granules is progressive with increased carbon dioxide absorption, from **pink** to **purple**.

(2) These indicators, **Peeramine brilliant yellow MN extra** dye concentrate and **ethyl violet,** are weak organic bases that form salts with weak acids, such as carbonic acid, and in so doing bring about the characteristic color changes.

(3) The **pink** color indicates the alkaline state, which is the active condition. As carbon dioxide is absorbed, the color eventually changes to **purple** when absorption becomes inefficient.

f. The color change does not supplant the need for observing physiologic signs of **carbon dioxide excess** in an anesthetized patient; it only provides an adjunct to the patient indications for the guidance of the anesthesiologist. False readings can be obtained if the anesthesiologist relies solely on color indicator changes. Complete hydration of each granule can block the chemical reactions previously described. A better indication of carbon dioxide absorption and molecule hydration is the degree of hardness or fragility (crumbling) of the soda lime or barium hydroxide lime particles. The fully hydrated molecule is very hard. The functioning molecule is readily crushed and relatively soft.

9. Trichloroethylene should not be administered with the carbon dioxide absorption technique, since it reacts with soda lime or barium hydroxide lime to form toxic substances, such as **phosgene** (a respiratory tract irritant) and especially dichloracetylene (explosive and neurotoxic to the Vth and VIIth cranial nerves).

10. Nitrous oxide usually is used in a semiclosed system.

F. Inspiratory and expiratory valves are necessary for all exhaled gases to pass through the carbon dioxide absorption system. These directional valves ensure unidirectional flow through the carbon dioxide absorber.

G. Escape valve. When the flow of gases is such that the reservoir bag contains more than the patient can breathe, the extra gases escape through the escape valve.

H. Reservoir bag. The anesthesia machine provides a constant flow of anesthetic gases into a reservoir bag. The bag fills when the flow from the anesthesia machine exceeds the inspiratory demands of the patient. Thus a readily available supply of anesthetic agents is provided to the patient constantly throughout the respiratory cycle. Also, the reservoir bag can be used to apply positive pressure to the airway for assisted or controlled respiration.

I. Breathing tubes and face masks. The gases from the anesthesia machine are delivered to the breathing system with a carbon dioxide absorption system or some other system and then to the patient.

1. Single-use, sterile, **disposable** breathing tubes, Y-pieces, face masks, and reservoir bags are available.
2. **The face mask** must provide a good, airtight fit with the patient's face. Excessive pressure of the mask on the face or eyes must be avoided.

II. Recommendations for machine operation

A. Prior to induction of anesthesia, **fill the reservoir bag** with oxygen, occlude the outflow of the breathing circuit, and compress the bag to check for leaks.

B. **Avoid allowing** oil, grease, or any combustible substance to come in contact with tanks, valves, gauges, or yokes. These substances may react with oxygen or nitrous oxide and explode.

C. **Do not lubricate** valves, regulators, or gauges.

D. **Open** cylinder valves slowly.

E. Always use oxygen from a cylinder through a pressure regulator.

F. **Defective equipment** must be repaired by an authorized technician.

G. **Avoid** using flammable and/or explosive anesthetics.

H. **Inform** the person(s) responsible for a defective machine to ensure that it is not used until repaired.

I. Have an authorized person check the anesthesia machine at regular intervals.

J. **Calibrate** machines on a routine, periodic basis.

Bibliography

Barton, P., and Nunn, J. F. Totally closed circuit nitrous oxide–oxygen anesthesia. *Br. J. Anaesth.* 47:350, 1975.

Bruce, D. L., and Bach, M. J. Psychological studies of human performance as affected by traces of enflurane and nitrous oxide. *Anesthesiology* 42:194, 1975.

Bruce, D. L., and Bach, M. J. Effects of trace anesthetic gases on behavioural performance of volunteers. *Br. J. Anaesth.* 48:871, 1976.

Newton, N. I., and Adams, A. P. Excessive airway pressure during anesthesia. Hazards, effects and prevention. *Anaesthesia* 33:689, 1978.

Nielsen, H., Vasegaard, M., and Stokke, D. B. Bacterial contamination of anesthetic gases. *Br. J. Anaesth.* 50:811, 1978.

Nott, M. R., and Norman, J. Resistance of Heidbrink-type expiratory valves. *Br. J. Anaesth.* 50:477, 1978.

Ping, F. C., Oulton, J. L., Smith, J. A., et al. Bacterial filters. Are they necessary on anesthetic machines? *Can. Anaesth. Soc. J.* 26:415, 1979.

Smith, G., and Shirley, A. W. Failure to demonstrate effect of trace concentrations of nitrous oxide and halothane on psychomotor performance. *Br. J. Anaesth.* 49:65, 1977.

Spurring, P. W., and Shenolikar, B. K. Hazards in anesthetic equipment. *Br. J. Anaesth.* 50:641, 1978.

Virtue, R. W. Minimal-flow nitrous oxide anesthesia. *Anesthesiology* 40:196, 1974.

Wilson, R. S., and Laver, M. B. Oxygen analysis. Advances in methodology. *Anesthesiology* 37:112, 1972.

10 General Anesthesia

I. General comments

A. General anesthesia is defined as a reversible state of unconsciousness produced by anesthetic agents, with loss of the sensation of pain over the whole body.

1. **The order of descending depression** of the central nervous system during general anesthesia is as follows:
   - **a.** Cortical and psychic centers.
   - **b.** Basal ganglia and cerebellum.
   - **c.** Spinal cord.
   - **d.** Medullary centers.
2. **General anesthetic drugs are administered:**
   - **a.** By inhalation.
   - **b.** Intravenously.
   - **c.** Intramuscularly.
   - **d.** Orally.
   - **e.** Rectally.
3. **In 1846 Oliver Wendell Holmes,** in a letter to Morton, recommended the word **anesthesia**: "The state should, I think, be called anesthesia. This signifies insensibility, more particularly to objects of touch." However, this word was mentioned by Plato in 400 B.C. to describe absence of emotions and by Dioscorides in the first century A.D. to denote absence of physical sensation.

B. Indications

1. Infants and young children.
2. Adults who prefer general anesthesia in spite of the recommendation that the surgery can be performed safely under local or regional anesthesia.
3. Extensive surgical procedures.
4. Patients with mental diseases.
5. Prolonged surgery (the duration of local anesthetics is limited).
6. Surgery for which local anesthesia is neither practical nor satisfactory.
7. Patients with a history of toxic or allergic reactions to local anesthetic drugs.
8. Patients on anticoagulant treatment.

C. Clinical signs of general anesthesia (using volatile anesthetics, particularly diethyl ether)

1. **First stage: analgesia.** From the start of induction of anesthesia to loss of consciousness.
2. **Second stage: excitement.** From loss of consciousness to the beginning of regular respiration. There may be coughing, breathholding, struggling, swallowing, and/or vomiting.
3. **Third stage: surgical anesthesia.** From the beginning of regular respiration to respiratory arrest. This stage is divided into four planes.

   Plane 1. From the onset of regular breathing to the cessation of eyeball movements.

   Plane 2. From the cessation of eyeball movements to the beginning of intercostal paralysis.

   Plane 3. From the beginning to the completion of intercostal paralysis.

   Plane 4. From complete intercostal paralysis to diaphragmatic paralysis.
4. **Fourth stage: overdosage.** From the onset of diaphragmatic paralysis to cardiac arrest.

D. **Theories** explaining the mechanism of general inhalation anesthesia include the following:

1. Colloid theory (1875).
2. Lipoid solubility theory (1899).
3. Surface tension or adsorption theory (1904).
4. Cell permeability theory (1907).
5. Biochemical theories (1952).
6. Neurophysiologic theories (1952).
7. Physical theories (1961).
8. Multiple mechanistic theory (1967).

II. Techniques of general inhalation anesthesia

A. Open-drop technique

1. **The liquid anesthetic** is vaporized on layers of gauze covering a wire open-drop mask. The vapor is mixed with oxygen and is inhaled. The open-drop method is useful for infants and children.

   a. **Advantages**

   (1) The respiratory system is open to the atmosphere at all times during inhalation and exhalation.

   (2) No reservoir of the anesthetic gases and vapors and very little rebreathing.

   (3) No resistance to inspiration.

   b. **Disadvantages**

   (1) Oxygen and carbon dioxide tensions are not controllable.

   (2) The concentration of anesthetics is controlled poorly.

   (3) Increased dead space, which could result in hypoxia and hypercapnia.

   (4) Lack of means to assist or control ventilation.

   (5) Possible skin irritation or burn from liquid anesthetic.

   (6) Possible injury to the eyes by mishandling of the liquid anesthetic or by direct trauma.

2. Because of these disadvantages, anesthetics that stimulate ventilation, such as diethyl ether and divinyl ether, are the safest ones to be used with the open-drop technique.

B. Insufflation technique

1. **Anesthetic gases and vapors** are mixed with oxygen delivered into the mouth by attachment of the rubber anesthesia tubing (a) to an oropharyngeal airway with a nipple, (b) to a catheter inserted into the nasopharynx, or (c) to a hook inserted at the corner of the mouth. Another technique is connection of the delivery tube to the nipple of the Crowe-Davis mouth gag.
2. **Expiration** occurs directly into the air. The dead space is smaller than with any other anesthesia technique, and there is no rebreathing and no way to assist or control ventilation. Spontaneous respiration can be adequately maintained by using anesthetic drugs, such as diethyl ether, that do not depress respiration.

C. Ayre T-piece system

1. The Ayre T-piece system is another example of an **open technique**. It has been recommended especially for general endotracheal anesthesia in infants and small children undergoing surgical repair of harelip and cleft palate.
2. **The T-piece (or Y-piece),** with a sidearm open to the atmosphere, is inserted between the delivery tube and the endotracheal tube.
3. **On inhalation,** the patient inhales air through the open sidearm of the T-piece together with some vapors and gases from the anesthesia machine through the other sidearm.
4. **On exhalation,** the gases go out into the air via the open sidearm of the T-piece.
5. **Advantages**
   a. No resistance to ventilation because of the absence of a reservoir bag and expiratory valve.
   b. Permits assisted or controlled ventilation by the intermittent closure of the open sidearm of the T-piece.
   c. Simple, safe, and useful for infants and small children.

D. Systems with nonrebreathing valves

1. **There is no rebreathing** of exhaled gases, and a reservoir bag is incorporated in the anesthesia system.
2. **A valve allows** inhalation only from the reservoir bag and directs exhaled gases completely to the ambient atmosphere.
3. **All nonrebreathing valves** should have insignificant resistance and produce minimal dead space.
4. **Carbon dioxide** cannot accumulate.
5. **Heat** is dissipated, and hyperthermia is prevented. To prevent a fall of body temperature, **infants and young children must be placed on a warming blanket** containing circulating water heated to normal body temperature and **monitored** with a rectal or esophageal thermometer.
6. **Ventilation** can be assisted by intermittent closing of the expiratory valve.
7. **The nonrebreathing valves** can be used with spontaneous, assisted, or controlled ventilation.

E. Semiclosed technique

1. **In a semiclosed technique** there is partial rebreathing of exhaled gases from a reservoir bag.
2. **Part of the expired gases** pass through the expiratory valve into the air, and part go into the reservoir bag.
3. **Closing the valve** allows positive-pressure ventilation.
4. **A chemical absorber** is usually placed in the anesthesia circle to avoid accumulation of carbon dioxide.
5. There is little loss of body heat and moisture.
6. The alveolar oxygen percentage more nearly approximates that delivered by machine.
7. **Disadvantages**
   a. Increased resistance to ventilation.
   b. Heat retention.
   c. These disadvantages can be corrected with assisted or controlled respiration.

F. Closed technique

1. There is no escape of gases and vapors.
2. There is complete rebreathing, and a reservoir bag is needed.
3. Oxygen is supplied for the metabolic demands, and carbon dioxide is absorbed chemically.
4. **There are two modifications of this method:**
   a. In the **to-and-fro method,** the gases and vapors pass back and forth through the canister without valves; soda lime or barium hydroxide lime is used for the carbon dioxide absorption.
   b. In the **circle method,** the flow of gases and vapors, directed by valves, passes through the carbon dioxide absorption system only once during each respiratory cycle.
5. **Advantages**
   a. Conservation of heat and moisture.
   b. No waste of drugs.
   c. Decreased hazards of fire and explosion.
   d. Ease of employing positive-pressure breathing for assisting or controlling respiration.
   e. Minimal pollution due to gaseous and volatile anesthetics.
6. **Disadvantages**
   a. Possible heat retention.
   b. Increased resistance to breathing due to valves, tubing, and the carbon dioxide absorption system.
7. The closed technique can be converted to the semiclosed method if excess gases and vapors are permitted to escape through the expiratory valve.

III. Uptake and distribution of inhalation anesthetics

A. The inhalation of the anesthetic drug produces a depth of anesthesia that depends on the **partial pressure** of the anesthetic within the brain. Changes in the mixture of the inspired gases result in changes of partial pressures in the alveoli, arterial blood, and brain.

B. When the **partial pressure of an anesthetic gas is higher** in the arterial blood than in the brain, the gas enters the brain and results in deeper anesthesia. The reverse happens when the partial pressure in the arterial blood is lower than in the brain.

C. The partial pressure of a gas in the brain always seeks an **equilibrium** with the gas in the arterial blood.

D. **The absorption and distribution** of the anesthetic gases and vapors in the brain depend on the inspired concentration of the drug and on respiratory, circulatory, and physical factors.

E. **The general laws** directing diffusion, solubility, and the interrelationship of volume, pressure, and temperature apply to the anesthetic vapors and gases.

F. **Minimal alveolar concentration.** The anesthetic potency of an anesthetic is defined as the **minimum alveolar concentration** necessary to prevent movement in an average patient in response to a painful stimulus.

IV. Gas laws

A. **Boyle's law.** At a constant temperature, the volume of a gas varies inversely with the pressure.

B. **Charles' (Gay-Lussac's) law.** At a constant pressure, the volume of a gas varies directly with its absolute temperature.

C. **Dalton's law of partial pressure.** The pressure exerted by a mixture of non-reacting gases is equal to the sum of the partial pressures of the individual gases.

D. **Henry's law of solution of gases.** At a constant temperature, the solubility of a gas in a liquid solution is proportional to the partial pressure of the gas.

E. **Graham's law of diffusion of gases.** The rate of diffusion of a gas through porous membranes is inversely proportional to the square root of the molecular weight.

F. **Avogadro's law.** At the same temperature and pressure, equal volumes of a gas contain an equal number of molecules.

G. **Poiseullle's law.** The volume flow in a tube is (1) directly proportional to the pressure drop along the length of the tube and to the fourth power of the radius of the tube, and (2) is inversely proportional to the length of the tube and to the viscosity of the fluid.

H. **Bernoulli's theorem.** The lateral pressure exerted by a liquid is least where velocity is greatest.

I. **Venturi principle.** The lateral pressure exerted by a liquid going through a tube of varying diameter is greatest in the widest portion; here the velocity is the least. Pressure is least at the narrowest part where velocity is greatest. Beyond the point of constriction, and as the diameter is restored to the original value, the pressure reverts to the original pressure.

V. Volatile liquid anesthetics

A. Chloroform

1. Chloroform is a clear, sweet-smelling liquid. The vapor is heavier than air.
2. **Advantages**
   - **a.** Rapid induction and recovery.
   - **b.** Nonirritating.

c. Good muscle relaxation.

d. Nonflammable and nonexplosive.

3. **Disadvantages**

a. **Myocardial depressant.**

b. **Hepatotoxic.**

4. **Biotransformation.** The hepatotoxicity of chloroform derives from its biotransformation by oxidation to the trichloromethyl radical, which, in sufficient concentration, acts as a destructive free radical.

B. **Diethyl ether**

1. Diethyl ether is a colorless, volatile liquid. The vapor is 2½ times heavier than air. The liquid contains 3% alcohol, and it is stored in sealed metal containers with a copper inner coating to retard oxidation.

2. The vapor is rapidly absorbed from the alveoli into the blood and carried to the brain, where it is taken up by the lipoid tissues; 85% of the diethyl ether is eliminated through the lungs, and the remainder is removed through the skin, urine, and secretions.

3. Diethyl ether anesthesia is associated with **release of endogenous catecholamines.** This accounts for the cardiovascular stability seen during clinical anesthesia.

4. **Advantages**

a. Reliable signs of anesthesia depth.

b. Respiration is stimulated.

c. Bronchodilator.

d. The circulation is not depressed.

e. Good muscle relaxation.

f. Relatively nontoxic and safe, with a lower death rate following its use than with any other anesthetic.

5. **Disadvantages**

a. Prolonged induction and recovery.

b. Irritating. Action causes secretion of mucus from the upper airway.

c. Emetic and thus dangerous in patients with full stomachs.

d. **Flammable and explosive.**

6. **Biotransformation.** Diethyl ether may be considered a safe anesthetic agent because of its biodegradation to nontoxic materials that are normally present.

C. **Divinyl ether**

1. Divinyl ether (Vinethene) is a clear, colorless liquid. The vapor is 2.2 times heavier than air. The liquid is highly volatile; to decrease volatility, 3.5% alcohol is added to the commercial product.

2. **Advantages**

a. Rapid induction and recovery.

b. Stimulates respiration.

c. Easy administration and maintenance of anesthesia.

3. Disadvantages

a. Irritant to upper airway and larynx.

b. May produce abnormal muscular movements.

c. Cannot be administered safely for long procedures; administration is limited to 15 min.

d. Hepatotoxic if anesthesia lasts more than 1 hr.

e. Flammable and explosive.

D. Ethyl vinyl ether (Vinamar) clinically resembles divinyl ether. It is **flammable and explosive.**

E. Ethyl chloride

1. Ethyl chloride is a clear liquid that smells like ether. Its boiling point, 12.5° C, is below room temperature. The vapor is heavier than air.

2. Advantages

a. Rapid induction and recovery.

b. Easy administration and control.

c. Local anesthesia by freezing.

3. Disadvantages

a. Myocardial depressant.

b. Hepatotoxic.

c. Explosive and flammable.

F. Fluroxene

1. Fluroxene (Fluoromar) is a clear, volatile liquid.

2. Advantages

a. Nonirritating.

b. No sensitization to catecholamines.

c. Nonexplosive. Lower limit of flammability in oxygen and in nitrous oxide–oxygen is 4% concentration. Fluroxene is **explosive** in a concentration **greater than 4%.**

3. Disadvantages

a. Poor relaxant.

b. Emetic.

4. Biotransformation. In humans, fluroxene is metabolized to the innocuous trifluoroacetic acid.

G. Halothane

1. Halothane (Fluothane) (Table 10-1) is a clear, colorless, potent volatile liquid. It has wide popularity, mainly because of its properties of smooth induction of anesthesia, comfortable recovery, easy maintenance of proper depth of anesthesia, and lack of flammability. Most of it is eliminated through the lungs.

2. It is not recommended for **obstetric anesthesia** or for patients with markedly increased intracranial pressure.

3. Fatal necrosis of the liver may occur following surgery carried out under general anesthesia in which halothane in its normally safe concentration is a major component. While there is overwhelming evidence that halothane is

Table 10-1. Characteristics of Some Inhalation Anesthetics

Anesthetic	Boiling Point (°C)	Vapor Pressure (torr at 20° C)	Inspired Vapor Concentration for Anesthesia (volume per 100 ml)			
					MAC	
			Induction	Maintenance	With O_2	With 70% N_2O
Nitrous oxide N_2O	−89	—	60–80	50–70	101	—
Halothane $CF_3CHBrCl$	50	243	2–4	0.5–2	0.77	0.28
Enflurane $CHF_2—O—CF_2—CHFCl$	56.5	175	2–5	1–2	1.68	0.56
Isoflurane $CHF_2—O—CHCl—CF_3$	48.5	250	2–4	1–2	1.3	0.66

not generally hepatotoxic, it is becoming clear that in rare instances some unusual hepatic effect occurs when it is administered for a second time within a short interval. Thus repeated exposures to halothane should be avoided.

4. **In children,** for unknown reasons, liver complications due to halothane anesthesia are extraordinarily rare.

5. **Advantages**
   a. Rapid, smooth induction and recovery.
   b. Pleasant.
   c. Nonirritating; no secretions.
   d. Bronchodilator.
   e. Nonemetic.
   f. Nonflammable and nonexplosive.

6. **Disadvantages**
   a. Myocardial depressant.
   b. It is an arrhythmia-producing drug.
   c. Sensitizes the myocardial conduction system to the action of catecholamines.
   d. It is a potent uterine relaxant.
   e. Possibly toxic to the liver.
   f. Recovery from anesthesia is occasionally accompanied by shivering or tremor. In most of the patients, body temperature is low.

7. **Biotransformation.** Metabolic degradation includes the appearance of bromide, chloride, and nontoxic trifluoroacetic acid in urine. Metabolites are slowly removed (in 2–3 weeks).

H. Methoxyflurane

1. Methoxyflurane (Penthrane) is a clear, colorless liquid with a characteristic fruity odor. It is **the most potent and least volatile inhalation anesthetic.** Following methoxyflurane anesthesia, some patients exhibit pallor of the skin, and prolonged somnolence occurs during the recovery period. A few patients complain of headaches during the postoperative period; others have expressed a dislike for the odor.

2. **The nephrotoxicity** associated with methoxyflurane is caused by the **free fluoride ions** formed during metabolic degradation of the drug and is usually manifested early as polyuria.

3. **Advantages**
   a. Great margin of safety.
   b. Good muscle relaxant.
   c. No sensitization to catecholamines.
   d. Nonflammable and nonexplosive.

4. **Disadvantages**
   a. Prolonged induction of anesthesia and prolonged recovery.
   b. **Nephrotoxic.**

5. **Biotransformation.** Metabolic biotransformation of methoxyflurane includes two major metabolic products, fluoride and oxalic acid. These are potentially

toxic to the kidney. Other products are carbon dioxide, dichloroacetic acid, and methoxyfluoroacetic acid. Metabolites are excreted in the urine within 10 days.

I. Trichloroethylene

1. Trichloroethylene (Trilene) is a colorless liquid. The vapor is heavier than air.

2. **Advantages**
   a. Nonirritating.
   b. Analgesic.
   c. Maintenance of stable blood pressure.
   d. Nonflammable and nonexplosive.

3. **Disadvantages**
   a. Myocardial depressant.
   b. Cardiac arrhythmias.
   c. Sensitizes the heart to catecholamines.
   d. Tachypnea.
   e. Poor muscle relaxant.
   f. Emetic.
   g. **Must not be used with carbon dioxide absorption system.** Reacts with soda lime or barium hydroxide lime to form toxic substances, such as phosgene (a respiratory tract irritant) and dichloracetylene (explosive and neurotoxic to the Vth and VIIth cranial nerves).

4. **Biotransformation.** Most of the drug is excreted unchanged by the lungs. A small amount changes in the body to form trichloroacetic acid, which is pharmacologically inert and is excreted by the kidney within several days.

J. Enflurane

1. Enflurane (Ethrane) (see Table 10-1) is a clear, colorless, stable volatile liquid with a pleasant ether-like odor.

2. It is a potent inhalation anesthetic (half as potent as halothane) and has physical, pharmacologic, and clinical properties similar to those of halothane.

3. **CNS excitation** may be noted as anesthesia is deepened, particularly in the presence of hypocapnia, but this may be terminated without complications by lightening the anesthesia.

4. **Enflurane and isoflurane** (Forane) are chemical isomers (see **K**). Both contain the same chemical elements, but they are arranged differently.

5. **Use of epinephrine** injections for hemostasis in humans is far less likely to produce arrhythmias during enflurane or isoflurane anesthesia than during halothane anesthesia. Ethrane has documented compatibility with epinephrine; a solution containing up to 10 ml of epinephrine 1:100,000 or 1:200,000 alone or in conjunction with local anesthetics may be injected subcutaneously—at a rate no greater than 10 ml/min, up to a maximum of 30 ml/hr. More dilute solutions and reduced dosages should be used in highly vascular areas.

6. **Advantages**
   a. Pleasant.
   b. Rapid induction and recovery.

c. Nonirritating; no secretions.

d. Bronchodilator.

e. Good muscle relaxation.

f. Maintenance of relative stability of the cardiovascular system. Cardiac rhythm extremely stable.

g. Nonemetic.

h. Nonflammable and nonexplosive.

i. Compatible with epinephrine.

7. **Disadvantages**

a. Myocardial depressant.

b. Progressive increase in depth of anesthesia produces a corresponding increase in hypotension.

c. Shivering on emergence.

d. **CNS irritant properties.** Enflurane may **irritate the CNS** if given in high concentrations, particularly if accompanied by hypocapnia.

e. As with all halogenated anesthetics, there is a possibility of liver damage.

f. May be harmful in patients with severely compromised renal function.

8. **Biotransformation.** Enflurane undergoes **limited biotransformation.** Only 2.4% of the administered enflurane is excreted in the urine as nonvolatile fluorinated metabolites (0.5% as inorganic fluoride). This indicates that enflurane is metabolized much less than trichloroethylene, methoxyflurane, fluroxene, and halothane. The levels of fluoride ion are much lower than those associated with evidence of nephrotoxicity following administration of methoxyflurane.

K. Isoflurane

1. Isoflurane (Forane) (**see** Table 10-1) is the **newest** inhalation anesthetic agent. It is a stable, volatile liquid that vaporizes easily at room temperature.

2. Isoflurane and enflurane are chemical isomers.

3. This fluorinated hydrocarbon is half as potent as halothane and has similar properties.

4. No abnormal motor activity, such as twitching or convulsions, is seen during isoflurane anesthesia.

5. **Advantages**

a. Good patient acceptance of the drug.

b. Rapid induction and recovery.

c. Nonirritating; no secretions.

d. Bronchodilator.

e. Excellent muscle relaxation.

f. Extremely stable cardiac rhythm.

g. Compatible with epinephrine. No arrhythmias with infiltration of epinephrine, 10–12 ml of a 1:100,000 solution.

h. Nonemetic.

i. Nonflammable and nonexplosive.

6. **Disadvantages**
   a. Depresses the cardiovascular system.
   b. Tendency of blood pressure to decline with the depth of anesthesia, with the pulse rate remaining somewhat elevated.
   c. Shivering.
   d. Possibility of acute or delayed injury to the liver.
   e. Isoflurane is metabolized, to a small extent, to fluoride ion and probably should not be used in patients with compromised renal function.
7. **Biotransformation.** Isoflurane degrades metabolically to organic fluoride compounds, such as trifluoroacetic acid. Fluoride ion, a potential nephrotoxin, is one product of the breakdown of isoflurane, although the amount formed is much smaller than from methoxyflurane.

VI. Gaseous anesthetic agents

A. Cyclopropane

1. Cyclopropane is a colorless, potent gas with a sweet smell. It is stored in orange metal cylinders as a pressurized liquid. It is 1½ times heavier than air.
2. **Advantages**
   a. Rapid induction of anesthesia and swift recovery.
   b. Nonirritating; no secretions.
   c. Blood pressure remains stable.
   d. Indicated in poor-risk patients.
3. **Disadvantages**
   a. Bronchoconstrictor.
   b. Sensitizes the myocardium to catecholamines.
   c. Cardiac arrhythmias.
   d. Emetic.
   e. Contraindicated in patients with toxic thyroid or pheochromocytoma.
   f. **Very explosive.**
4. **Biotransformation.** Data are not available.

B. Ethylene

1. Ethylene is similar to nitrous oxide in its anesthetic properties. This gas is slightly more potent than nitrous oxide and must be administered in the same concentrations. Because of its explosive properties and its unpleasant odor, it has never gained much popularity. It is **lighter than air.**
2. **Advantages**
   a. Nonirritating.
   b. Analgesic.
   c. No effect on metabolism.
   d. Rapid induction and emergence.
3. **Disadvantages**
   a. The high concentration required for surgical anesthesia produces hypoxia.
   b. Poor muscle relaxation.
   c. **Explosive.**

C. Nitrous oxide

1. Nitrous oxide (N_2O) (see Table 10-1), the least potent of the anesthetic gases, is the most frequently administered inhalation anesthetic. It is the only inorganic gas used in clinical anesthesia.
2. **It is compressed to a liquid** and stored in steel **cylinders colored blue** for identification. Nitrous oxide returns to the gaseous state when released from the cylinder. The gas is colorless and tasteless and has a faintly sweet odor. The cylinder becomes cold and can accumulate a deposit of frost when heat for vaporization is received from the tank's wall and surrounding atmosphere.
3. **Nitrous oxide is 1½ times heavier than air.** It passes rapidly through the alveolar membranes. Nitrous oxide does not combine with hemoglobin; it circulates in the plasma in physical solution only. The greater portion of it is removed unchanged through the lungs **within 2–3 min.** Small amounts escape through the skin.
4. **The molecule of oxygen in N_2O** is not available for cell ventilation because N_2O does not decompose within the body.
5. Nitrous oxide is a **weak anesthetic** that is widely administered as a supplementary agent with one or more other general anesthetics. Narcotics, with or without muscle relaxant drugs, are often used with it.
6. **In the absence of hypoxia,** there is little effect on the heart rate, myocardial contractility, respiration, blood pressure, liver, kidney, or metabolism. Postoperative emesis is rare.
7. **Changes occur in air-filled cavities** because nitrous oxide is 35 times more soluble in the blood than nitrogen. During induction of anesthesia, nitrous oxide invades a closed, air-filled space 35 times more rapidly than nitrogen leaves the cavity, increasing the enclosed pressure or volume. It diffuses into closed gas spaces (such as the ventricles, during diagnostic pneumoencephalography, causing an increase in cerebrospinal fluid pressure; the intestines, intensifying distention of intestinal obstruction; and the pleural space, aggravating a pneumothorax).
8. Nitrous oxide is not employed with the closed technique.
9. Oxygen 100% must be given at the termination of surgery to prevent **diffusion anoxia** on emergence.
10. Nitrous oxide is a **very safe anesthetic** if oxygen is supplied in sufficient concentration.
11. Many hospitals supply nitrous oxide and oxygen to wall outlets in their operating rooms from remote central supply areas.
12. **Advantages**
    a. Rapid induction of anesthesia and emergence.
    b. Does not sensitize the myocardium to epinephrine.
    c. Nonirritating.
    d. Intense analgesia.
    e. Nonemetic.
    f. **Nonflammable and nonexplosive but supports the combustion of other agents** even in the absence of oxygen.
13. **Disadvantages**
    a. Requires low oxygen concentration for the surgical level of anesthesia.
    b. Weak anesthetic.

c. No muscular relaxation.

d. Possible bone marrow aplasia and fatal agranulocytosis from prolonged administration.

e. Changes in middle ear mechanics (due to differential solubility of nitrous oxide and nitrogen, causing pressure changes), which are believed to have contributed to postoperative hearing loss.

14. **Biotransformation.** At the present time, there is no evidence to indicate that metabolism of this anesthetic drug occurs.

Bibliography

Black, G. W. Enflurane. *Br. J. Anaesth.* 51:627, 1979.

Blitt, C. D., Gandolfi, A. J., Soltis, J. J., et al. Extrahepatic biotransformation of halothane and enflurane. *Anesth. Analg.* (Cleve.) 60:129, 1981.

Brum, H. R., and Sipes, I. G. Biotransformation and hepatotoxicity of halothane. *Biochem. Pharmacol.* 26:209, 1977.

Cohen, E. N., Trudell, J. R., Edmunds, H. N., et al. Urinary metabolites of halothane in man. *Anesthesiology* 43:392, 1975.

Cormack, R. S. Awareness during surgery. A new approach. *Br. J. Anaesth.* 51:1051, 1979.

Cousins, M. J., Greenstein, L. R., Hitt, R. A., et al. Metabolism and renal effects of enflurane in man. *Anesthesiology* 44:44, 1976.

Eger, E. I., Calverley, R. K., and Smith, N. T. Changes in blood chemistries following prolonged enflurane anesthesia. *Anesth. Analg.* (Cleve.) 55:547, 1976.

Fabian, L. W. Should we continue to use nitrous oxide? *Surv. Anesth.* 24:335, 1980.

Inman, W. H. W., and Mushin, W. W. Jaundice following halothane. *Br. Med. J.* 2:1455, 1978.

Kawamura, R., Stanley, T. H., English, J. B., et al. Cardiovascular responses to nitrous oxide exposure for two hours in man. *Anesth. Analg.* (Cleve.) 59:93, 1980.

Knill, R. L., Manninen, P. H., and Clement, J. L. Ventilation and chemoreflexes during enflurane sedation and anaesthesia in man. *Can. Anaesth. Soc. J.* 26:353, 1979.

Mazze, R. I., Calverley, R. K., and Smith, N. T. Inorganic fluoride nephrotoxicity: Prolonged enflurane and halothane anesthesia in volunteers. *Anesthesiology* 46:265, 1977.

Peter, S. R. M. Pulmonary physiologic studies of the perioperative period. *Chest* 76:576, 1976.

Roth, S. Mechanism of anaesthesia. A review. *Can. Anaesth. Soc. J.* 27:433, 1980.

Sharp, J. H., Trudell, J. R., and Cohen, E. N. Volatile metabolites and decomposition products of halothane in man. *Anesthesiology* 50:2, 1978.

Smith, N. T., Calverley, R. K., Prys-Roberts, C., et al. Impact of nitrous oxide on the circulation during enflurane anesthesia in man. *Anesthesiology* 48:345, 1978.

Sonntag, H., Donath, U., Hillebrand, W., et al. Left ventricular function in conscious man and during halothane anesthesia. *Anesthesiology* 48:320, 1978.

Wabba, W. M. Analysis of ventilatory depression by enflurane during clinical anesthesia. *Anesth. Analg.* (Cleve.) 59:103, 1980.

Wade, J. G., and Stevens, W. C. Isoflurane. An anesthetic for the eighties? *Anesth. Analg.* (Cleve.) 60:666, 1981.

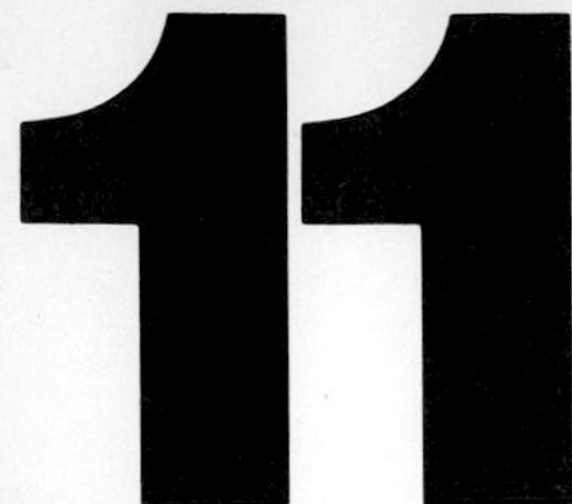

11 Intravenous Anesthesia

I. **The ultrashort-acting barbiturates** are administered to provide a rapid, pleasant induction of anesthesia. In sufficient amounts, these drugs can accomplish all the anesthetic stages, but they may produce serious cardiovascular depression. Thus, their usefulness as primary anesthetics is limited to short, minor procedures that do not require muscle relaxation and do not involve the interior organs of the great cavities of the body, especially the abdomen. They are commonly used in combination with nitrous oxide and oxygen.

A. **Thiopental and thiamylal**

1. Thiopental (Pentothal) and thiamylal (Surital) are **similar** in their pharmacologic actions, and so they are described together.
2. Aqueous solutions are **strongly alkaline, pH 11** (pH of blood is 7.4), and therefore are not compatible with acidic substances.
3. Their initial hypnotic action is intense, rapidly induced (within 30–40 sec of IV injection), and of short duration. This is followed by mild hypnosis or heavy sedation.
4. Like the inhalation anesthetic agents, the ultrashort-acting barbiturates produce unconsciousness mainly by blocking the central brainstem core (reticular activating system), which subserves wakefulness.
5. **For induction and maintenance** of anesthesia, they are frequently supplemented with nitrous oxide.
6. **For continuous administration**, a 0.4% solution is infused by IV drip. An initial fast drip rate is used for **induction** of anesthesia, followed by a slow rate for **maintenance. For intermittent administration,** a 2–2.5% aqueous solution is used. Stronger solutions are irritating to veins and tissues.
7. Following an **IV test dose** of 25–75 mg (1–3 ml of a 2.5% solution), **induction of IV anesthesia** is carried out slowly by injection of thiopental, 4–7 mg/kg over 30–45 sec.
8. **Intubation** is facilitated with IV succinylcholine (80–100 mg), and **maintenance** of anesthesia is begun with nitrous oxide, oxygen, narcotics, halothane, or enflurane. Muscle relaxant agents are administered as indicated. Supplemental doses of barbiturates are given as needed.
9. **Intraarterial infusion**. Every effort must be made to avoid intraarterial infusion, which can lead to arterial occlusion and gangrene of the extremity, and **extravascular infiltration,** which may cause tissue necrosis.
10. Once prepared, unused portions of solutions should be discarded after 24 hr.
11. **Indications**
    a. Induction of anesthesia prior to administration of other anesthetic agents.
    b. Supplement to regional anesthesia.

c. Providing hypnosis during balanced anesthesia with other drugs.

d. Control of convulsive conditions during or following inhalation anesthesia, local anesthesia, or other causes.

e. In psychiatry, narcoanalysis and electroconvulsive treatment.

12. **Contraindications.** Barbiturates are absolutely contraindicated in patients with:

a. **Status asthmaticus.**

b. **Latent or manifest porphyria.** This is a congenital metabolic disease characterized by a marked increase in the production and excretion of porphyrins and their precursors. A very serious complication may occur in patients with **acute intermittent porphyria.** This rare disease is exacerbated by the administration of barbiturates, which causes a marked increase of porphyrin synthesis. Symptoms include acute attacks of abdominal pain, muscle paralysis, psychiatric manifestations, and the passage of reddish urine. The course is very rapid and fatal.

13. **Advantages**

a. Induction of anesthesia is rapid and pleasant.

b. If supplemented, these drugs are suitable for maintenance of anesthesia.

c. No secretions.

d. Nonemetic.

e. No sensitization of the autonomic tissues of the heart to catecholamines.

f. Nonexplosive.

14. **Disadvantages**

a. Can cause respiratory depression or apnea.

b. Little analgesia.

c. Poor muscle relaxation.

d. Increased danger of laryngospasm.

e. Cardiovascular depression, particularly in hypovolemic or debilitated patients.

f. Shivering may occur.

g. Parasympathomimetic.

h. May cause prolonged depression.

i. There is no antagonist. Once given, these agents cannot be removed.

B. Methohexital

1. Methohexital (Brevital), a rapidly induced, ultrashort-acting barbiturate anesthetic agent, differs chemically from thiopental and thiamylal in that it contains no sulfur; however, its pharmacologic properties are similar.

2. Methohexital is administered IV (1 mg/kg in a 1% solution with pH 11). It is $2\frac{1}{2}$ times more potent than the thiobarbiturates, and recovery is quicker.

3. It is useful for induction of anesthesia in the dental chair, for outpatient surgery, for electroconvulsive therapy, and for minor gynecologic or orthopedic operations.

C. Uptake, distribution, and elimination of IV barbiturates

1. The barbiturates have a high fat solubility, which permits them to enter all parts of the body rapidly. The tissue uptake is a function of both local blood circulation and concentration of the drug in the arterial blood.

2. Because the brain receives a great proportion of the cardiac output, a high percentage of the infused drug reaches the brain rapidly, with resulting CNS depression.

3. The duration of unconsciousness depends on the rate of redistribution of the drug from the brain to the other parts of the body.

4. Repeated IV doses lead to prolonged anesthesia because fatty tissues act as a reservoir, accumulating thiopental or thiamylal in concentrations 6 to 12 times greater than the plasma concentration and then releasing the drug slowly. For this reason, the thiobarbiturates are administered as the sole anesthetic agent only for brief (15-min) procedures.

5. The elimination process depends on what fraction of the agent is inactivated with each pass through the hepatic or renal blood circulation.

D. Biotransformation

1. The IV barbiturates are completely metabolized in the body, and the products of their metabolism are excreted; 10–15% of each of these drugs is metabolized in the body each hour. It is not biotransformation that terminates their effects but their redistribution in the body.

2. The thiobarbiturates undergo metabolic degradation by desulfuration and oxidation, mainly in the liver. Excretion of inactive metabolites takes place through the kidney. Biotransformation of the oxybarbiturates occurs only in the liver.

E. Hazards of IV barbiturates

1. The solution of thiamylal or thiopental used for IV anesthesia must have a concentration of 2.5% or less. Stronger solutions may result in **thrombophlebitis** due to chemical irritation of the vein wall, particularly in old, chronically ill patients with poor or obstructed venous circulation.

2. **Extravascular infiltration** of strong solutions of thiopental or thiamylal may lead to sloughing and tissue necrosis due to the alkaline pH of the solution. **Treatment of extravasation** includes application of hot, moist towels and injection of the area with 10 ml of 1% procaine for dilution of the alkaline solution, prevention of vasospasm, and relief of pain.

3. **Accidental intraarterial injection** of thiopental or thiamylal is a rare but very serious complication. This catastrophe is especially likely to happen **in the region of the elbow**, where the brachial artery is located in close proximity to the cubital veins. **Arteries** may be very superficial in unusual locations at the elbow, and the pulsation may be eliminated by the tourniquet. Struggling, obesity, darkness of the skin, and lack of good light during venipuncture predisposes to error. Such accidents can be avoided by an **IV test dose** of 25–75 mg (1–3 ml of 2.5% solution) and asking the patient whether there is any pain.

   a. Occurrence of this complication is extremely unlikely if the veins of the dorsum of the hand are used for venipuncture.

   b. When intraarterial injection happens, the patient complains of a **severe burning pain over the forearm and hand,** and this is followed by blanching or cyanosis and disappearance of the pulse. There may be massive edema. Severe spasm will be followed by intravascular thrombosis.

   c. When the injection is at the elbow, **gangrene of the fingers, hand, or forearm** follows.

   d. **Therapy** includes intraarterial injection of 10 ml of 1% procaine, sympathetic block, anticoagulants, antibiotics, and surgical exploration and removal of the clot. Amputation may be necessary.

II. Neuroleptanalgesia

A. **A neuroleptic drug** (another term for tranquilizer) and a **narcotic analgesic drug,** when administered together, produce a psychophysiologic state with the following characteristics:

1. Somnolence without total unconsciousness.
2. Psychological indifference to the environment.
3. No voluntary movements.
4. Analgesia.
5. Satisfactory amnesia.

B. Due to predominance of the neuroleptic and analgesic effect, the state produced is referred to as **neuroleptanalgesia.** This term is still used to describe the method, although an inhalation anesthetic (nitrous oxide) and a muscle relaxant agent are added.

C. Droperidol-fentanyl (Innovar)

1. Innovar is a premix of 50:1 droperidol (Inapsine) and fentanyl (Sublimaze), each milliliter comprising 2.5 mg of droperidol and 0.05 mg of fentanyl.
2. Innovar is used as preanesthetic medication and as an adjunct to the induction and maintenance of general anesthesia.
3. The pharmacologic effects of Innovar are most easily discussed by describing those produced by its individual components.

D. Droperidol

1. A tranquilizer, droperidol acts in 5–10 min following IM or IV injection. The effects are detectable 6–12 hr after a single injection.
2. **Advantages**
   a. Droperidol produces sleepiness and mental detachment for several hours.
   b. It is antiemetic.
   c. It has a weak blocking effect on alpha-adrenergic receptors.
3. **Disadvantages**
   a. There is no antagonist for droperidol; once given, it cannot be removed.
   b. It is a peripheral vasodilator that may produce hypotension.
   c. Large doses may cause muscle movements simulating extrapyramidal effects (dystonia, akathisia, oculogyric crisis). These can be controlled or reversed by antiparkinsonism drugs.
4. **Metabolism**. Droperidol is mostly broken down in the liver; 10% is excreted in the urine.

E. Fentanyl

1. Fentanyl is a powerful narcotic analgesic agent. It acts within 3–5 min following IV injection, and the effects of analgesia last 30–60 min.
2. Fentanyl in a dose of 0.1 mg (2 ml) has the analgesic potency of 10 mg of morphine or 75 mg of meperidine.
3. The combination of nitrous oxide, oxygen, fentanyl, and a muscle relaxant is gaining in popularity as the halogenated agents become increasingly suspected as causative agents of postoperative liver toxicity.
4. **Advantages**
   a. The action of fentanyl **can be reversed** by a narcotic antagonist (nalorphine, levallorphan, or naloxone).

b. Fentanyl does not release histamine.

c. It causes euphoria.

d. It has minimal effects on the cardiovascular system.

5. Disadvantages

a. Fentanyl can cause respiratory depression.

b. It can cause bradycardia.

c. It can cause bronchoconstriction.

d. It is an emetic.

e. It produces miosis.

f. Large doses may lead to muscle rigidity (muscles of the thorax, abdomen, and extremities). During surgery, the use of muscle relaxants reverses any muscle rigidity that fentanyl may produce.

6. Metabolism. Most of the drug is destroyed in the liver; 10% is excreted in the urine.

F. Neuroleptanesthesia with nitrous oxide, oxygen, droperidol, fentanyl, and muscle relaxants.

1. Advantages

a. There are no secretions.

b. There is no venous or tissue irritation.

c. The cardiovascular system is stable.

d. There is no sensitization of the myocardial conduction system to the action of catecholamines.

e. There are no toxic effects on liver or kidney function.

f. Cerebrospinal fluid pressure and intraocular pressure are reduced.

g. It is nonemetic.

h. It is nonexplosive.

i. Recovery is prompt.

j. Long periods of analgesia and amnesia are induced.

k. In the recovery room, the patient tolerates the endotracheal tube for a prolonged period.

2. Disadvantages

a. Respiratory depression and apnea can be caused by fentanyl and muscle relaxants.

b. Assisted or controlled ventilation is necessary.

c. Action of muscle relaxants must be reversed.

III. Dissociative anesthesia

A. Ketamine

1. Ketamine (Ketalar, Ketaject) is a parenterally administered phencyclidine derivative that is used to produce a state called **dissociative anesthesia.** Following administration of ketamine, the patient rapidly becomes mentally dissociated from the environment.

2. A nonbarbiturate anesthetic, ketamine produces rapid anesthesia and profound analgesia.

3. **Analgesia** and unconsciousness are produced within 30 sec following IV injection and within 5–8 min following IM administration.
4. **Ketamine and barbiturates** are chemically incompatible because of precipitate formation, so they should not be injected from the same syringe.
5. **Induction of anesthesia** is accomplished with IV dosage of 1–2 mg/kg and maintenance of anesthesia with supplementary doses of 0.5 mg/kg.
6. **Metabolism.** Ketamine is metabolized quickly to alcohols, which are excreted in the urine.
7. **Indications**
   a. Induction agent for general anesthesia.
   b. Sole anesthetic agent for short diagnostic and surgical procedures that do not require skeletal muscle relaxation, particularly in children.
   c. Procedures in which control of the airway is difficult, especially for correction of burn scars of the neck, which render extension and intubation difficult or impossible. Even with ketamine, the possibility of upper airway obstruction exists.
8. **Contraindications**
   a. Intraocular surgery.
   b. A history of increased cerebrospinal pressure, cardiovascular accident, or psychiatric problems.
   c. Hypertension.

B. Advantages

1. The solution is not irritating to veins or tissues.
2. Profound analgesia is induced.
3. **Laryngeal and pharyngeal reflexes** may be obtunded. Thus a patent airway can be maintained without endotracheal intubation.
4. Muscle tone is preserved.

C. Disadvantages

1. **Heart rate,** BP, and intraocular pressure are increased.
2. **Diplopia, eye movements, and nystagmus** may occur. It is because of the possibility of nystagmus that intraocular surgery under ketamine is hazardous and contraindicated.
3. **Confused states,** with unpleasant dreams and frightening or upsetting hallucinations, may occur in adults during the recovery period. They are less intense in children.
4. There is no antagonist. Once given, ketamine cannot be removed.

Bibliography

Heisterkamp, D. V., and Cohen, P. J. The use of naloxone to antagonize large doses of opiates administered during nitrous oxide anesthesia. *Anesth. Analg.* (Cleve.) 53:12, 1974.

Hug, C. C. Pharmacokinetics in drugs administered intravenously. *Anesth. Analg.* (Cleve.) 57:704, 1978.

Johnstone, R., Jobes, D., Kennell, E., et al. Reversal of morphine anesthesia with naloxone. *Anesthesiology* 41:361, 1974.

Kaniaris, P., Batrinos, M., Varonos, D., et al. Cholinergic action of thiopental on the hypothalamohypophyseal axis. *Anesth. Analg.* (Cleve.) 60:310, 1981.

Kripke, B. J., Finck, A. J., Shah, N. K., et al. Naloxone antagonism after narcotic-supplemented anesthesia. *Anesth. Analg.* (Cleve.) 55:800, 1976.

Lanning, C. F., and Harmel, M. H. Ketamine anesthesia. *Annu. Rev. Med.* 26:137, 1975.

Metcalf, I. R., and Holland, A. J. C. Inadvertent intra-arterial injection of thiopentone. *Can. Anaesth. Soc. J.* 27:395, 1980.

Waxman, K., Shoemaker, W. C., and Lippmann, M. Cardiovascular effects of anesthetic induction with ketamine. *Anesth. Analg.* (Cleve.) 59:355, 1980.

Zsigmond, E. K., and Domino, E. F. Ketamine. Clinical, pharmacology, pharmacokinetics and current clinical uses. *Anesth. Rev.* 7:13 (April), 1980.

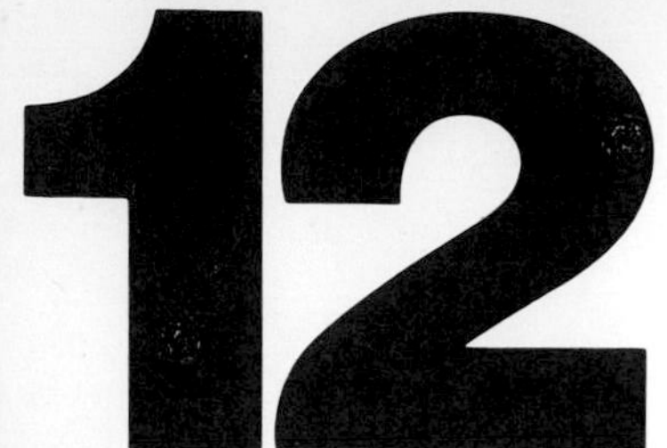

Muscle Relaxants

I. Mechanism of neuromuscular transmission

A. Acetylcholine. On the arrival of the nerve impulse (action potential electrical current) at the neuromuscular junction, the motor nerve releases acetylcholine.

1. **The liberated acetylcholine** reacts with receptors in the motor end-plate membrane and permits entrance of Na^+, which causes a sudden depolarization (electrically positive). The entry of Na^+ is followed by an outward migration of K^+. **The motor end-plate** is the flattened terminal expansion at the end of the motor nerve fiber, on the muscle fiber.

2. **The current of depolarization** constitutes the motor end-plate action potential, which is propagated along the membrane of the muscle fiber and causes it to contract.

B. Within a few milliseconds of its liberation, **acetylcholine is hydrolyzed by acetylcholinesterase** (true cholinesterase), in the area of the motor end-plate, to totally inactive choline and acetic acid. The cell membrane regains its original impermeability to Na^+, which is extruded from the cell and partially replaced by K^+, and the motor end-plate and muscle fiber become repolarized.

II. Mechanism of neuromuscular block.

Interference with the physiology of the neuromuscular transmission will interrupt nerve impulses arriving at the end-plate. The four types of neuromuscular block are as follows:

A. Deficiency block

1. Deficiency block occurs when drugs interfere with the synthesis and/or transmission of acetylcholine.

2. The following agents decrease the liberation of acetylcholine on arrival of the nerve impulse and may increase clinical block produced by competitive receptor blocking agents:

   a. Local anesthetics (such as procaine).

   b. Neomycin, kanamycin, streptomycin.

   c. The toxin of *Clostridium botulinum.*

   d. Calcium deficiency.

   e. Magnesium excess.

B. Nondepolarizing block (competitive block)

1. In nondepolarizing block, the drug is preferentially bound to cholinergic receptors. The drug does not have the action of acetylcholine but prevents the union of acetylcholine to the receptor, resulting in prevention of depolarization and contraction. It acts by competitive inhibition.

2. Drugs causing neuromuscular block by this mechanism include **tubocurarine, gallamine, and pancuronium.** Their effect can be opposed by increasing the local concentration of acetylcholine, which can be accomplished by ad-

ministering anticholinesterases (neostigmine). Their action can be increased when there is a decrease in the liberation of acetylcholine, as in myasthenia gravis.

3. These drugs do not cause muscular contractions (fasciculations) when injected IV.

C. Depolarizing block

1. In depolarizing block (phase I), the drug acts similarly to acetylcholine but for a longer period of time, thus causing a persistent depolarization that produces fasciculations, followed by flaccidity.

2. Agents causing depolarizing block include **succinylcholine and decamethonium.** These drugs differ from the nondepolarizing drugs in that, once attached to these receptors, they act similarly to acetylcholine in producing **depolarization.** This depolarization (unlike that caused by acetylcholine) lasts for several minutes instead of a few milliseconds.

3. Following IV administration of the depolarizing relaxants, the initial depolarization produces a contraction of the muscle, observed as a short period of muscular fasciculations.

D. Dual block (desensitization block)

1. In dual block, the membrane is depolarized first (phase I) and then is slowly repolarized. The drug enters into the fiber and acts as a nondepolarizing agent (phase II), even though the membrane potential is restored.

2. During the early stage, when the block is mainly depolarizing, anticholinesterases may increase the block or have no effect.

E. A peripheral nerve stimulator may be used to ascertain the type of neuromuscular block.

1. **The needle electrodes** of a nerve stimulator are placed subcutaneously over the distribution of the ulnar nerve at the elbow or wrist. A supramaximal stimulus is used, and movements of the fingers and the adductor effect of the thumb are observed. The stimulus is either a single surge of electric current delivered every few seconds, resulting in **twitch**, or a current delivered 50–100 times per second, resulting in **tetanus.**

2. **In the presence of nondepolarizing blockade,** there is posttetanic facilitation and fade of successive stimuli on both fast (tetanic) and slow (twitch) rates of nerve stimulation.

3. **In the presence of a depolarizing blockade,** both fast (tetanic) and slow (twitch) rates of nerve stimulation are well sustained, and posttetanic facilitation is absent.

4. **The nerve stimulator** can be used to prevent overdosage with neuromuscular blocking drugs. Skeletal muscle relaxant agents should be avoided when there is no muscle response to nerve stimulation.

III. Differences between nondepolarizing and depolarizing relaxant drugs

A. Nondepolarizing drugs

1. **They do not produce muscular fasciculations** following IV administration.

2. **Their effects are increased** by diethyl ether, halothane, enflurane, and isoflurane.

3. **Their effects are decreased** by anticholinesterase agents, lowered body temperature, depolarizing relaxant drugs, epinephrine, and acetylcholine.

4. **Both a twitch stimulus** (a single electrical stimulus delivered every few seconds) and tetanic stimulation (a rapid rate of electric stimuli) produce a

gradual fading of the response. Following tetanic stimulation there is an increased response to a twitch stimulus (posttetanic facilitation).

5. **The block produced** by nondepolarizing drugs is reversed by anticholinesterase drugs (such as neostigmine).

B. Depolarizing drugs

1. **They produce muscular fasciculations** following IV administration.
2. **Their effects are increased** by anticholinesterase agents, lowered body temperature, and acetylcholine.
3. **Their effects are decreased** by nondepolarizing relaxant drugs.
4. **Twitch** and tetanic electrical impulses produce no fading of the response. Following tetanic stimulation, there is no increase in response to a twitch impulse (no posttetanic facilitation).
5. **The depolarizing block** (phase I) cannot be reversed by presently known antagonists.

IV. Muscle relaxants used in anesthesia

A. General comments

1. **All neuromuscular blocking agents** impair pulmonary respiration and can produce **apnea.** These drugs are given IV and must be used only by those skilled in performing endotracheal intubation and with administration of artificial ventilation with equipment providing adequate respiration under positive pressure. Artificial respiration must not be discontinued until the muscle tone of the patient is adequate with a satisfactory spontaneous respiration.
2. **Muscle relaxants** are administered routinely in major surgical procedures and very frequently for minor surgery because, with the help of muscle relaxants, general anesthesia can be maintained in light planes.
3. **The nondepolarizing agents** are more often administered for **major surgery** because their effects last longer (20–45 min).
4. **The depolarizing drugs** are used more often for **short surgical procedures,** such as endotracheal intubation, laryngoscopies, bronchoscopies, esophagoscopies, and manipulations of short duration.
5. **The sensitivity of different groups of muscles** to muscle relaxants varies considerably. The muscles of the eyelids are paralyzed first; then the extremities, jaws, and intercostal and abdominal muscles; and finally, the diaphragm.
6. **For intubation,** it is common practice to use succinylcholine and later to administer a long-acting agent, such as pancuronium, for maintenance of muscle relaxation during surgery.
7. **Succinylcholine** has been employed following use of nondepolarizing agents to provide muscular relaxation for **suturing of the peritoneum;** this may create difficulties if neostigmine is administered to reverse the competitive block either before succinylcholine metabolism or before the motor end-plate regains its physiologic sensitivity. **This practice is not recommended.**
8. **Temperature.** A lowered body temperature increases the action of depolarizing muscle relaxants but decreases the action of nondepolarizing muscle relaxants.
9. Muscle relaxants are employed to decrease the convulsions in **electroconvulsive therapy** and in the therapy of **tetanus.**

10. **All muscle relaxants should be administered with great caution** in patients with **myasthenia gravis.** The sensitivity of these patients to nondepolarizing blockers is markedly increased, and they usually require only one-tenth the average dose. They may occasionally be somewhat resistant to depolarizing agents.

11. **The placental barrier**

    a. **Tubocurarine and succinylcholine** do not cross the placental barrier readily. A single dose of succinylcholine 300–500 mg can be injected into the mother without detection in the child.

    b. **Gallamine** crosses the placenta, but the infant's respiration is not affected significantly.

    c. **Pancuronium** can be detected in the fetal blood, but no clinical effects have been reported.

B. **Effects on respiration**

1. In normal doses, muscle relaxants are **nontoxic,** with few side effects. However, their action on ventilation must be monitored carefully. Assisted or controlled ventilation is always necessary. A patient may receive enough oxygen from the mixture of the anesthetic gases, but if alveolar ventilation is not satisfactory, carbon dioxide retention will occur. At the end of surgery, it must be established that respiration is adequate.

2. In a few patients, **a mechanical respirator** may be needed in the recovery room for a period of time before a patient can be permitted to breathe spontaneously.

3. **Respiratory depression due to nondepolarizing drugs** must be treated with **neostigmine** (or pyridostigmine) **and atropine** (or glycopyrrolate). When depression is due to **depolarizing** agents, assisted or controlled ventilation must be continued until respiration is satisfactory.

C. **Techniques for measuring adequacy of respiration**

1. Ability to develop a negative pressure of 30 torr against an obstructed airway (inspiratory force).

2. Ability to develop sustained muscle tension (handgrip or head lift) for 5 sec.

3. Ability to create an expired vital capacity of at least 15 ml/kg.

4. The ultimate criterion for satisfactory spontaneous ventilation is the maintenance of normal values of the arterial blood gases for several hours.

V. **Nondepolarizing muscle relaxant drugs**

A. **Tubocurarine**

1. **General considerations**

    a. A purified extract of *Chondodendron tomentosum,* tubocurarine acts by preventing acetylcholine from reaching the receptor area of the muscle cell membrane at the neuromuscular junction.

    b. The average initial dose in adults is 15–20 mg. Given **IV**, the **drug acts** within 3 min, and the effect may last 30–40 min. Supplemental doses may be required for long surgical procedures.

    c. **The dose of tubocurarine** required to produce skeletal muscle relaxation depends on many factors:

        (1) Physical fitness.

        (2) Muscle development.

        (3) The patients's age.

(4) Body temperature.

(5) Concomitant diseases.

(6) The anesthetic agent.

(7) The depth of general anesthesia.

d. Tubocurarine precipitates with alkaline solutions.

e. **Skeletal muscle relaxation** is profound, dose-dependent, and without muscular fasciculations. Muscle pains are absent. There is no effect on smooth muscles. The order of muscle relaxation is similar to that with any other muscle relaxant drug. The eye muscles are the first to be affected, then the face and limb muscles, and finally the trunk muscles. In a patient with an electrolyte imbalance, the paralyzing action may be abnormally prolonged.

f. **Relaxation of the extraocular muscles** is followed by a decrease in intraocular pressure.

g. There is no effect on the heart, but **hypotension** may follow IV infusion of tubocurarine because of **ganglionic blockade, histamine release,** or dilation of the network of the capillaries.

2. **Indications**

a. To induce skeletal muscle relaxation during light anesthesia.

b. To facilitate mechanical ventilation.

c. To control convulsions.

3. **Contraindications**

a. Myasthenia gravis or myasthenic syndrome (associated with carcinoma of the lung).

b. Renal diseases.

c. Bronchial asthma. Bronchoconstrictor action may follow due to histamine release.

4. **Tubocurarine is antagonized** by anticholinesterases as follows:

a. Neostigmine 2.5 mg with atropine 1 mg IV.

b. Edrophonium, 10 mg IV.

c. Pyridostigmine 10 mg with atropine 1 mg IV.

5. **Biotransformation.** In normal persons, tubocurarine is excreted unconjugated by the kidney. In the presence of renal failure, biliary excretion in the liver may occur.

B. **Gallamine**

1. **Gallamine** (Flaxedil) is a synthetic drug that acts by preventing the depolarizing effect of acetylcholine at the neuromuscular junction. It is one-sixth as potent as tubocurarine.

2. It has no direct action on the heart but has a **vagal blocking effect** that produces a **sinus tachycardia.** There is no histamine-like effect, and fasciculations are not produced.

3. **The IV dose** in adults is 80–120 mg. The effect may last 20–40 min. Supplementary doses of gallamine (20–40 mg) are given as required. The solution is precipitated by alkaline solutions.

4. **Gallamine is antagonized** by anticholinesterases as follows:

a. Neostigmine 2.5 mg with atropine 1 mg IV.

b. Edrophonium, 10 mg IV.

c. Pyridostigmine 10 mg with atropine 1 mg IV.

5. It is excreted entirely unchanged by the kidney, so it is **contraindicated in patients with kidney failure.**

C. **Pancuronium**

1. **Pancuronium** (Pavulon) is a synthetic nondepolarizing neuromuscular blocking agent, about 5 times as potent as tubocurarine. It acts by preventing acetylcholine from reaching the receptor area of the muscle cell membrane at the neuromuscular junction.

2. **The onset of action** is within 3 min, and the duration of effect is about 30–40 min.

3. There is a slight **rise in pulse rate, BP, and cardiac output.**

4. There are **no muscle contractions** and no postoperative muscle pain.

5. There is **no histamine release** or bronchospasm.

6. Pancuronium is **antagonized** by acetylcholine, anticholinesterases, and potassium.

7. **The action of pancuronium is increased** by inhalation anesthetics, magnesium, hypokalemia, and certain antibiotics (neomycin, streptomycin, kanamycin, and bacitracin).

8. **Pancuronium is indicated** as an adjunct to general anesthesia to induce skeletal muscle relaxation. It also may be employed to facilitate endotracheal intubation and the management of patients undergoing mechanical ventilation. In patients with **myasthenia gravis,** even small amounts of pancuronium may have profound effects.

9. **Prior injection of succinylcholine,** as for endotracheal intubation, enhances the relaxant action of pancuronium and the duration of effect, so the administration of pancuronium must be delayed until the succinylcholine shows signs of wearing off.

10. In adults, the **initial IV dose** range is 0.04–0.1 mg/kg. Supplemental injections may be required for long procedures.

11. **Pyridostigmine** (Regonol) or **neostigmine** in conjunction with **atropine** will antagonize the skeletal muscle relaxant effect of pancuronium.

12. **Metabolism.** The method of detoxification and route of elimination of pancuronium are not yet completely known. Renal elimination is the major excretory pathway, but biliary excretion may also be significant.

D. **Persistence of a nondepolarizing neuromuscular block** can be detected by a **peripheral nerve stimulator.** Tetanic fade and posttetanic facilitation are characteristic of a residual action of the muscle relaxant drug, which can be abolished by IV injection of neostigmine. However, this must always be preceded by IV atropine to prevent bradycardia, cardiac arrest, and/or excessive secretions. As a rule, atropine and neostigmine must be injected each time a nondepolarizing muscle relaxant agent has been used, even in the presence of a spontaneous ventilation that seems to be satisfactory.

VI. Antagonists to nondepolarizing muscle relaxant drugs

A. **Acetylcholine**

1. The nondepolarizing relaxant drugs compete with acetylcholine for the cholinergic receptor. Thus **acetylcholine is an effective antagonist** to these relaxants.

2. **Acetylcholine injected IV is not effective** because it is hydrolyzed before reaching the neuromuscular junction.

3. The concentration of acetylcholine can be increased at the neuromuscular junction by inhibition of the enzyme **acetylcholinesterase.** This enzyme hydrolyzes acetylcholine.

B. Anticholinesterase drugs

1. **The anticholinesterase drugs** antagonize a nondepolarizing neuromuscular block by inhibition of acetylcholinesterase.

2. **Neostigmine** (Prostigmin) is a cholinergic stimulant that enhances the cholinergic effect by facilitating the transmission of impulses across the neuromuscular junction. It inhibits the destruction of acetylcholine by acetylcholinesterase. Neostigmine has effects similar to those of physostigmine (eserine), but it is less likely to cause disturbing side effects. **Dose:** Neostigmine, 2.5–5 mg, with atropine, 1–2 mg, IV; 1–2 mg of atropine is sufficient to prevent bradycardia. Neostigmine and atropine can be injected IV at the same time because the vagolytic action of atropine precedes the cardiac muscarinic effect of neostigmine. The effects of neostigmine last 1–2 hr.

   a. **Adverse reactions** related to overdosage:

      (1) **Muscarinic effects.** Bradycardia, increased salivary and bronchial secretions, bronchospasm, vomiting, peristalsis, diarrhea, contraction of the bladder, miosis, and diaphoresis. These side effects can be counteracted by **atropine.**

      (2) **Nicotinic effects:** muscle cramps, fasciculations, and weakness.

   b. **The 5-mg dose of neostigmine should not be exceeded.** If the patient is not able to sustain a tetanic contraction after this amount of neostigmine has been given, ventilation should be supported until the relaxant has had time to be eliminated.

3. **Edrophonium** (Tensilon) forms a reversible complex with acetylcholinesterase. When the concentration of edrophonium is decreased, the complex dissociates, freeing acetylcholinesterase to continue hydrolyzing acetylcholine. Edrophonium has a short duration of action and must be reserved for diagnostic rather than therapeutic use. **The dose** is 10 mg IV. Its effect lasts 5–10 min; 20 mg is equivalent to 2.5 mg of neostigmine.

4. **Pyridostigmine** (Mestinon, Regonol) acts by inhibition of acetylcholinesterase. Pyridostigmine is one-fifth as potent as neostigmine. It lasts longer than neostigmine and takes longer to achieve peak effectiveness. **The dose** is 10 mg (the equivalent of 2.5 mg of neostigmine). Atropine usually is required.

5. **Glycopyrrolate** (Robinul) is an **anticholinergic** synthetic agent. It is administered SQ, IM, or IV. It can be injected in place of atropine in the reversal of nondepolarizing muscle blockade with neostigmine or pyridostigmine. The dose is half that of atropine.

VII. Depolarizing muscle relaxants

A. Succinylcholine

1. **General considerations**

   a. **Succinylcholine** is a synthetic short-acting depolarizing drug that produces relaxation of skeletal muscles. Paralysis is produced by a block of the nerve impulse transmission at the neuromuscular junction. It prevents the access of acetylcholine to the cholinergic receptors of the endplate.

   b. The drug may be **administered by a single IV injection** of a small dose (60–80 mg for a 70-kg adult); relaxation results within 1 min. Recovery of muscle tone is rapid and is complete within 5–15 min.

c. **For prolonged relaxation,** the drug may be administered by continuous or intermittent infusion. The rate of administration for continuous IV infusion varies markedly. Solutions containing succinylcholine 0.1–0.2% (1–2 mg/ml) are used for continuous drip.

d. **Intubation.** The average IV dose of succinylcholine for endotracheal intubation in adults is 60–80 mg and in children, 20 mg. **Infants** show an increased tolerance to succinylcholine; its use in infants and children should be preceded by atropine to prevent the occurrence of bradycardia. In contrast, infants vary markedly in response to tubocurarine. In the absence of an available IV route in infants and children, succinylcholine may be injected IM in a single dose: 1–1.5 mg per kilogram of body weight in children 3 years old and younger and 1 mg per kilogram of body weight in children 4 years old and older.

2. **Indications**

   a. For skeletal muscle relaxation during endotracheal intubation.

   b. Abdominal operations.

   c. Electroconvulsive treatment.

   d. Regarded as an essential drug for the emergency therapy of laryngospasm. Relaxation of the spastic laryngeal muscles follows IV or IM administration within 1 min.

3. **Contraindications**

   a. Patients who have sustained **thermal trauma** or extensive muscle trauma and those who have neurologic disorders involving motor deficits, including tetanus.

   b. Patients with a **penetrating injury of the eye** or while the globe is open.

   c. Patients with **myotonia** in whom a rigidity develops that renders inflation of the lungs impossible.

4. **Succinylcholine is hydrolyzed by alkaline solutions.** It loses potency if mixed with thiopental (Pentothal), thiamylal (Surital), or methohexital (Brevital). Therefore separate administrations of the drugs are indicated. Succinylcholine solutions are stable when stored under refrigeration, but potency slowly decreases on standing at room temperature.

5. **Strong skeletal muscle contractions (fasciculations)** are seen following IV injection of succinylcholine and before relaxation. Subsequently the patient may complain of severe muscle pains persisting for several days. These contractions are observed in the eyebrow and eyelid muscles, then in the shoulder girdle and abdominal muscles, and finally in the muscles of the hands and feet. These muscular fasciculations are the result of the depolarization process and can be **minimized** by administering the injection slowly. They are rarely observed following a second injection. These twitchings can be **prevented** by the prior IV injection of tubocurarine (3–6 mg) or pancuronium (0.5–1 mg). Fewer fasciculations are observed if succinylcholine is given IM.

6. **Postoperative muscle pain** may follow the administration of succinylcholine. The patient notices these pains on the day following surgery, particularly when the surgical procedure was short.

   a. Among the influencing factors are:

      (1) **Sex.** Women are most affected.

      (2) **Age.** Children are relatively unaffected.

      (3) **Time of ambulation** following sugery.

b. Efforts have been made to **prevent** or **decrease** this pain by decreasing the amount of the drug administered, by reducing the rate of infusion, and by changing the route of injection. The following drugs injected IV before the injection of succinylcholine may decrease the degree of muscle pain.

(1) Tubocurarine, 3–6 mg IV.

(2) Pancuronium, 0.5–1 mg IV.

(3) Gallamine, 20 mg IV.

7. Succinylcholine causes **myoglobinemia in children.**

8. **Miotics,** such as echothiophate (Phospholine) and isoflurophate (Floropryl), are cholinesterase inhibitors. They may increase the duration of action of succinylcholine. Drops of echothiophate solution in the eyes of glaucoma patients may depress both plasma and red cell pseudocholinesterase levels. In these patients, the administration of succinylcholine may be followed by prolonged **apnea.**

9. **Intraocular pressure** is increased following the administration of succinylcholine. This effect is of short duration, occurring during the fasciculatory phase and subsiding as complete paralysis supervenes. The extraocular muscles develop a tetanic state that constricts the globe, resulting in a rise in intraocular pressure.

a. Succinylcholine **must not be used during intraocular surgery,** especially when the eye is incised for extraction of a cataractous lens or in a patient with a penetrating wound of the eyeball.

b. The increase in intraocular pressure following administration of succinylcholine can be **prevented** by IV injection of tubocurarine 3 mg or pancuronium 0.5 mg 3 min before administering succinylcholine.

c. Succinylcholine is **not contraindicated** in extraocular surgery of the eye or for facilitation of endotracheal intubation in patients undergoing cataract extraction under general anesthesia.

10. **Intragastric pressure.** Succinylcholine may provoke regurgitation of gastric contents by producing fasciculations of abdominal skeletal muscles, which in turn may increase intragastric pressure. This increase in pressure can be prevented by the IV administration of tubocurarine 3 mg or pancuronium 0.5 mg 3 min before succinylcholine administration.

11. **Cardiac arrhythmias, bradycardia, hypertension, and increased salivation** are frequently associated with the administration of succinylcholine, especially during endotracheal intubation and laryngoscopic examination. Atropine appears to be a satisfactory agent for rapidly restoring normal heart rhythm when bradycardia or premature ventricular contractions occur. When atropine is given IV before succinylcholine, heart arrhythmias are not so frequent; but when it is administered during laryngoscopy and endotracheal intubation, marked heart irregularities may be observed.

12. **Bradycardia and heart arrhythmias** are more common following repeated doses of succinylcholine. These may be prevented by previous IV injection of atropine (0.3–0.5 mg in the adult). The appearance of cardiac irregularities is less frequent with continuous than with intermittent succinylcholine administration.

13. **Succinylcholine-induced hyperkalemia**

a. **Cardiovascular collapse** and **cardiac arrest** may follow the IV injection of succinylcholine in patients with:

(1) Severe burns.

(2) Massive trauma.

(3) Tetanus.

(4) Spinal cord injury.

(5) Brain injury.

(6) An upper or lower motor neuron lesion.

(7) Uremia with increased serum potassium.

b. These patients release a significant amount of potassium following the injection of succinylcholine.

14. **Malignant hyperthermia.** Succinylcholine has been incriminated in the malignant hyperthermic reaction. The **abnormal response** to the drug is exaggerated fasciculations followed by rigidity and difficulty with intubation. Body temperature then increases at an alarming rate. **Malignant hyperthermia during anesthesia must be regarded as a life-threatening condition that requires rapid, vigorous therapy if the patient is to survive.**

15. **Prolonged apnea**

a. **Prolonged apnea due to succinylcholine** may be caused either by decreased pseudocholinesterase activity or (rarely) by a change in the response of the motor end-plate (dual block) in patients who have received large amounts of succinylcholine. One out of 3000 patients will have a prolonged response to succinylcholine.

b. **In dual block,** the motor end-plate is altered so that it becomes insensitive to further action by drugs or acetylcholine (desensitization block, or phase II block).

c. **An atypical pseudocholinesterase should be considered** when spontaneous respiration has not returned within 15 min following the administration of succinylcholine.

d. **A peripheral nerve stimulator** must be used for diagnosis whether the depression is of central or peripheral origin. A strong response in the muscles stimulated indicates that the neuromuscular function is intact and that the depression is of central origin.

e. **If the neuromuscular block is not complete,** a sustained response without posttetanic facilitation or fading suggests that a **depolarizing block** is still present. Posttetanic facilitation and fading indicate that a **nondepolarizing block** is present, a **dual block** having supervened.

f. **If apnea** has been proved to be due to a neuromuscular block, **therapy** will depend on the type of block.

(1) **If a depolarizing block** is present:

(a) Continue controlled ventilation until spontaneous respiration returns.

(b) Administer fresh-frozen plasma or blood to restore the pseudocholinesterase level of the plasma.

(2) **If a dual block** is present, controlled ventilation must be continued, and an anticholinesterase may be administered IV: edrophonium 10 mg or neostigmine 2.5 mg with atropine 1 mg.

16. **Metabolism.** Succinylcholine is destroyed by a plasma enzyme, **pseudocholinesterase.** The enzymatic hydrolysis occurs in two steps: The products of the first stage are succinylmonocholine and choline; in the second step, the succinylmonocholine is split so that the end products are succinic acid

and choline. The end products then are excreted by the kidney or enter normal metabolic pathways.

B. Decamethonium

1. **Decamethonium** (Syncurine) is a synthetic depolarizing drug that acts by persistent depolarization of the postsynaptic membrane of skeletal muscle.
2. **Its action is similar to succinylcholine** but is of longer duration.
3. Decamethonium has **no cardiac effect,** and there is no evidence of any effect on the spinal cord, brain, or autonomic ganglia.
4. **Fasciculations** may occur, but these are not as marked as those following succinylcholine.
5. **The IV dose in adults is 3 mg** (equivalent to tubocurarine, 15 mg). The effect may last 20 min. The drug is compatible with alkaline solutions. Neostigmine and edrophonium do not antagonize decamethonium—on the contrary, they may prolong its action.
6. **It is excreted** mainly unchanged in the urine. It is not hydrolyzed, which explains why its duration of action is longer than that of succinylcholine.

C. Antagonists to the action of depolarizing blocking agents are not available.

Bibliography

Baraka, A. Self-taming of succinylcholine-induced fasciculations. *Anesthesiology* 46:292, 1977.

Blitt, C. D., Moon, B. J., and Kartchner, C. D. Duration of action of neostigmine in man. *Can. Anaesth. Soc. J.* 23:80, 1976.

Duke, P. C., Fung, H., and Gartner, J. The myocardial effects of pancuronium. *Can. Anaesth. Soc. J.* 22:680, 1975.

Eisenberg, M., Balsley, S., and Katz, R. L. Effects of diazepam on succinylcholine-induced myalgia, potassium increase, creatine phosphokinase elevation, and relaxation. *Anesth. Analg.* (Cleve.) 58:314, 1979.

Fogdall, R. P., and Miller, R. D. Neuromuscular effects of enflurane, alone and combined with d-tubocurarine, pancuronium, and succinylcholine in man. *Anesthesiology* 42:173, 1975.

Forbes, A. R., Cohen, N. H., and Eger, E. I. Pancuronium reduces halothane requirement in man. *Anesth. Analg.* (Cleve.) 58:49, 1979.

Lee, C., Yang, E., and Katz, R. L. Predetermination of dose requirement of pancuronium. *Anesth. Analg.* (Cleve.) 59:722, 1980.

Miller, R. D., and Roderick, L. Pancuronium-induced neuromuscular blockade and its antagonism by neostigmine at 29, 37, and 41°C. *Anesthesiology* 46:333, 1977.

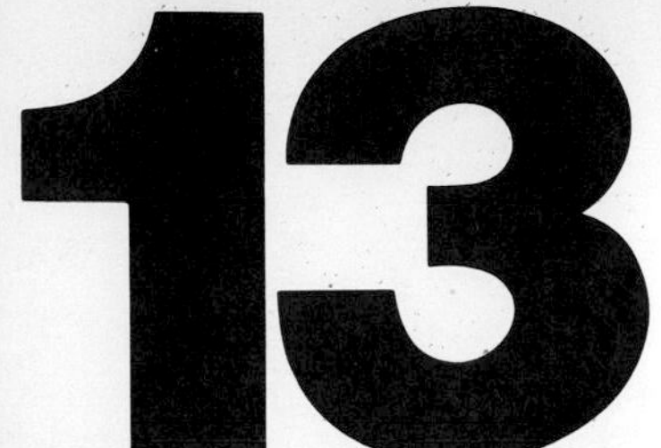

13 Laryngoscopy and Endotracheal Intubation

I. The laryngoscope

A. In anesthesia, **the laryngoscope** is used for exposure and direct viewing of the larynx and its surrounding structures, with the main purpose of insertion of the tube through the glottis and into the trachea.

1. The laryngoscope is usually L-shaped, so that **the handle,** with batteries, is at a right angle to **the blade.**
2. **The blade,** which is inserted into the mouth, consists of the **spatula,** the **flange**, and the **tip.** It also has a light source.
   - **a.** The long axis of the spatula may be **straight** or **curved.**
   - **b. The tip of the blade** contacts the **epiglottis** or **vallecula** (the angle made by the tongue and epiglottis) and directly or indirectly raises the epiglottis.

B. There are anatomic variations and pathologic conditions that make laryngoscopy difficult. This has led to the development of a great variety of laryngoscope blades, each with its own claimed advantages (MacIntosh, Fink, Bizarri-Guiffrida, Polio, Miller, Wisconsin, Snow, Flagg, Guedel, Bennett, Eversole, Siker, Huffman, Hipple, Whitehead, etc.).

C. The most significant recent development is the flexible **fiberoptic laryngoscope.** Prior to intubation, the endotracheal tube is slipped over the flexible part of the laryngoscope. During insertion of the tube, the laryngoscope acts as an introducer.

II. Laryngoscopy

A. Larynx

1. **The larynx consists** of four major cartilages: two arytenoids, one thyroid, and one cricoid; and five accessory cartilages: two corniculate, two cuneiform, and the epiglottis.
2. **The superior laryngeal nerve** is the **sensory nerve** of the larynx, and it serves as the motor nerve of the cricothyroid muscle. It is under the floor of the pyriform sinus, which is located on each side of the pharynx.
3. **The inferior laryngeal nerve** is the **motor nerve** of the larynx. The superior and inferior laryngeal nerves belong to the vagus nerve.

B. Laryngoscopy

1. **Examination** of the larynx is carried out by:
   - **a. Indirect laryngoscopy** with a laryngeal mirror inserted into the mouth.
   - **b. Direct laryngoscopy** with a laryngoscope.
2. **The structures to be visualized** are the vallecula, epiglottis, true and false vocal cords, glottis, anterior commissure, posterior commissure, pyriform sinuses, and the posterior pharyngeal wall down to the esophageal introitus.

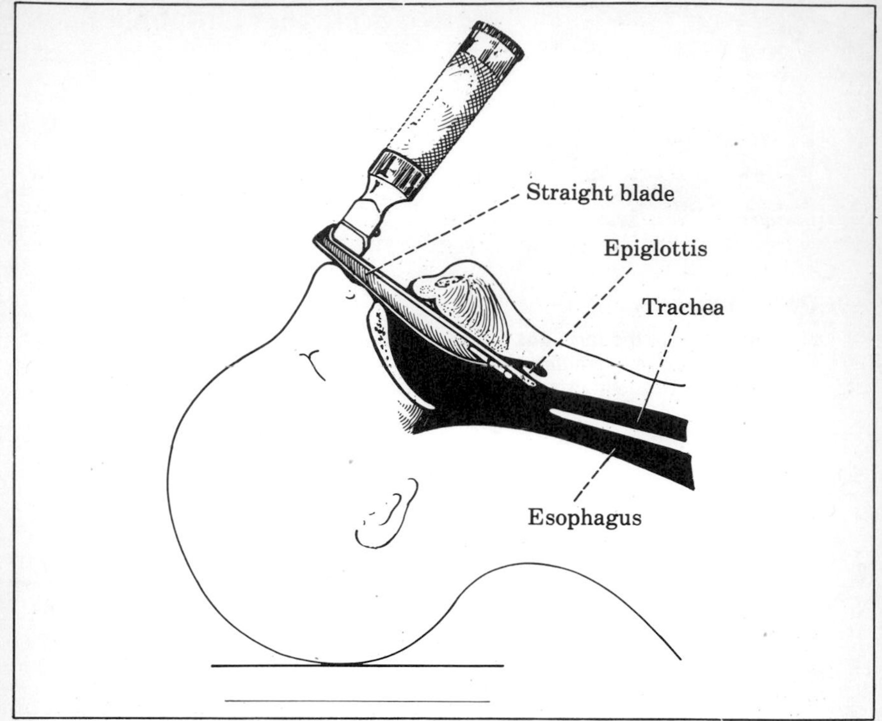

Fig. 13-1. Direct laryngoscopy with a straight blade. The straight blade is inserted beyond the epiglottis to raise it. The vocal cords are coming into view. (From J. C. Snow. *Anesthesia in Otolaryngology and Ophthalmology*. Springfield, Ill.: Charles C Thomas, 1972. Reproduced by permission.)

C. Direct laryngoscopy includes: (1) positioning the head, (2) insertion of the laryngoscope blade, (3) visualization of the epiglottis, (4) elevation of the epiglottis, and (5) exposure and viewing of the larynx, and related structures.

1. **Position of the head.** The head may rest on a pillow. **The right hand** is placed on the patient's forehead to extend the head at the atlanto-occipital joint.

2. **Insertion of the laryngoscope blade.** The handle of the laryngoscope is held with **the left hand.** With the fingers of **the right hand,** the patient's jaw is opened and the lips are spread apart, the lower lip being pushed out of the path of the laryngoscope blade, which is inserted between the teeth at the right side of the mouth.

3. **Visualization of the epiglottis.** The blade is advanced inward and toward the midline until the **uvula** and then the **epiglottis** come into view.

4. **Elevation of the epiglottis.** There are two techniques to raise the epiglottis:

   a. **The straight blade** is inserted beyond the epiglottis, which is raised by the tip of the blade. Under the epiglottis, the glottis comes into view (Fig. 13-1).

   b. **The curved blade** is inserted into the angle made by the tongue and the epiglottis (vallecula). By lifting the base of the tongue, the epiglottis is also raised and the glottis comes into view (Fig. 13-2). The superior aspect

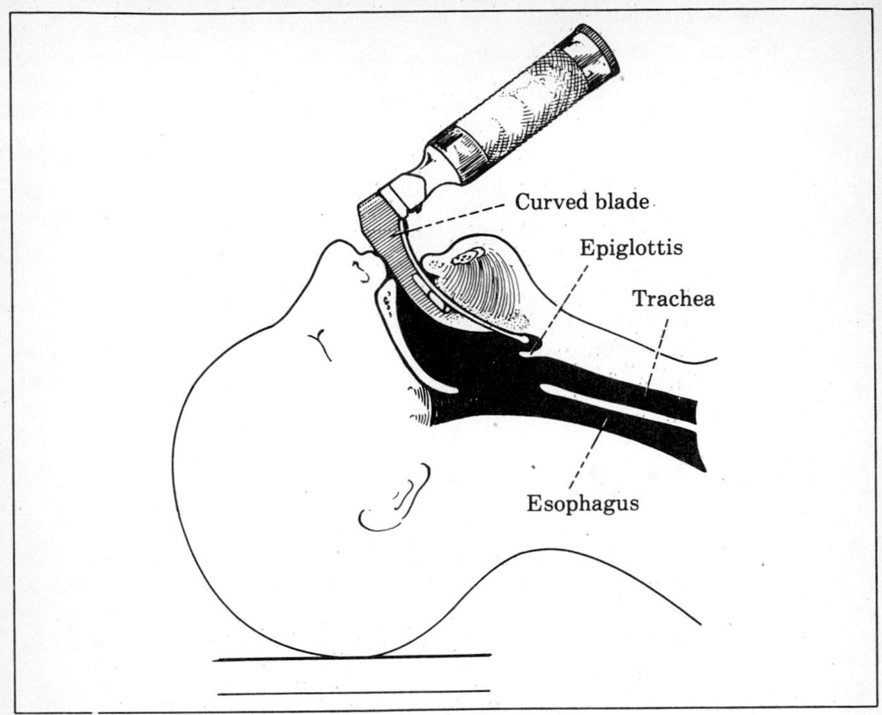

Fig. 13-2. Direct laryngoscopy with a curved blade. The curved blade is inserted into the angle made by the base of the tongue and the epiglottis. Lifting the base of the tongue also raises the epiglottis, and the vocal cords come into view. (From J. C. Snow. *Anesthesia in Otolaryngology and Ophthalmology*. Springfield, Ill.: Charles C Thomas, 1972. Reproduced by permission.)

of the epiglottis is supplied by the IXth cranial (glossopharyngeal) nerve, and the inferior (posterior) aspect is supplied by the internal laryngeal nerve. Thus, because the inferior part of the epiglottis is not touched and not stimulated, the curved blade can be used at a lighter plane of anesthesia than the straight blade, without producing spasm of the larynx.

D. **During laryngoscopy,** the laryngoscope must be lifted upward and forward. **It should not be used as a lever** with the upper teeth acting as a fulcrum.

III. Complications during laryngoscopy

A. **Bruises, abrasions, and lacerations** of the mouth, pharynx, larynx, and esophagus may occur.

1. **Edentulous patients** are less likely than others to present these complications.
2. **The lips** may be traumatized if they are compressed between the laryngoscope blade and the teeth. This may cause considerable postoperative discomfort during eating.

B. **Damage to the teeth, gums, or dental prostheses** may occur.

1. **The teeth** may be chipped or knocked out if they are used as the fulcrum for the laryngoscope blade.

2. **In children and older people,** loose teeth are easily dislodged.

3. **Knocked out, chipped, or fractured teeth** should be recovered. Otherwise, an x-ray examination of the head, neck, lungs, and stomach should be carried out immediately. Bronchoscopic removal of a tooth from the lung is mandatory as an emergency procedure, and this should be followed by prophylactic treatment with corticosteroids and antibiotics.

C. **Circulatory changes** in BP and cardiac rhythm are common during laryngoscopy. Prior oxygenation and rapid, atraumatic laryngoscopy will reduce the possibility of these changes.

IV. **Endotracheal intubation**

A. **Endotracheal anesthesia** is produced by introduction of the anesthetic gases into the trachea by way of a tube inserted through the larynx (or tracheotomy) into the trachea. This can be carried out through the nose, mouth, or tracheal stoma. The difficulties encountered in inserting a tube into the trachea are obviated by use of direct laryngoscopy.

B. **Indications**

1. **Head and neck surgery.** The anesthesiologist or nurse-anesthetist and anesthesia equipment are located at a distance from the patient's airway, and a free airway can only be maintained by an endotracheal tube in place.

2. **Intrathoracic surgery.** The problem of **pneumothorax,** which outweighs all other considerations, is most easily overcome by respiration through an endotracheal tube.

3. **Intraperitoneal surgery.** Utilization of muscle relaxants and artificial respiration is required.

4. **Surgery with the patient in a lateral or prone position.** In these positions, normal access to the airway is impossible.

5. **A patient with an obstructed airway** that cannot be handled by simple means.

6. **A patient with a full stomach** who nevertheless requires general anesthesia. Here the endotracheal tube cuff serves to protect the lower respiratory tract from aspirates.

7. Surgical procedures requiring **the anesthesiologist to be remote** from the patient.

8. Operations in which **major hemorrhage** can be anticipated.

9. **Severely ill patients.**

10. **Complicated techniques of anesthesia,** such as hypothermia or hypotension.

11. **Instances in which intermittent positive-pressure breathing** is to be employed.

12. **Pediatric surgery.**

13. **Certain nonsurgical conditions,** including:

    a. Grave asphyxia neonatorum.

    b. Resuscitation.

    c. Grave laryngeal obstruction.

    d. Patients with atelectasis and signs of exudate in the lungs.

C. **Advantages**

1. Endotracheal intubation ensures a patent airway as long as the tube remains open.

2. The normal anatomic dead space (150 ml) is decreased to 75 ml.
3. Ventilation can be assisted or controlled without inflating the stomach and intestines.
4. The possibility of aspiration of secretions, blood, tissues, and vomitus is diminished drastically.
5. Ventilation can be assisted or controlled with the patient in the prone, lateral, or other unusual positions.
6. Respiration can be controlled during use of skeletal muscle relaxant drugs.
7. Suctioning of the lungs is facilitated.
8. The anesthesiologist or nurse-anesthetist and anesthesia equipment are kept away from the surgical field during head and neck procedures.

D. Disadvantages

1. **The endotracheal tube** increases resistance to respiration. To keep resistance at a minimum, use of the widest internal diameter endotracheal tube that will fit the larynx is recommended.
2. **Trauma** to the lips, teeth, nose, throat, and larynx can occur, resulting in hoarseness, pain, and dysphagia. Abrasion of the mucosa may result in extensive **surgical emphysema.** Perforation of the membrane at the decussation of the cricopharyngeal muscle can lead to mediastinitis.

E. Endotracheal tubes

1. **Endotracheal tubes,** whether disposable or reusable, are manufactured from synthetic rubber or other synthetic materials, such as polyethylene and polyvinyl chloride. Another type of tube is made of a spiral coil of nylon or wire embedded in latex to prevent kinking. The tubes, with or without cuffs, may be opaque or transparent.
2. **Polyvinyl chloride.** Polyvinyl chloride is the most widely used material for plastic endotracheal tubes.
   a. Polyvinyl chloride endotracheal tubes are soft and do not irritate the trachea.
   b. They have little tendency to kink.
   c. They tend to mold to the curves of the mouth and larynx at body temperature.
   d. Due to its smooth surface, a suction catheter can be passed through the tube with ease.
   e. The tubes are damaged by heat.
   f. Many polyvinyl chloride endotracheal tubes are intended for single use only.
3. It is preferable to use an **unkinkable** tube, with a spiral coil of nylon or wire embedded in latex, in the following situations:
   a. Head and neck surgery.
   b. When the anesthesiologist has to be placed toward the patient's feet.
   c. When the patient has to be turned over.
   d. In neurosurgical procedures.
4. **The following types of tubes** are used:
   a. **Cole.** Narrow at the distal end; useful in infants.
   b. **Davol.** White or translucent; manufactured from plasticized polyvinyl chloride.

c. **Murphy.** Blunt bevel with an extra opening on the side (Murphy eye).

d. **Portex.** Manufactured from special nontoxic polyvinyl chloride.

e. **Tovell (armored tube).** Latex, with an embedded metal spiral and a cemented cuff.

f. **Sanders.** Latex tube with a continuous spiral of nylon monofilament embedded in the wall, making it light, flexible, and resistant to collapse. An eccentric pocket in the tip holds the end of the special nylon-rod stylet in place during intubation.

g. **The Carlens double-lumen tube** has a double lumen and two cuffs. One cuff, on the distal end, is positioned in the left bronchus. The second cuff is on the portion that remains in the trachea, proximal to the opening for the right bronchus.

5. The **size of the endotracheal tube** is the internal diameter (ID) in millimeters, which is marked on each tube.

6. **Inflatable balloon cuff with a pilot balloon.** Endotracheal tubes used in adults are equipped with an inflatable balloon cuff to achieve a gas-tight fit when seated in the trachea.

   a. **The cuff is tested before use,** and inflation of the cuff following intubation is done slowly with 5–10 ml of air.

   b. **Cuffs must not be inflated** to a pressure greater than that needed to prevent audible leakage of gas when the breathing bag is compressed.

   c. **The inflated cuff is useful** in intermittent positive-pressure ventilation and is extremely effective in eliminating aspiration of gastric contents from the pharynx into the lungs.

7. **Stylets** must be well lubricated before being inserted into the endotracheal tube. **The stylet must never protrude beyond the end of the tube:** Serious injury to the pyriform fossa, cricothyroid membrane, or cricopharyngeal membrane, with resulting subcutaneous emphysema, mediastinitis, or even pneumothorax, can be produced by neglect of this simple precaution.

F. **Other equipment**

1. **Oropharyngeal airway**

   a. **During induction of anesthesia,** insertion of an oropharyngeal airway prevents respiratory obstruction from a relaxed tongue and soft pharyngeal tissues.

   b. **It prevents biting and obstruction** of the endotracheal tube.

   c. **It facilitates suctioning** of the pharyngeal liquid materials.

   d. **A nasopharyngeal airway** offers an alternative to the oropharyngeal airway in providing an open airway.

   e. **Complications**

      (1) **Airway obstruction** may develop from an oropharyngeal airway if it is inserted improperly, because the tongue is pressed into the hypopharynx.

      (2) **Nasal bleeding** may start during insertion of a nasopharyngeal airway.

      (3) **Loosening or breakage of the teeth** may result from the patient's biting on the oropharyngeal airway.

      (4) **Laryngospasm and coughing** may be caused by a long oropharyngeal airway that touches the epiglottis or vocal cords.

2. **Throat pack.** The inflatable cuff can be replaced by a throat pack. A strip of gauze saturated in water is laid along both sides of the endotracheal tube into the pharynx (a portion of the throat pack, 10–15 cm, must be left outside the mouth). The pharyngeal pack is a satisfactory replacement for the cuff in infants and children.

3. **Lubricants.** A thin coat of a water-soluble lubricant may be used to lubricate the endotracheal tube; more lubrication is needed for insertion of a nasotracheal tube. If a stylet is used, lubrication is necessary to aid in its removal.

4. **Atomizer for topical anesthesia.** An atomizer is very satisfactory for topical anesthesia of the pharynx and larynx.

5. **Suction catheters.** There are different sizes of disposable plastic suction catheters for cleaning the pharynx, larynx, trachea, and bronchi. The adapter connecting the suction catheter to the main suction tubing has an opening regulated by the thumb, and the distal end of the catheter has a minimum of two openings.

V. Techniques of endotracheal intubation

A. The trachea may be intubated through the:

1. **Mouth** under direct laryngoscopy.
2. **Nose** under direct laryngoscopy or by blind insertion.
3. **Mouth or nose with a fiberoptic laryngoscope** (see **VI.I**).
4. **Tracheal stoma** without a laryngoscope.

B. Orotracheal intubation

1. **Intubation through the mouth** performed under general anesthesia.

   a. **Under light general anesthesia,** muscle relaxation with succinylcholine or pancuronium, and hyperventilation with oxygen, the laryngoscope blade is inserted into the relaxed mouth both for exposure and visualization of the larynx and for insertion of the endotracheal tube through the glottis into the trachea.

   b. **The tube is inserted** into the larynx and trachea **until the cuff goes out of sight** behind the vocal cords. If the tube is uncuffed, it must be inserted 3–4 cm beyond the vocal cords in adults and not more than 1–2 cm in children.

2. **Awake intubation**

   a. **Indications.** Awake intubation is indicated in patients with upper airway obstruction, extensive maxillofacial deformities, anatomic or pathologic situations that make intubation difficult, or obesity, as well as in patients who are in coma or who come to surgery with full stomachs.

   b. **The awake patient's** cooperation is needed for an orotracheal intubation. Exposure of the larynx can be performed by spraying the mouth, tongue, pharynx, epiglottis, pyriform sinuses, and larynx with a topical anesthetic.

      (1) **Topical anesthesia** with 4% cocaine, spray with Cetacaine (2% tetracaine) or lidocaine 4%, together with small amounts of IV diazepam, fentanyl-droperidol (Innovar), ketamine, or thiopental, is a satisfactory technique.

      (2) **Superior laryngeal nerve block** can be done by applying cotton swabs soaked in a topical anesthetic solution (4% lidocaine) to the left and right pyriform sinuses, with the curved Jackson forceps. Blocking of the superior laryngeal nerve is confirmed by the onset of hoarseness. Two methods of applying the solution are:

(a) **Under direct vision** with a laryngoscope.

(b) **Under indirect vision** with a reflected light and laryngeal mirror.

(3) **Topical anesthesia** of the trachea and larynx can also be performed by translaryngeal injection of 2 ml of topical anesthetic (2% lidocaine) into the trachea through the **cricothyroid membrane.** The solution spreads as the patient coughs.

c. **If there are movements of the vocal cords,** the moment of greatest abduction must be selected for introduction of the tube.

C. Nasotracheal intubation

1. Indications

a. **Certain intraoral procedures** and certain plastic operations around the face.

b. **Maxillofacial operations.**

c. **Ankylosis** of the temporomandibular joint.

d. Repair of **fractured jaws.**

e. Conditions that make **direct laryngoscopy impossible.**

f. **Conditions that make oral intubation impossible,** as in the patient with the jaws wired together.

g. **Pierre Robin syndrome,** in which there is a hypoplastic mandible (micrognathia) in association with cleft palate, backward displacement of the tongue (glossoptosis), and a small epiglottis.

2. Nasotracheal intubation is performed **under general or topical anesthesia.**

a. One method is **through the nose under direct laryngoscopy.** The nostrils are examined to determine which has the better patency. Phenylephrine (Neo-Synephrine) 0.5%, 4% cocaine, or 4% lidocaine with 0.5% phenylephrine is applied to the mucosa of the nose. Following **light general anesthesia,** muscle relaxation, and hyperventilation with oxygen, the nasotracheal tube is inserted through the selected nostril. Then the laryngoscope blade is introduced into the mouth for exposure of the larynx. Under direct vision, the tube is directed into the larynx, with or without the aid of a Magill intubating forceps.

b. Another method is **by blind insertion through the nose.** This technique is attempted in the **awake patient** or when nasotracheal intubation under direct laryngoscopy fails. **When the patient is breathing,** the breath sounds can be heard through the tube as the distal end approaches the glottis. When the sounds suddenly cease but the patient continues to breathe, the tube has entered the esophagus.

3. When nasotracheal intubation is attempted, the patient's head must be placed **on a small pillow 8 cm high** with the chin extended.

4. Nasal intubation may be complicated by **nasal bleeding,** so this technique must be avoided in patients with a history of hypertension or blood dyscrasias and in patients on anticoagulant therapy.

5. Although **dental operations** are easier in the patient who is intubated through the nose, there are few such operations that cannot be carried out with an orotracheal tube.

D. Intubation through a tracheal stoma

1. **Intubation through a tracheal stoma** is much easier than through the mouth or nose. It can be carried out without general anesthesia, muscle relaxants, or the laryngoscope.

2. The patient is advised to clean the tracheobronchial tree by coughing. Then the stoma and trachea are sprayed with **Cetacaine (2% tetracaine)** or **4% lidocaine,** and a lubricated tube is inserted through the tracheotomy.

3. **If general anesthesia** is indicated, the endotracheal tube is connected with the anesthesia machine for the administration of oxygen and the anesthetic gases.

E. Intubation in children

1. **Most surgical operations** in children are performed under general endotracheal anesthesia.

2. **There are anatomic differences** between a child's and an adult's larynx.

   a. **The infant larynx** is located more cephalad than in the adult, with the larynx at the level of the third to fourth cervical vertebra, as compared to its location at the fifth to sixth vertebra in the adult.

   b. **The tongue** in children is larger and the epiglottis is shorter, so it may slip more easily from the laryngoscope blade. **The epiglottis** is stiff and U-shaped, in contrast to the flexible, flat epiglottis of the adult.

   c. **The loose areolar tissue of the larynx** may react to irritation and trauma by formation of **edema in children,** whereas adult tissue predominantly reacts by creation of granulation tissue.

   d. **The cricoid ring** is the narrowest point in the upper airway in children.

3. **The endotracheal tube** may be inserted easily through the larynx of a child, but with some difficulty through the cricoid ring. Any force or pressure can lead to formation of **subglottic edema.**

4. **In children below the age of 12 years,** the narrow trachea and the possibility of subglottic edema preclude the use of cuffed endotracheal tubes.

F. The proper placement of the tube must be checked following intubation:

1. **By visualization of the tube** and its cuff just distal to the vocal cords.

2. **By watching for chest movements** during assisted ventilation, particularly the left upper chest.

3. **By comparative auscultation** of both lung fields, particularly the left chest. The stethoscope must be placed well out over the lower lobes in the midaxillary line. Breath sounds created by short, sharp inflations of the lungs are the most easily heard. If there is any concern that the tube may have entered a mainstem bronchus, the tube is withdrawn 2–3 cm and the auscultation is repeated.

4. **If any speculation exists** as to possible esophageal placement of the tube, the epigastrium must be auscultated. If this does not allay all doubt, a laryngoscope must be reinserted into the mouth for visualization of the larynx. If necessary, the tube is completely withdrawn and a new one is inserted.

5. When an endotracheal intubation is performed in an area other than the operating room, the **correct placement** of the tube must be **checked by x-ray.**

G. Extubation

1. **On completion of surgery,** the mouth and trachea are suctioned carefully.

2. While monitoring clinical signs with the aid of a peripheral nerve stimulator, **the neuromuscular block** produced by the nondepolarizing muscle relaxant agents is reversed with IV administration of 2.5 mg of neostigmine and 1 mg of atropine.

3. **Respiratory depression** due to narcotics is reversed with naloxone, 0.2–0.4 mg IV.

4. **Extubation is carried out** at the peak of inspiration under light anesthesia and with adequate spontaneous respiration. Extubation in extremely light planes of anesthesia may lead to a severe paroxysm of cough, laryngospasm, and bronchospasm. These can be treated with 60 mg of succinylcholine IV and/or intermittent positive pressure with oxygen.

5. **Extubation must not be done** with a suction catheter within the tube. This will decrease the PO_2 within the lungs and is not effective in preventing aspiration.

VI. Laryngoscopy and intubation in difficult cases

A. In certain patients, **direct laryngoscopy** to expose the larynx for intubation may prove difficult, traumatic, and even unsuccessful.

1. **These patients may exhibit:**

   a. **Anatomic variations,** such as a receding mandible; deep throat; short, muscular neck, and a full set of teeth; protruding upper incisor teeth; enlarged tongue; Pierre Robin syndrome (micrognathia, cleft palate, and glossoptosis); and extreme anterior position of the larynx.

   b. **Pathologic situations,** such as large tumors of the larynx or pharynx; enlarged thyroid gland; limited motion of the mandible or cervical spine; ankylosis of the temporomandibular joint; and deformity of the head or neck due to trauma, surgery, or congenital malformations.

2. **In children,** micrognathia and macroglossia are the most frequent problems.

3. **Edentulous patients** may present fewer difficulties in exposing the larynx.

B. **Direct laryngoscopy for oral or nasal intubation** can be handled with any straight or curved blade, but for persons with anatomic and pathologic variations, a variety of blades and tubes—and a functioning suction tube—must be readily available.

1. **A Sanders tube** is very useful. To direct the tube correctly, the distal end of the stylet must be in the pocket of the tube, and the proximal end should be kept fastened. When this tube is in place, the stylet cannot be removed unless it has been very well lubricated beforehand.

2. **The presence of a functioning suction tube** is necessary in all situations, particularly in cases of repeated injections of succinylcholine with increased secretions of thick saliva and mucus.

C. When the laryngoscope blade is introduced into the mouth (preferably a straight blade rather than a curved one), **following the uvula and epiglottis,** the free (right) hand can be used to exert external **pressure on the thyroid cartilage** of the larynx. This enables the glottis or arytenoid cartilages to come into view. An assistant can do this under the direction of the anesthesiologist.

D. **During laryngoscopy,** if the anatomy of the pharynx and larynx is distorted and the patient has respiratory obstruction or is in apnea due to muscle relaxant drugs, **intermittent compression of the chest** by the assistant will produce audible breath sounds and visible air bubbles or secretions. These may help in directing the laryngoscope blade and insertion of the tube into the trachea.

E. Endotracheal intubation may be aided by introducing the **straight laryngoscope blade** through **the right corner of the mouth** and directing it into the pharynx over the molar teeth, with the tongue at the left side of the blade. The endotracheal tube is then placed in the right corner of the mouth after the assistant has retracted the lips outward.

1. **The right lateral route** becomes a very easy route for insertion of the tube if one or two of the patient's right molar teeth are missing.

2. **When the tip** of the laryngoscope blade is forced too far to the left in the hypopharynx, external pressure on the larynx toward the tip of the laryngoscope blade is necessary.
3. In a very rare instance, **the left lateral route** with the channel of the blade opened to the left may be indicated.

F. **In a few pathologic situations** with large malignant lesions in the pharynx and larynx or gross swelling of the neck as a result of trauma, hematoma, or previous x-ray treatment, the landmarks for direct laryngoscopy are absent.
   1. **The anesthesiologist must familiarize** himself or herself with the situation of the pharynx when the patient is conscious via the indirect laryngoscope and x-ray studies of the upper airways. Intubation must be performed with the patient awake.
   2. **In patients with absent laryngoscopy landmarks,** the use of succinylcholine is contraindicated. This drug relaxes the vocal cords, but a malignant tumor is unaffected and tends to obscure the larynx.
   3. **General anesthesia** with partial respiratory obstruction may precipitate complete obstruction. **A tracheotomy set** must be readily available.

G. **In patients with trismus,** endotracheal intubation must be carried out **in the conscious patient** either through the nose blindly or by direct viewing with a laryngoscope.

H. When **only the arytenoid cartilages can be seen,** it may be possible to pass a tube anterior to the arytenoids and enter the trachea. External pressure on the thyroid cartilage may be necessary.

I. **The flexible fiberoptic laryngoscope** is a very useful instrument for direct viewing in difficult intubations.
   1. **The flexible length** of the fiberoptic laryngoscope passes through an endotracheal tube.
   2. **The right hand** controls the end-tip deflection. With the patient under topical anesthesia and sedation, **the left hand** inserts the flexible part of the laryngoscope **through the mouth** and advances it in midline over the upper teeth and base of the tongue until the tip of the laryngoscope touches the posterior wall of the pharynx. The deflected portion of the laryngoscope is then curved forward.
   3. By advancing the fiberoptic laryngoscope slightly, the anesthesiologist is able to visualize the tip of the epiglottis and vocal cords.
   4. When the end-tip is well in place within the trachea, the operator simply advances the endotracheal tube. The laryngoscope acts as a stylet for the tube, facilitating a successful endotracheal intubation.
   5. When intubation is completed, the fiberoptic laryngoscope is removed, and the tube is left in place.
   6. The oral route is preferable to the nasal route to avoid nasal bleeding.

J. **The fiberoptic bronchoscope** also may be used for difficult intubation. It is a more elaborate instrument than the fiberoptic laryngoscope and has better optic features.

VII. Complications of endotracheal intubation

A. Trauma during intubation

1. **Nasotracheal intubation** is associated with a high incidence of **bleeding.**
2. The endotracheal tube and/or stylet may injure the mucosa of the mouth, pharynx, or larynx.

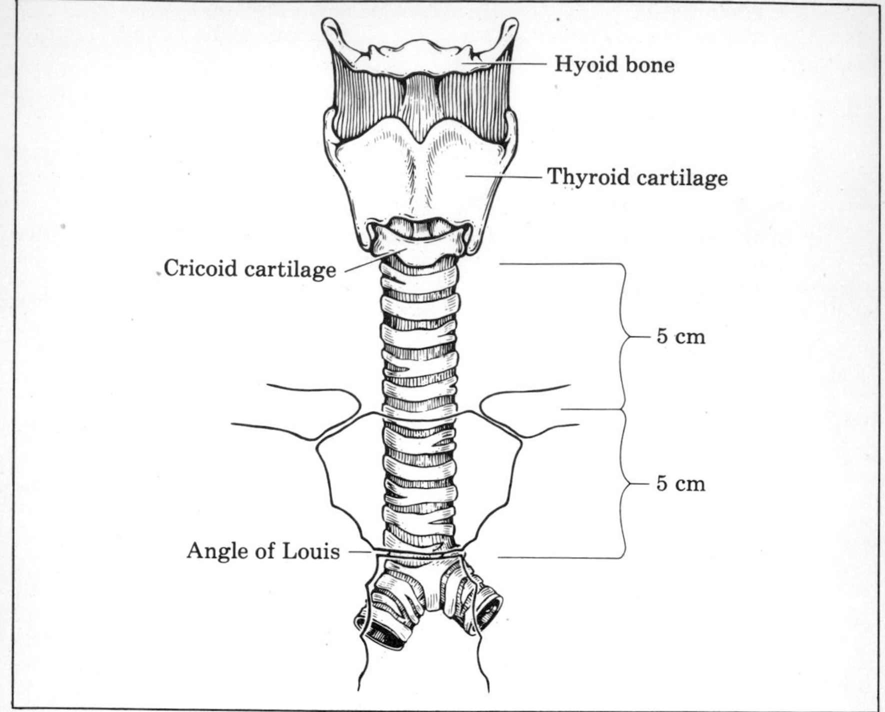

Fig. 13-3. Larynx, trachea, and bifurcation. The bifurcation of the trachea into the left and right bronchi corresponds to the angle of Louis. The right bronchus is more nearly vertical than the left bronchus.

B. Endobronchial intubation

1. **A long tube** may enter the right main bronchus because of its size and the lesser angle it forms with the trachea. **Right endobronchial intubation** will result in obstruction, atelectasis, or collapse of the left lung and, possibly, of the right upper lobe of the right lung.

2. **Prevention**

   a. **The length** of the endotracheal tube should be estimated for each patient by placing it externally alongside the mouth and neck, from the tip of the chin to the suprasternal notch.

   b. The chest should be inspected and auscultated.

3. **The bifurcation** of the trachea into the left and right bronchi corresponds to the sternal angle of Louis, or the second costal cartilage (Fig. 13-3). The stem of the right bronchus is shorter and wider, with its first branch arising 2.5 cm from the bifurcation (carina).

C. Esophageal intubation must be recognized as early as possible by observation and auscultation of the chest and epigastrium. **The tube should be removed immediately.**

D. Endotracheal tube obstruction

1. **Causes**

   a. Kinking. This may be prevented by using a spiral embedded tube in cases where kinking is likely to occur.

b. Biting.

c. A foreign body, such as mucus, blood, pus, debris, or granulation tissue, may obstruct the tube.

2. **Prevention** of endotracheal tube obstruction requires the constant alertness of the anesthesiologist or nurse-anesthetist.

E. **Laryngospasm** may follow extubation in a patient under extremely light anesthesia. **Therapy** includes administration of oxygen under positive pressure with a bag and tight-fitting mask. If laryngospasm persists, 60 mg of succinylcholine should be given IV.

F. **Subglottic edema**

1. **Laryngeal or subglottic edema,** due to mechanical trauma, may follow within 1 hr of extubation, with signs of respiratory obstruction, particularly in children. This condition results from the development of a transudate in the areolar tissue just below the vocal cords. It frequently is due to an acute inflammation superimposed on a slight trauma during intubation.

2. **In infants and children,** the slight edema of the mucosa will reduce the size of the larynx considerably. Croupy cough, hoarseness, expiratory stridor, and, as swelling increases, signs of ventilatory obstruction (dyspnea, tachypnea, tachycardia, and suprasternal retraction) develop.

3. **Therapy** includes a cold, moist, oxygen-enriched atmosphere, dexamethasone (Decadron) 4–8 mg IV, diphenhydramine (Benadryl) 25–50 mg IV, hydration, antibiotics, and mild hypothermia (35° C) by use of a plastic canopy tent (Croupette) with a circulating ice-water mattress. If all these fail and the patient is still restless and hypoxic, **intubation and/or tracheotomy** should be performed immediately.

G. **Postintubation sore throat**

1. This is the most common complication of endotracheal intubation. **The reported incidence** varies from 20 to 100%, and it occurs more often in females. **Note:** It has also been reported in 10% of nonintubated patients.

2. **Pharyngeal injury may** be associated with discomfort on swallowing and **laryngeal trauma,** with hoarseness or dysphonia.

3. **Trauma** is considered to be the main cause; the soreness can be produced during laryngoscopy. Other causes are static pressure, excessive friction between the tube and the posterior wall of the pharynx and larynx, the effects of surgery in the throat area, and the use of an indwelling esophagogastric tube.

4. The sore throat is usually self-limiting, lasting only 2–3 days, and does not need treatment.

H. **Postintubation granuloma of the larynx**

1. **Granuloma of the larynx** due to endotracheal intubation is a rare complication. The lesion appears most frequently on the posterior one-third of the vocal cords. It has been observed only in adults and more often in women than in men.

2. **Laryngeal granuloma or ulceration** must be suspected when hoarseness, sore throat, dysphonia, or dysphagia persists for days or weeks.

3. **Many patients tolerate endotracheal intubation for days** without clinical signs and symptoms of chronic injury to the larynx, but others, following a short period of intubation, may show granuloma of the larynx in spite of the best prophylactic measures.

4. **The following factors** may contribute to the formation of postintubation granuloma of the larynx:

a. **Head position.** The incidence is increased following head and neck surgery.

b. **Infection.** Preexisting respiratory tract infection may be a contributing factor.

c. **Trauma.** The vocal cords may be injured during intubation, either by a tube or by static pressure of the tube in place.

5. **Symptoms.** Hoarseness, fullness or tension in the throat, sensation of a foreign body, or pain radiating to the ear. In the presence of persistent dysphonia, difficult breathing, or persistent sore throat or hoarseness, the anesthesiologist should request a consultation with an otolaryngologist.

6. **Prophylaxis** includes avoidance of trauma, direct viewing for intubation, use of muscle relaxant agents, avoidance of excessive flexing or extending of the head and neck, and use of clean, sterile anesthesia equipment.

7. **Therapy** consists of surgical excision of the pedunculated granuloma under direct laryngoscopy, followed by vocal rest until healing is complete. The use of electrocautery creates intractable perichondritis because there is bare cartilage under the base of the ulcer.

I. **Tracheal stenosis**

1. **Tracheal stenosis is a very serious complication;** it is more common in adults and is associated with prolonged intubation.

2. **It occurs at the area** of the inflatable cuff and consists of a circumferential fibrous stricture of the trachea.

3. **The stenosis begins** as mucosal edema and ulceration, and eventually the cartilaginous rings are exposed. The rings then soften and finally disappear. Subsequently, scar tissue changes the trachea into a fibrous stenosis.

4. **Symptoms**

a. Early symptoms consist of a dry cough and inability to remove sputum, which may result in an attack of pneumonia. The symptoms later may progress to dyspnea and signs of respiratory obstruction.

b. Examination must include x-ray and bronchoscopy.

5. **Therapy.** In severe fibrous tracheal stenosis, surgical intervention is necessary.

Bibliography

Barako, A. Intravenous lidocaine controls extubation laryngospasm in children. *Anesth. Analg.* (Cleve.) 57:506, 1978.

Baron, S. H., and Kohlmoos, H. W. Laryngeal sequelae of endotracheal anesthesia. *Anesth. Analg.* (Cleve.) 54:767, 1975.

Blanc, V. F., and Tremblay, N. A. G. The complications of tracheal intubation: A new classification with a review of the literature. *Anesth. Analg.* (Cleve.) 53:202, 1974.

Gold, M. I., and Muravchick, S. Arterial oxygenation during laryngoscopy and intubation. *Anesth. Analg.* (Cleve.) 60:316, 1981.

Holinger, P. H., Schild, J. A., Kutnick, S. L., et al. Subglottic stenosis in infants and children, *Ann. Otol. Rhinol. Laryngol.* 85:591, 1976.

Ikeda, S., Yanai, N., and Ishikawas, S. Flexible bronchofiberscope. *Keio J. Med* 17:1, 1968.

Klainer A. S., Turndor, H., Wu, W. H., et al. Surface alterations due to endotracheal intubation. *Am. J. Med.* 58:674, 1975.

Koka, B. V., Jeon, I. S., Andre, J. M., et al. Postintubation croup in children. *Anesth. Analg.* (Cleve.) 56:501, 1977.

Lindholm, C. E., Ollman, B., Snyder, J. V., et al. Cardiorespiratory effects of flexible fiberoptic bronchoscopy in critically ill patients. *Chest* 74:362, 1978.

Mulder, D. S., Wallace, D. H., and Woolhouse, F. M. The use of fiberoptic bronchoscope to facilitate endotracheal intubation following head and neck trauma. *J. Trauma* 15:638, 1975.

Murphy, P. A fiberoptic endoscope used for nasal intubation. *Anaesthesia* 22:489, 1967.

Raj, P. P., Forestner, J., Watson, T. D., et al. Techniques for fiberoptic laryngoscopy in anesthesia. *Anesth. Analg.* (Cleve.) 53:708, 1974.

Salem, M. R., Mathrubhutham, M., and Bennet, E. J. Difficult intubation: Current concepts. *N. Engl. J. Med.* 295:879, 1976.

Stanley, T. H., Kawamura, R., and Graves, C. Effects of nitrous oxide on volume and pressure of endotracheal cuffs. *Anesthesiology* 41:256, 1974.

Taylor, P. A., and Towley, R. M. The bronchofiberscope as an aid to endotracheal intubation. *Br. J. Anaesth.* 44:611, 1972.

Westley, G. R., Cotton, E. K., and Brooks, J. G. Nebulized racemic epinephrine by IPPB for the treatment of croup. *Am. J. Dis. Child.* 132:484, 1978.

Wright, R. B., and Manfield, F. F. V. Damage to teeth during the administration of general anesthesia. *Anesth. Analg.* (Cleve.) 53:405, 1974.

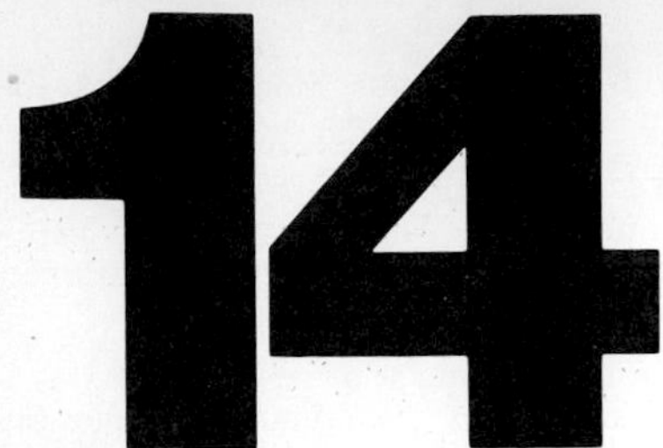

Local and Regional Anesthesia

I. General considerations

A. The local anesthetic drugs are **capable of blocking nerve conduction** of impulses in all nervous tissues. This action is reversible, and there is complete recovery of nerve physiologic function.

B. The extent of the anesthetized field depends on the site of application of the local anesthetic solution, the total volume administered, the concentration of the agent, and the penetrating ability of the agent.

C. Most local anesthetic drugs constitute a hydrophilic amino group connected by an intermediate chain to a lipophilic aromatic residue.

1. These drugs are **synthetic** (with the exception of cocaine), contain nitrogen, are basic in reaction, and have a bitter taste.
2. They are **prepared as salts** of hydrochloric or sulfuric acid.
3. These salts **form strong acid solutions,** but tissue irritation is minimized by the high buffer capability of the body.

D. The local anesthetics **affect all cells,** but have a special predilection for nerve tissue. Their main pharmacologic property is the **blocking of nerve conduction** when applied at any site on a neuron.

1. **They have a vasodilating effect** (with the exception of cocaine).
2. **Infiltration into an inflamed area does not produce satisfactory anesthesia** because the increased acidity of the infected tissues decreases the activity of the local anesthetic drugs. The pH of pus is 5.

E. Absorption

1. **Skin.** The local anesthetic agents **do not penetrate the skin,** and they are ineffective when applied to intact skin.
2. **Subcutaneous tissue.** Absorption in the subcutaneous tissue depends on the vascularity of the tissue unless epinephrine is added to the solution.
3. **Eyes.** In the eye, absorption is effective through the conjunctival membrane by means of externally applied aqueous solutions or subconjunctival injection.
4. **Mucous membranes.** Absorption from surface application to the mucous membranes of the nose, pharynx, trachea, bronchi, and alveoli is as rapid as IV injection.
5. **IM injection.** Absorption from IM injection is less rapid than from either IV injection or surface application to the mucous membranes of the tracheobronchial tree.
6. **Vasoconstrictors** do not delay absorption from mucous membranes.
7. **Esophagus.** There is no significant absorption from the mucous membranes of the esophagus.

8. **Stomach and urethra.** Absorption by the mucous membranes of the stomach and urethra is rapid.

9. **Spinal canal.** Absorption into blood is slow, and blood levels seldom are detectable following doses for spinal anesthesia. Vasoconstrictors (epinephrine, phenylephrine) delay absorption and increase the duration of the anesthetic effect by 60%.

10. **Peridural space.** Local anesthetics diffuse along the nerves through intravertebral foramina. Absorption is similar to that of subcutaneous tissues. Vasoconstrictors delay absorption.

F. **Detoxification.** Degradation rate varies with the particular agent and is carried out by **enzymes of the blood and liver.** The **kidney** eliminates the breakdown products and a portion of the local anesthetics unchanged.

II. **Nerve blocks.** The following nerve blocks occur when local anesthetics are applied at specified anatomic sites.

A. **Surface (topical) anesthesia** results from the application of certain local anesthetics to damaged skin or mucous membranes.

1. Certain local anesthetics are effective when applied to **inflamed or diseased skin and mucous membranes** as solutions, aerosols, creams, jellies, ointments, or suppositories.

2. **The following drugs** (see sec. **V** and Table 14-1) are administered to produce surface anesthesia of the conjunctiva, cornea, mouth, nose, pharynx, esophagus, larynx, trachea, urethra, or anus: benzocaine, butyl aminobenzoate, cocaine, dibucaine (Nupercaine), hexylcaine (Cyclaine), lidocaine (Xylocaine), piperocaine (Metycaine), proparacaine (Ophthaine), and tetracaine (Pontocaine).

B. **Infiltration and block anesthesia**

1. **Infiltration anesthesia** is carried out by injecting the local anesthetic solution into the area to be anesthetized.

2. **Block anesthesia** is accomplished by injecting the local anesthetic solution around the nerve trunk at a distance from the area to be operated on. The procedure is named according to the area injected (for example, paravertebral block, brachial plexus block).

3. **The drugs and doses used for infiltration and block** anesthesia are given in Table 14-2.

C. **Spinal anesthesia**

1. Spinal anesthesia (subarachnoid or intrathecal block) (see Chap. 15) is carried out by injecting the local anesthetic into the **spinal subarachnoid space** below the level of the spinal cord (second lumbar vertebra in adults).

2. The term **saddle block** designates spinal anesthesia limited to the sacral and caudal dermatomes. This is achieved by injection of a small amount of

Table 14-1. Doses of Local Anesthetics for Topical Anesthesia

Drug	Concentration	Duration	Maximal Dose
Cocaine	4%	30 min	200 mg
Lidocaine (Xylocaine)	2–4%	15 min	200 mg
Tetracaine (Pontocaine)	0.5%	45 min	50 mg
Benzocaine	2–10%	Several hours	

Table 14-2. Doses of Local Anesthetics for Infiltration and Nerve Blocks

Drug	Concentration	Duration	Maximal Dose
Procaine (Novocain)	2–4%	½ hr	1000 mg
Lidocaine (Xylocaine)	1–2%	1–2 hr	500 mg
Mepivacaine (Carbocaine)	1–2%	1–2 hr	500 mg
Tetracaine (Pontocaine)	0.1–0.25%	2–3 hr	75 mg
Chloroprocaine (Nesacaine)	1–2%		1000 mg
Piperocaine (Metycaine)	1–2%		750 mg
Hexylcaine (Cyclaine)	1–2%		500 mg
Bupivacaine (Marcaine)	0.5%	5–7 hr	200 mg
Etidocaine (Duranest)	0.5–1%	4–6 hr	300 mg

hyperbaric anesthetic solution, commonly with the patient in the sitting position.

3. **The nerves anesthetized** by the local anesthetic drug are determined by the degree of the drug's upward passage in the spinal subarachnoid space. This is influenced by:
   a. **The site and rate** of injection.
   b. **The specific gravity, volume, and concentration** of the solution.
   c. **The curvature** of the spine.
   d. **The patient's position** during and after injection and **his or her movements.**
   e. **The size** of the subarachnoid space.
4. **Spinal block takes effect** in a specific order: Autonomic nerves are anesthetized first, followed by those mediating cold, warmth, pain, and touch, and then by those mediating somatic motor function and proprioception. **Function is regained** in the reverse order.
5. **Spinal anesthesia may be achieved** either by a single injection through a needle or through a catheter threaded into the subarachnoid space via a large-bore needle. The amount of local anesthetic drug required is minimal, because the nerve roots are bare.
6. **The patient is conscious.**
7. **The duration of spinal anesthesia** depends on the rate at which the anesthetic drug leaves the affected nerve roots. **The greatest amount diffuses** into the spinal fluid and leaves the subarachnoid space through venous drainage. A smaller amount leaves through the lymphatics. The duration of block tends to be longer in the elderly.
8. **The duration of spinal anesthesia is prolonged** by:
   a. Increasing the concentration of a single dose.
   b. Repeated fractional administrations through a catheter in place **(continuous spinal anesthesia).**
   c. Adding a vasoconstrictor to the solution.
9. Local anesthetic solutions injected for spinal anesthesia are **hyperbaric, isobaric,** or **hypobaric,** depending on whether their specific gravity is

Table 14-3. Doses of Local Anesthetics for Spinal Anesthesia, Single-Dose Technique

Drug	Concentration	Duration	Maximal Dose
Procaine (Novocain)	10%	1 hr	150 mg
Lidocaine (Xylocaine)	5%	1½ hr	150 mg
Mepivacaine (Carbocaine)	4%	1–2 hr	150 mg
Tetracaine (Pontocaine)	1%	1½–2 hr	20 mg

higher than, the same as, or lower than that of cerebrospinal fluid (CSF). The specific gravity of CSF is 1.003–1.007.

10. **Tetracaine** is the most widely used spinal anesthetic. It acts for 1½–2 hr. Other drugs used are procaine, lidocaine, and mepivacaine. Doses are given in Table 14-3.

D. Epidural and caudal anesthesia

1. Epidural or caudal anesthesia (see Chap. 16) is accomplished by injecting the local anesthetic solution into the epidural space of the lumbar area or sacral canal.

   a. Continuous epidural anesthesia is carried out by placing a fine catheter through a needle into the space between the dura and the ligamentum flavum for repeated injections of the local anesthetic solution. The injection is ordinarily made below the level of the second lumbar vertebra. It can be done at other sites, but this requires great expertise.

   b. **In caudal anesthesia,** the local anesthetic solution is administered through the **sacral hiatus** into the epidural space of the **sacral (caudal) canal.** Continuous caudal anesthesia is carried out by placing a fine catheter through a needle into the caudal canal for repeated injections of the local anesthetic.

2. In epidural or caudal anesthesia, **the area of action** is determined by the particular nerves that the local anesthetic comes into contact with, and it may include the nerves in the paravertebral, epidural, and subarachnoid spaces or the spinal cord itself.

3. **The factors that influence** the extent and duration of the anesthesia produced are the same as for spinal anesthesia, but the total volume of anesthetic required is greater.

4. **The possibility of toxicity** is high because of the large doses required, the vascularity of the epidural space, and the difficulty of the method.

5. **The main advantage** of epidural anesthesia compared to the spinal technique is that it produces extensive regional anesthesia without dural puncture and injection of foreign substances into the CSF, and it eliminates post-lumbar-puncture headache.

6. **The drugs of choice** for epidural and caudal anesthesia are lidocaine, mepivacaine, and bupivacaine. Doses are given in Table 14-4.

E. Intravenous regional anesthesia. See Chapter 17, section **VII.**

F. Hyaluronidase (Wydase)

1. **Hyaluronic acid** is found in the interstitial spaces. It holds the cells together and delays diffusion.

2. **Hyaluronidase** is an enzyme that hydrolyzes hyaluronic acid and thus permits more rapid spread of solutions into the tissues. It is added to local

Table 14-4. Doses of Local Anesthetics for Epidural (Peridural) Anesthesia (Lumbar or Caudal Area), Single-Dose Technique

Drug	Concentration	Duration	Maximal Dose
Procaine (Novocain)	1–2%	1 hr	1000 mg
Lidocaine (Xylocaine)	1–2%	1½ hr	500 mg
Mepivacaine (Carbocaine)	1–2%	1–2 hr	500 mg
Tetracaine (Pontocaine)	0.1–0.25%	2–3 hr	75 mg
Bupivacaine (Marcaine)	0.5–0.75%	3½–5 hr	225 mg
Etidocaine (Duranest)	0.5–1%	4–6 hr	300 mg

anesthetic solutions to facilitate their diffusion in infiltration and block anesthesia. It decreases the duration of the block.

3. Due to an increased incidence of toxic systemic reactions caused by the local anesthetic drugs when hyaluronidase is used, hyaluronidase is not recommended for infiltration and block anesthesia.

4. Hyaluronidase is standardized in turbidity reducing units.

G. Vasoconstrictors

1. The local anesthetic drugs (except cocaine) **dilate the blood vessels,** resulting in an increased rate of absorption and decreased duration of anesthetic action.

2. **Vasoconstrictor drugs** may be added to injectable local anesthetic solutions. Their hemostatic action prolongs and increases the anesthetic effect and therefore may decrease the danger of toxic systemic reactions.

3. **Epinephrine** (Adrenalin) is the most often used vasoconstrictor drug.

   a. Epinephrine counteracts the depressing action of the local anesthetics on the heart and circulation.

   b. It is used in concentrations of 1:100,000 (1 mg/100 ml) or 1:200,000 (1 mg/200 ml). Stronger epinephrine solutions may cause tissue injury due to ischemia. The total quantity injected with a local anesthetic should not exceed 1 mg (1 ml of 1:1000 solution). When it is administered into the subarachnoid space, 0.2–0.3 mg of epinephrine provides the greatest increase in duration of the block.

   c. **The addition of epinephrine to a surface anesthetic** solution applied to mucous membranes does not affect the duration of surface anesthesia.

   d. **Epinephrine should be omitted** from local anesthetic solutions:

      (1) In patients with a history of hypertension, thyrotoxicosis, diabetes, or heart disease.

      (2) In surgical procedures on the fingers or toes, because severe vasospasm and ischemia of the extremities may occur.

4. Another vasoconstrictor used is **phenylephrine** (Neo-Synephrine), but this is used in concentrations 2 to 10 times higher than epinephrine.

III. Advantages

A. Local anesthesia is sometimes preferable to general anesthesia for the following reasons:

1. The technique is simple, and minimal equipment is required.

2. The drugs are nonflammable.

3. There is less bleeding.
4. There is less nausea and vomiting.
5. There is less disturbance to body functions.
6. It can be used when general anesthesia is contraindicated because of recent ingestion of food by the patient.
7. There is no pollution of the environment.
8. Less postoperative observation and care of the patient are required.
9. There is a lower incidence of pulmonary complications.
10. It is less expensive.

B. **Regional anesthesia produces complete sensory block,** which prevents harmful impulses from the area of surgery. This is not the case with general anesthesia, which ordinarily does not prevent impulses caused by surgery from reaching the CNS and creating a stress response and sometimes abnormal reflexes.

C. **Regional anesthesia is indicated** in the following special circumstances in which the patient's alert cooperation is required:
1. Identification of lacerated hand tendons.
2. Thalamotomy.
3. Cordotomy.

IV. Complications due to local anesthetics

A. **The systemic and local adverse reactions** are similar for all local anesthetic agents.
1. Many of the adverse reactions are mild and easily treated, but **catastrophes may occur.** Most often these reactions are due to overdosage or errors of technique. Equipment for cardiopulmonary resuscitation must be readily available at all times. If correct treatment is rapidly undertaken, even catastrophic reactions are reversible.
2. **Therapy** is directed to the maintenance of adequate ventilation and circulation.

B. **Systemic reactions due to local anesthetics**
1. Systemic reactions are associated with high blood levels of local anesthetic drugs, which ordinarily result from overdoses, rapid systemic absorption, or inadvertent IV administration.
   a. **IV administration** is the most dangerous technique.
   b. **Absorption from the mucosa of the nose, pharynx, and respiratory tract** is rapid, similar to the absorption rate from IV administration. The reasons for this are the rich vascularity of these areas and the rapid absorption of the anesthetic solution from the alveoli. The absorbed anesthetic agent circulates directly to the heart, which explains why many sudden deaths have followed topical application of local anesthetics to the mucosa of the tracheobronchial tree.
   c. **Other factors** accounting for toxic reactions are (1) the rate of metabolism and detoxification of the local anesthetic drugs and (2) the presence or absence of epinephrine and hyaluronidase in solutions. **Epinephrine** delays absorption and **hyaluronidase** increases absorption.
   d. Interaction with other drugs.
2. The adverse reactions mainly affect the heart, circulation, respiration, and central nervous system.

a. **The effects on the heart and vessels** are the result of direct myocardial depressant and vasodilatory action of the local anesthetics. Hypotension, bradycardia, thready pulse, pallor, clammy skin, sweating, and cardiac arrhythmias possibly leading to cardiac arrest characterize these effects.

b. **The medullary centers** may be affected, resulting in depressed respiration, apnea, and vascular collapse.

c. **The CNS reactions** are characterized by nausea, emesis, talkativeness, euphoria, restlessness, dizziness, anxiety, excitement, and disorientation. These may be followed by muscle twitching, convulsions, coma, respiratory failure, and heart failure, leading to cardiac arrest.

3. **Therapy**

a. **For convulsions.** Diazepam (Valium), ultrashort-acting barbiturates (thiopental, thiamylal), and artificial ventilation with or without skeletal muscle relaxants.

b. **For respiratory depression.** Oxygen and artificial ventilation.

c. **For cardiovascular collapse.** Vasopressors, IV fluids, and external cardiac massage.

C. **Reactions due to epinephrine added to solutions of local anesthetics**

1. Most of the reactions to epinephrine are due to overdoses or interaction with other drugs (thyroid, digitalis). **The systemic signs and symptoms of epinephrine overdose** are apprehension, palpitations, tremors, tachycardia, tachypnea, hypertension, sweating, restlessness, fainting, weakness, headache, and skin pallor. **Hypertension** may precipitate a cerebral hemorrhage, arrhythmias, or coronary occlusion. **In extreme overdosage,** tachycardia may develop into pulmonary edema and ventricular fibrillation.

2. The reactions due to epinephrine differ from the systemic reactions produced by the local anesthetics in that **epinephrine produces tachycardia and does not ordinarily cause convulsions.**

3. **Treatment** consists of administration of barbiturates, propranolol, vasodilators, and oxygen.

D. **Systemic allergic reactions**

1. Allergic reactions due to local anesthetics **are rare.** Probably less than 0.5% of all reactions are truly allergic.

2. **Signs and symptoms** progress from urticaria, pruritus, angioneurotic edema, asthmatic breathing, syncope, and respiratory arrest to renal shutdown and even death.

3. **Treatment** includes epinephrine, antihistamines, bronchodilators, and oxygen.

E. **Local reactions due to local anesthetics**

1. Swelling, abscess, ulceration, and skin sloughing may follow infiltration and nerve blocks by local anesthetic drugs. **Skin sloughs** may follow the injection of dibucaine and hexylcaine.

2. **Therapy** includes antibiotics and sympathetic blocks.

F. **Precautions**

1. **If a patient is allergic** to a particular local anesthetic, the use of a drug from another chemical group is recommended. **Skin, conjunctiva, and patch tests** are not reliable for predicting the possibility of allergic reactions.

2. **The derivatives of aminobenzoic acid** inhibit the effects of **sulfonamides,** so it is advisable to avoid combining these two types of drugs.

3. **Local anesthetics with epinephrine** should not be injected during inhalation anesthesia with cyclopropane, halothane, or other halogenated anesthetics, because serious ventricular arrhythmias may occur.

4. **Epinephrine must be omitted** from local anesthetic solutions used for:

   a. Nerve block anesthesia in areas with **end-arteries,** since it may cause sloughing.

   b. Infiltration and nerve block **in patients in labor.** Epinephrine may produce vasoconstriction of the blood vessels of the uterus, with resulting decreased placental circulation, diminished uterine contractions, and prolonged labor.

   c. Nerve block anesthesia in **elderly patients** with a history of hypertension, cardiovascular diseases, diabetes, or thyrotoxicosis.

5. **Single-dose vials** of local anesthetic drugs should be used during spinal, epidural, and caudal blocks.

6. **For therapy of possible toxic reactions** and complications, the following should be available at all times:

   a. An endotracheal tube and laryngoscope.

   b. Equipment for administration of oxygen and artificial positive ventilation, as well as for maintenance of a pharyngeal airway.

   c. Diazepam, ultrashort-acting barbiturates, skeletal muscle relaxant drugs, IV fluids, and vasopressors.

G. **Cardiac arrest and cardiopulmonary resuscitation.** See Chapter 8.

V. Local anesthetic drugs

A. Cocaine

1. Cocaine is a benzoic acid ester that **produces surface anesthesia** with strong vasoconstricting effects when applied topically to damaged skin or mucous membranes.

2. **It is considered a standard** in comparing the potency and toxicity of other local anesthetics used for surface anesthesia.

3. **It shrinks mucous membranes** and decreases bleeding, and thus prevents its own fast absorption in the blood circulation.

4. Cocaine is used extensively as a topical anesthetic for operations in the **nasal cavity.** It is not ingested or injected.

5. When cocaine is applied on the **eye,** the cornea may become clouded and pitted, and ulceration may result.

6. **Heat decomposes** cocaine solution, and boiling causes rapid hydrolysis of it.

7. **Absorption is slow,** but toxic reactions may occur because cocaine is eliminated and detoxified slowly.

8. **Acute poisoning** produces **cortical stimulation** with excitement, restlessness, confusion, tremor, hypertension, tachycardia, rapid shallow respiration, nausea, emesis, abdominal pain, exophthalmos, and mydriasis. The stimulation is followed by depression and cardiac arrest from respiratory depression.

9. Cocaine presents **drug abuse problems,** because prolonged use can bring about a psychic dependence.

10. **Dosage.** Cocaine is used in 4% solution **for surface anesthesia** of the nose, pharynx, larynx, and tracheobronchial tree. The **onset of action** is immediate, and the duration of action is 45 min. The **maximal dose** is 200 mg.

B. Procaine

1. Procaine (Novocain) is an aminobenzoic acid ester used in infiltration, block, spinal, epidural, and caudal anesthesia.

2. **It is considered a standard** in comparing the potency and toxicity of other local anesthetics used for injections.

3. It is administered IV for therapy of chemically or mechanically induced **arrhythmias** during general anesthesia, heart surgery, or induced hypothermia.

4. Procaine is absorbed with ease from the site of injection. To decrease absorption and prolong local anesthesia, **epinephrine** 1:200,000 is added to the procaine solution. Following absorption, **rapid hydrolysis** occurs from the enzyme in the plasma (procaine esterase), a factor that accounts for its relative safety.

5. IV use is contraindicated in persons with **myasthenia gravis** because it produces a degree of neuromuscular block. Procaine should not be given with sulfonamides.

6. **The yellow discoloration** in a 1–2% solution indicates the presence of amines, which are harmless.

7. **Procaine does not penetrate the skin or mucous membranes** and is therefore of no value for surface anesthesia.

8. **Dosage**

   a. **For infiltration and block anesthesia,** 2–4% with or without epinephrine 1:200,000. Surgical local anesthesia is obtained within 2–5 min and lasts for 45–60 min. The maximal dose is 1000 mg.

   b. **For epidural anesthesia,** 25 ml of a 1.5% solution.

   c. **For caudal anesthesia,** 25 ml of a 1.5% solution.

   d. **For spinal anesthesia,** 50–200 mg, depending on the effect desired. The duration of effect is less than 1 hr.

   e. **For IV anesthesia** a 0.1–0.2% solution injected slowly (10–15 ml/min) for 1–4 hr. Injection of 1000 mg IV over 1 hr is easily tolerated.

C. Chloroprocaine

1. Chloroprocaine (Nesacaine) is a halogenated **analog of procaine** with similar pharmacologic properties.

2. It is available in solution for infiltration, block, caudal, and epidural anesthesia. It is not effective for surface anesthesia. The drug is twice as potent as procaine, has a fast onset of action, and is 4 to 5 times more rapidly metabolized.

3. **Dosage**

   a. **For infiltration and block anesthesia** a 1–2% solution with or without epinephrine 1:100,000 or 1:200,000. The maximal dose is 1000 mg.

   b. **For caudal and epidural anesthesia,** 15–25 ml of a 2–3% solution with epinephrine 1:200,000.

D. Piperocaine

1. Piperocaine (Metycaine) is a benzoic acid ester used for surface, infiltration, block, spinal, and caudal anesthesia. Its toxicity and potency are slightly greater than those of procaine. As a surface anesthetic, it has half the potency of cocaine.

2. **Dosage**

   a. **For infiltration and block anesthesia,** a 1–2% solution. The effect is immediate and lasts 1 hr. The maximal dose is 750 mg.

   b. **For caudal anesthesia,** 35 ml of a 1.5% solution.

   c. **For spinal anesthesia** using the saddle block method, 1 ml of a 3% solution containing 5% dextrose is sufficient to produce anesthesia lasting 75 min. The maximal dose is 100 mg.

   d. **For surface anesthesia,** a 2–4% solution is used in the nose, throat, and urethra.

E. Hexylcaine

1. Hexylcaine (Cyclaine) is a benzoic acid ester used for infiltration, block, and surface anesthesia. Toxicity and potency are slightly greater than those of procaine, but it has a longer duration of action. When it is used for surface anesthesia, its potency is equal to that of cocaine.

2. **Dosage**

   a. **For infiltration and block anesthesia,** a 1–2% solution with a maximal dose of 500 mg. The onset of action is within 5–15 min, and its duration is 1–1½ hr. Local irritation and necrosis of the skin have been reported following injection. **Sloughs of the skin** have occurred following intradermal injection.

   b. **For surface anesthesia,** a 5% solution with a maximal dose of 250 mg. The onset of action is within 2–3 min, and its duration is 30 min.

F. Tetracaine

1. Tetracaine (Pontocaine) is a para-aminobenzoic acid ester used to produce surface, infiltration, block, caudal, and spinal anesthesia. It is the **most popular anesthetic for spinal anesthesia.** Its potency and toxicity are 10 times those of procaine. Tetracaine should not be given with sulfonamides. The onset of action occurs in 5–10 min, and its duration is 2 hr.

2. **Dosage**

   a. **For infiltration and block anesthesia,** a 0.1–0.25% solution with or without epinephrine 1:200,000. The maximal dose is 100 mg.

   b. **For caudal anesthesia,** 35 ml of a 0.15% solution with epinephrine 1:200,000.

   c. **For spinal anesthesia** of the perineum, 5 mg; the perineum and lower limbs, 10 mg; and up to the costal margin, 10–12 mg. Anesthesia lasts 1½–2 hr. Epinephrine, 0.2–0.3 mg, may be added.

   d. **For surface anesthesia**

      (1) **Eye,** 0.1 ml of a 0.5% solution.

      (2) **Nose, throat, and trachea,** 1 ml of a 1–2% solution.

      (3) **Damaged skin or rectum,** 0.5–1% ointment.

      (4) **The maximal dose** is 50 mg.

G. Lidocaine

1. Lidocaine (Xylocaine) is an amide that is commonly employed for surface, infiltration, block, spinal, epidural, and caudal anesthesia. It is also used IV to treat chemically or mechanically induced arrhythmias during general anesthesia, heart surgery, or induced hypothermia.

2. **Compared with procaine,** the onset of effect is more rapid, more intense, more extensive, and longer in duration. Potency and toxicity are twice those

of procaine, and it is a local vasodilator. When the concentration is increased, the toxicity also increases, because the drug is more rapidly absorbed.

3. Anesthesia with lidocaine lasts 1–1½ hr. With epinephrine, the duration is 2 hr.

4. The initial effect of an **overdose** is depression rather than excitation. Drowsiness and amnesia may occur, especially when lidocaine is used without epinephrine. Hypotension, sweating, nausea, emesis, muscle twitches, and **convulsions** also may occur. Hypersensitivity reactions to lidocaine are exceedingly rare.

5. **Dosage**

   a. **For infiltration and block anesthesia,** 2–60 ml of a 0.5–2% solution with or without epinephrine 1:200,000. The maximal dose is 300 mg without epinephrine and 500 mg with epinephrine.

   b. **For epidural anesthesia,** 15–30 ml of a 1–2% solution with or without epinephrine 1:200,000.

   c. **For spinal anesthesia,** a 5% solution with 7.5% dextrose. For obstetric use, in normal vaginal delivery, 50 mg (1 ml) provides perineal anesthesia for 2 hr.

   d. **For surface anesthesia,** a 2–4% solution can be applied to the cornea, pharynx, larynx, and tracheobronchial tree. The maximal dose is 250 mg. A 2% jelly is used in urethral endoscopy.

   e. **For therapy of arrhythmias.** A dose of 50–100 mg and/or 1–2 mg/min (1 mg/ml) in a slow IV drip is recommended for therapy of **ventricular arrhythmias** during general anesthesia and cardiac arrest. The drug is superior to procainamide (Pronestyl) because it decreases the irritability of the heart without depressant action on the cardiac output and peripheral vascular system.

H. Mepivacaine

1. Mepivacaine (Carbocaine), like lidocaine, is an amide used for infiltration, block, spinal, epidural, and caudal anesthesia. It is not effective for surface anesthesia. Potency and toxicity are **similar to those of lidocaine.**

2. The onset of action is rapid, and its duration is 2 hr. Mepivacaine produces **less vasodilation** than lidocaine and can be used without epinephrine, which, if added, does not increase the duration.

3. **Mepivacaine is indicated** (a) in patients with a history of hypertension, cardiovascular disease, diabetes, or thyrotoxicosis; (b) in nerve blocks in the ears, fingers, toes, and penis; and (c) during labor. In these patients, a vasoconstrictor is undesirable.

4. **Dosage**

   a. **The maximal dose** should not exceed 1000 mg in 24 hr or more than 8 mg per kilogram of body weight in a single dose.

   b. **For infiltration and block anesthesia,** 5–40 ml of a 1–2% solution.

   c. **For caudal anesthesia,** 15–30 ml of a 1–2% solution.

I. Bupivacaine

1. Bupivacaine (Marcaine) is related chemically and pharmacologically to mepivacaine and lidocaine. Its toxicity is equal to that of tetracaine.

2. **For infiltration and peripheral nerve blocks,** the solution used is 0.25–0.75%. The maximal dose is 200 mg, and the duration of effect is 3–8 hr. Epinephrine in 1:200,000 concentration is added to the solution when indicated.

3. **For epidural or caudal anesthesia,** 15–30 ml of a 0.25–0.75% solution is used.

J. Etidocaine

1. Etidocaine (Duranest) is the **newest** local anesthetic agent.
2. It is a long-acting local anesthetic of the amide type, similar to lidocaine structurally. It is 4 times as potent as lidocaine while only twice as toxic.
3. **For infiltration, peripheral nerve blocks, epidural anesthesia, and caudal anesthesia (except spinal),** the solution used is 0.5–1.5% with epinephrine 1:200,000. The maximal dose is 300 mg, and the duration of effect is 4–6 hr.

Bibliography

Backer, C. L, Tinker, J. H., Robertson, D. M., et al. Myocardial reinfarction following local anesthesia for ophthalmic surgery. *Anesth. Analg.* (Cleve.) 59:257, 1980.

Covino, B. G. Local anesthesia. *N. Engl. J. Med.* 286:975, 1035, 1972.

De Jong, R. H. Toxic effects of local anesthetics. *J.A.M.A.* 239:1166, 1978.

Foster, A. H., and Carlson, B. M. Myotoxicity of local anesthetics and regeneration of the damaged muscle fibers. *Anesth. Analg.* (Cleve.) 59:727, 1980.

Mather, L. E., and Tucker, G. T. Pharmacokinetics and biotransformation of local anesthetics. *Int. Anesthesiol. Clin.* 16:23, 1978.

Moore, D. C., Bridenbaugh, L. D., Thompson, G. E., et al. Bupivacaine. A review of 11,080 cases. *Anesth. Analg.* (Cleve.) 57:42, 1978.

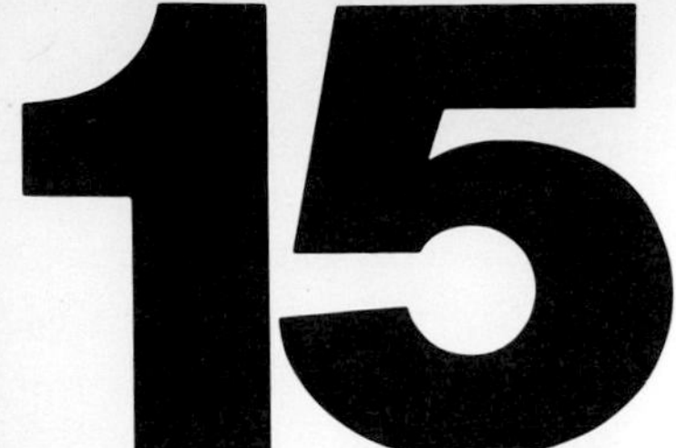

Spinal Anesthesia

I. Definition

A. **Spinal anesthesia** (subarachnoid nerve block and spinal analgesia) results from the deposition of a local anesthetic drug within the subarachnoid space at a lumbar interspace. A reversible nerve block of the anterior and posterior roots, posterior root ganglion, and portions of the spinal cord occurs, leading to loss of autonomic, sensory, and motor activity.

B. **Various functions** are carried within the mixed spinal nerve, including mediation of sensation (temperature, pain, touch, pressure, touch localization, proprioception), autonomic activity, and motor function. In a general way, each function is controlled by nerve fibers that differ in their resistance to local anesthesia, thereby allowing for differential blockage.

C. **Block of the spinal cord** begins caudally and proceeds in a cephalad direction for each modality. This process is reversed on dissipation.

1. **The heavy, myelinated fibers** (motor function and proprioception) are the most resistant to block and the first to which function returns. They thus require the highest drug concentration.

2. On the average, the **level of autonomic block** is two or more dermatomes cephalad to the level of skin analgesia, while the level of motor block lies two to three segments caudal to the analgesia site.

II. Indications

A. Surgery

1. **Lower extremity procedures** that involve soft tissue, vasculature, or bone.

2. **Perineum,** including anal, lower rectal, vaginal, and urologic surgery.

3. **Lower abdomen,** involving either the wall (hernia) or intraperitoneal operations (distal small intestine, appendix, rectosigmoid, bladder and lower ureter, and gynecologic procedures).

4. **Upper abdomen,** including cholecystectomy, closure of a perforated gastric ulcer, and transverse colostomy. Spinal anesthesia for upper abdomen surgery is not indicated for all patients because of the marked physiologic changes that it causes.

B. Obstetrics

1. Vaginal delivery.

2. Cesarean section.

C. **Diagnostic and therapeutic** procedures that are painful.

III. Contraindications

A. Absolute

1. **Bleeding disorders.** There is danger of piercing the abundant venous plexuses with the spinal needle, which could result in spinal cord compression.

2. **Septicemia.** Meningitis may supervene.
3. **Increased intracranial pressure.** Shifts of the brain may occur with cerebrospinal fluid (CSF) loss.
4. **Patient refuses consent.** Spinal anesthesia without consent is assault.
5. **Chronic dermatitis or a skin infection** near the puncture site. Pathogens may be introduced.
6. **Systemic diseases** with neurologic sequelae, e.g., pernicious anemia, neurosyphilis, or porphyria.
7. **Preexisting spinal cord disease** (amyotrophic lateral sclerosis and multiple sclerosis).
8. **Hypotension.** Sympathetic blockade removes the major compensatory mechanism.

B. Relative

1. **Hemorrhage.** Use a low saddle block anesthesia only when it is needed for surgery and if the vital signs are compensated.
2. **Back problems** due to muscle strain, facet syndrome, arthritis, or disc degeneration. Recurrent back pain in these patients may be associated with lumbar puncture. Nevertheless, despite such back problems, should spinal anesthesia be the only indicated procedure, a recent report would support its use on patients who had previous surgery on the lumbar spine. The authors consider that radiologic assessment of the vertebral column for the actual surgical site and a careful neurologic examination are mandatory for a successful outcome. The lumbar puncture is performed in the sitting position to widen the interspaces, and the needle is usually inserted above the scar.
3. **Respiratory disease.** Do not use spinal anesthesia if a middle to high spinal level is required, because respiratory inadequacy will occur.
4. **Extremely tense or psychotic** patients may become uncooperative during surgery, leading to management problems.
5. **Children** are upset by numbness and paresis.
6. **Acute upper respiratory disease.** A viral meningitis with upper respiratory symptoms may be present and progress to CNS signs later. The use of spinal anesthesia may confuse the cause of the problem and delay treatment.
7. **Abdominal distention.** Spinal anesthesia leads to an increase in gastrointestinal tone with a constricted bowel. Theoretically, there is a possibility of perforation, but this complication is rare in practice.
8. **Presence of a full stomach.** High spinal anesthesia will impair coughing, thus reducing the patient's ability to clear vomitus and more readily permit aspiration.

IV. Anatomy

A. General considerations

1. **There are 33 vertebrae:** 7 cervical, 12 thoracic, 5 lumbar, 5 sacral, and 4 coccygeal.
2. **The spinal cord ends at the second lumbar (L_2) vertebra.**
3. **The dural sac** (the outer investing layer of the spinal cord) **ends at the second sacral (S_2) vertebra.**
4. **Puncture for spinal anesthesia** can be made safely at the interspaces between L_2 and L_3, L_3 and L_4, or L_4 and L_5.
5. **Landmarks are established** when a line connecting the iliac crests intersects the lumbar spine. The L_4 spinous process or the $L_{4\text{-}5}$ interspace is

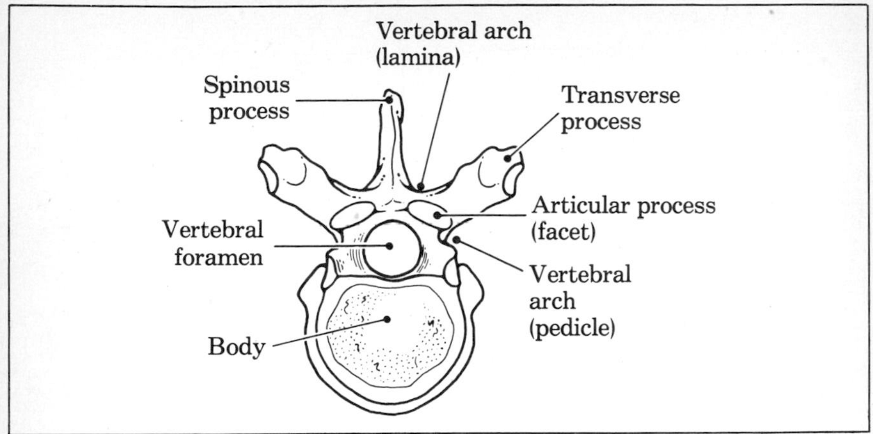

Fig. 15-1. A typical lumbar vertebra.

identified. Count up or down to identify the other spaces. The needle is positioned and the drug is injected below the spinal cord proper, and the original, or highest, concentration of solution bathes the **cauda equina** before diffusion and dilution.

B. **Lumbar vertebra.** A typical lumbar vertebra (Fig. 15-1) is composed of the following parts.

1. **Body.**
2. **Vertebral arch** (pedicles compose the anterior portion and laminae compose the posterior portion).
3. **Transverse processes** arise at the site of fusion of the pedicles with laminae.
4. **Spinous process,** which arises at the site of fusion of the laminae.
5. **Superior and inferior articular process (the facets).** Attachment to the adjoining vertebra completes the boundaries of the intravertebral foramen.

C. **Ligaments** hold the vertebral column together and protect the spinal cord. Proceeding in an anterior-to-posterior direction, they are (Fig. 15-2):

1. **The anterior longitudinal ligament,** which runs from the atlas (C_1) to the sacrum on the anterior surface of the vertebral bodies. It is not important in the technique of lumbar puncture.
2. **The posterior longitudinal ligament,** which runs the entire length of the vertebral column on the posterior surface of the vertebral bodies. It supports the intervertebral discs. It may be injured during the placement of the spinal needle.
3. **The ligamentum flavum,** which is a thick, yellow-appearing ligament connecting the adjoining laminae. It is thinned out in the posterior midline of the arch, permitting an entrance for veins. It offers distinct resistance to the passage of the needle.
4. **The interspinous ligament,** which is a dense ligament connecting adjoining spinous processes. It fuses anteriorly with the ligamentum flavum and posteriorly with the supraspinous ligament.
5. **The supraspinous ligament,** which connects the tip of the spinous processes. Together with the interspinous ligament, it offers minimal resistance to the exploring spinal needle.

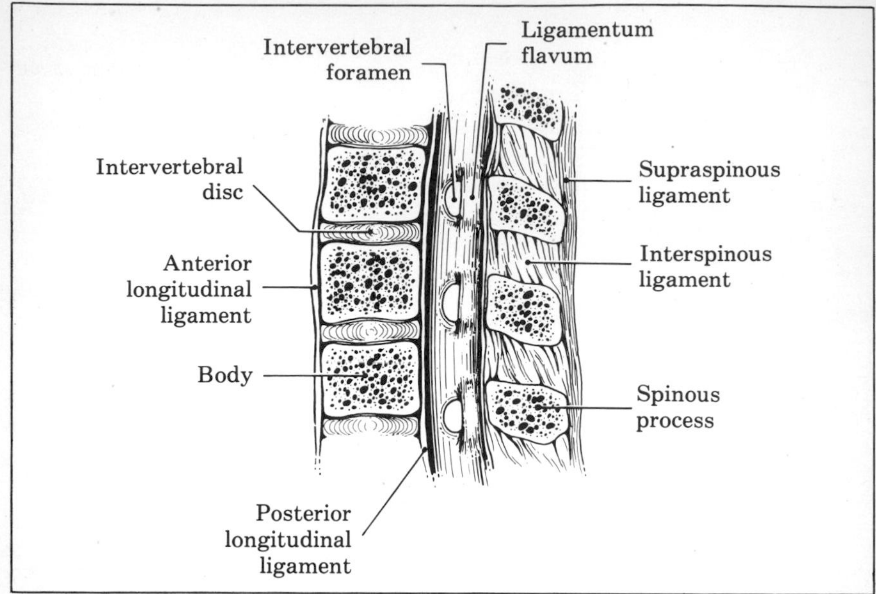

Fig. 15-2. The ligaments of the vertebral column.

D. Vasculature

1. **The following arteries** supply blood to the spinal cord and surrounding structures:
   a. **Spinal branches** of the vertebral and the ascending cervical artery of the inferior thyroid artery in the neck.
   b. **The intercostals** in the thorax.
   c. **The lumbar,** iliolumbar, and lateral sacral arteries in the abdomen and pelvis.
   d. **The arterial branches** enter the vertebral canal by the intervertebral foramen and join both the **anterior spinal artery,** which lies within the pia mater in the anterior median fissure of the spinal cord, and the **posterior spinal arteries,** which lie bilaterally in front of the posterior roots of the spinal cord.
   e. **Each spinal artery** extends the entire length of the spinal cord. The branches of the posterior spinal artery freely anastomose and communicate with the vessel on the opposite side.
   f. **Injury to the lumbar arteries,** as may occur in aortic manipulations, can result in **paraplegia.** T_{10} appears to be most important, since it is the major supplier of the lumbar enlargement of the spinal cord.
2. **The veins** that drain blood from the vertebral column form intricate plexuses that extend the entire length of the spinal cord. The veins are divided into external and internal groups, depending on their position outside or inside the vertebral canal, and anastomose freely with one another.
   a. **The external vertebral venous plexus** surrounds and drains the body and arches of the vertebrae.
   b. **The internal vertebral venous plexus** consists of four longitudinal veins, two located anteriorly in the peridural space (on the posterior surface of

the vertebral body) and two located posteriorly in the peridural space, in front of the lamina.

c. **A series of venous rings** at each vertebral level allows free intercommunication.

d. **The spinal cord itself** has six longitudinal veins situated within the pia.

(1) **An anterior median longitudinal vein** in the anterior median fissure.

(2) **A posterior median longitudinal vein** in the posterior sulcus of the spinal cord.

(3) **Four lateral longitudinal veins,** which run behind the nerve roots.

e. **The plexuses** freely anastomose and drain into the intervertebral veins, which leave the vertebral canal through the intervertebral foramina.

f. **The vertebral system of veins** parallels the caval system and offers an alternate route for the return of blood in the presence of increased intrathoracic or abdominal pressure. The extensive vasculature can be pierced during lumbar tap. Thus **any bleeding disorder contraindicates the procedure.**

3. **Vertebral (spinal) canal**

a. The **contents** are bounded anteriorly by the vertebral body and the posterior longitudinal ligament; laterally by the pedicles, attached facets, and ligamentum flavum; and posteriorly by the laminae and ligamentum flavum (Fig. 15-3).

b. **The vertebral canal contains** the spinal cord and its three investments (the pia, arachnoid, and dura mater); subarachnoid fluid; spinal nerves with their anterior and posterior roots and posterior root ganglion; vasculature; and an epidural space that is several millimeters deep in the lumbar region. The vertebral canal is practically circular, with a diameter of 15 mm.

V. Technique

A. Inspection and palpation of the lumbar site should be done at the time of the **preoperative visit,** since technical problems or infection observed at this time may contraindicate the planned use of spinal anesthesia.

B. Patient position

1. **The lateral position** is most comfortable for the patient.

a. **The head** is supported on a 7.5–10 cm pad, the chin is flexed on the upper sternum, the lower arm is extended at a right angle to the body, the thighs and knees are flexed maximally against the abdomen, and the upper arm and hand hold the upper thigh at the knee.

b. **The upper shoulder** must not be drawn forward but, rather, should remain in the plane of the back. This is an essential point that must be checked continually, because it will permit the best vertebral column alignment.

c. The lateral position allows **maximal flexion of the lumbar spine** and, by opening up the interspaces, facilitates the midline approach for lumbar puncture. If a paramedian approach is used, less flexion is needed.

2. **The sitting position** makes it easier for the anesthesiologist to identify the landmarks. However, premedicated patients may become dizzy in the upright position, and an assistant is required to support the patient and to ensure that the chin is placed on the upper sternum and that the arms are folded on the lap. This position is recommended for saddle block anesthesia or for a grossly obese patient whose landmarks are not distinct.

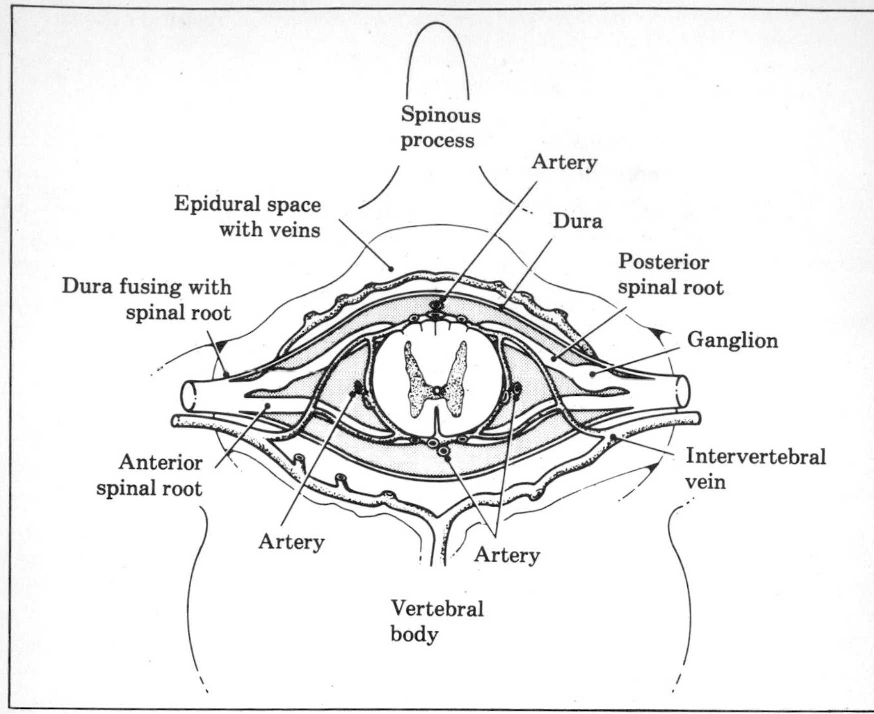

Fig. 15-3. The vertebral (spinal) canal and its contents.

3. **The prone position** is utilized if the surgeon desires the jackknife (Buie) or prone position. Thus the anesthesiologist may accomplish the block with **hypobaric saddle block anesthesia** in the definitive surgical position, with preparation for surgery beginning immediately after injection of the spinal anesthetic. More technical skill than usual is demanded in this situation because:

   a. **The back muscles** are not relaxed, which hinders the identification of landmarks.

   b. **The spinal fluid** will not appear because it has insufficient pressure to flow against gravity. It must be aspirated for accurate identification.

   c. **A paramedian approach** is required because the lumbar spine, unable to be flexed maximally, offers very narrow interspaces.

C. **Skin preparation**

1. **Aseptic technique** is mandatory. The operator wears sterile gloves, mask, and cap. The lumbar site is shaved and prepared with a wide application of an antiseptic solution—povidone-iodine (Betadine) is preferred. The site is wiped dry after 2–3 min, allowing time for good antisepsis. Drapes border the skin site and limit the potential for contamination. Do not allow the gloves to contact the skin, the antiseptic, the anesthetic solution, or the lumbar puncture needle shaft.

2. **Palpate the skin** through a thin sterile gauze and infiltrate the selected site with an intracutaneous injection of local anesthetic. This permits continual identification and analgesia for repeated taps if necessary.

3. **A 3.8-cm, 19-gauge needle** is introduced through the analgesic zone and is used for both a deeper infiltration of local anesthetic and introduction of the lumbar puncture needle. Note that in adults the distance from the skin to the ligamentum flavum is more than 4 cm.

D. Approach

1. **Midline approach**

   a. **The needle,** a 22-gauge or finer needle (24, 25, or 26), is passed through the **introducer** (which has penetrated the skin, subcutaneous fat, and supraspinous ligament) into the interspinous ligament. The introducer is passed in a cephalad direction at an angle of 80 degrees from the plane of the back at the caudal end of the $L_{2\text{-}3}$, $L_{3\text{-}4}$, or $L_{4\text{-}5}$ interspace. If bone is encountered, both the lumbar puncture needle and the introducer must be withdrawn to the subcutaneous fat and redirected at a slightly different angle.

   b. **The successfully inserted needle** will traverse the remainder of the interspinous ligament; the ligamentum flavum, which will offer some resistance; and the dura, where a distinct "pop" is felt when it is pierced. Removal of the stylet from within the lumbar puncture needle permits free flow of spinal fluid.

2. **Paramedian (lateral) approach**

   a. **The paramedian approach does not require** as much lumbar flexion, but, most importantly, the upper shoulder and arm must remain in a plane parallel to that of the back.

   b. **Infiltration** is made at a site approximately 1 finger's breadth lateral to the midline and adjacent to the caudal end of the interspace selected.

   c. **The 19-gauge introducer needle** permits an infiltration tract through the skin, subcutaneous fat, and paraspinous fascia and muscle. It is directed with two planes in mind: one direction will bring the lumbar puncture needle-tip to a midline position approximately 4 cm deep; the second direction is similar to the midline approach described in **1**, with the needle advancing in a cephalad direction 80 degrees from the plane of the back. The successfully directed needle enters the subarachnoid space after piercing the ligamentum flavum and dura.

E. Problems during lumbar puncture

1. **Paresthesias**

   a. **A properly placed needle** lies within a dense nerve network, the **cauda equina.** It is remarkable that the needle does not impale a spinal nerve very often. However, this must be considered as a possible cause for pain that persists after entrance into the subarachnoid space or during injection of the local anesthetic. If it occurs, the spinal anesthesia approach is abandoned.

   b. **More commonly, pain occurs** on entrance to the space and is the result of brushing of the nerve fibers against the needle shaft. This discomfort is transient and will not lead to pain or complications after injection.

2. **Spinal fluid**

   a. **Spinal fluid must be inspected** and found clear and colorless. If it is not clear, a sample is taken for analysis, and the procedure is abandoned.

   b. **The bloody tap.** The vasculature is plentiful within the vertebral canal, and the exploring needle may pierce a vessel, especially if the needle is not in the midline when piercing the ligamentum flavum. If blood appears, a few milliliters are allowed to run out. If the blood does not disappear, the stylet is replaced. If after about a minute the spinal fluid still has not cleared, the needle is removed, and another site is selected.

c. **Most of the blood-tinged spinal fluid** is allowed to run out prior to injection, since blood might cause a foreign body reaction (meningismus).

F. **Duration of surgery**

1. **For a single dose,** each drug has an average effective duration of action (see sec. **VI**). Since dissipation of block proceeds in a caudad direction, the effective duration for each drug will be shortest for abdominal operations and longest with surgery on the perineum, with intermediate times for abdominal wall and leg procedures. Selection of the appropriate safe drug will permit satisfactory conditions for surgery for 1–2½ hr, depending on the incision site.

2. **For some cases** in which spinal anesthesia would be the preferred technique, either the time for surgery is longer than 2–2½ hr or the duration cannot be anticipated because of either a diagnostic or a procedural uncertainty. These situations may be dealt with in the following two ways:

a. **Use of subarachnoid vasoconstrictors,** such as 0.2 mg of epinephrine will prolong a block by 50% (phenylephrine, 5 mg, by 100%), while ephedrine, 50 mg, will not significantly prolong the duration of anesthesia.

(1) **The subarachnoid deposition of the vasoconstrictor** has only a local effect on the vasculature and impairs the removal of the subarachnoid-deposited local anesthetic. Therefore a higher spinal fluid concentration of drug permits a greater uptake by the nerve, leading to the prolonged effect.

(2) **Controversy exists** regarding the potential of vasoconstrictors to cause prolonged spinal cord ischemia, with resultant neurologic sequelae. This may occur when higher doses bathe the nerve roots for prolonged periods, but it has not been shown with the doses recommended. However, if a patient has a significant small-vessel sclerosing disease (e.g., diabetes) that might affect the spinal cord, it is preferable to use the catheter technique for repeated injections, because it avoids the risk of ischemia associated with vasoconstrictor prolongation.

b. **The catheter technique** is indicated whenever the extent of the surgical procedure is in doubt or when the spinal cord vasculature may be impaired.

(1) **A Tuohy needle** with a Huber point (directionally curved bevel) and a short bevel is used in a manner similar to that used for a peridural catheter placement. A dural puncture is made, and the catheter is passed. Only 3 cm of catheter need be retained within the subarachnoid space. The remainder is taped in position along the midline of the back, ending at the shoulder for ease of repeat injections by the anesthesiologist.

(2) **The lowest anesthetic dose** recommended for the procedure (see sec. **VI**) is given and, if satisfactory, is repeated when necessary (usually within 1 hr) with half the original loading dose.

(3) **Disadvantages**

(a) Increased incidence of **postspinal headache** due to larger-gauge (18-gauge) needles.

(b) Fear of **cutting the catheter** on the needle tip within the subarachnoid space.

(c) **Sepsis** introduced either alongside the catheter or by contamination of the local anesthetic.

VI. Drugs

A. Three drugs—tetracaine, lidocaine, and procaine—have provided safe, consistent spinal anesthesia.

B. Tetracaine is a fully potent anesthetic producing autonomic, sensory, and motor block. It is supplied in two forms for spinal anesthesia: (1) a 1% solution and (2) niphanoid, a soluble form of the drug that consists of fine particles resembling snow.

1. **Sterilization** of the ampules is by autoclave at 755 torr and 121° C for 15–20 min. It is recommended that the ampules not be reautoclaved.
2. **Onset of action** is within 5–10 min, and **effective duration** for intraabdominal anesthesia is 1½ hr, with epinephrine, 2 hr, while perineal and lower extremity anesthesia lasts 2–2½ hr, with epinephrine, 3–4 hr.
3. **Tetracaine may be administered** as a 0.4–0.5% solution by the addition of sterile 10% D/W, producing a specific gravity of 1.022 for **hyperbaric** spinal anesthesia. It may be administered as a 0.1% solution when combined with sterile distilled water for **hypobaric** spinal anesthesia.
4. **Recommended doses** for the average-size patient are 4–5 mg for vaginal delivery, 8–10 mg for lower extremity and low abdominal wall surgery, and 10–14 mg for intraabdominal surgery. If epinephrine is used, the tetracaine dose is reduced by 1 mg.

C. Lidocaine is a fully potent anesthetic that results in block of autonomic, sensory, and motor function. It is supplied as a 5% solution in 7.5% D/W and has a specific gravity of 1.030–1.035 for hyperbaric spinal anesthesia. Ampules are sterilized by autoclaving in a manner similar to that for tetracaine.

1. **The onset of action** is rapid, with complete anesthesia within 2 min. **Effective duration** is 1½ hr and with epinephrine, 2 hr.
2. **Average doses** are 40–50 mg for vaginal delivery, 75–100 mg for lower extremity and lower abdominal surgery, and 100–150 mg for high spinal levels.

D. Procaine is a fully potent anesthetic supplied in an ampule as a dry powder or as a 10% solution. It is sterilized by autoclave in the same manner as tetracaine and should not be reautoclaved.

1. **The onset of action** is within 5 min. **Its duration** is 1 hr.
2. **Average doses** are 60–70 mg for vaginal delivery or dilatation and curettage and 100 mg for a cesarean section.

E. Bupivacaine is a fully potent anesthetic that is currently undergoing clinical trials as an agent for spinal anesthesia. A recently published double-blind comparison of bupivacaine with tetracaine employed on a milligram-to-milligram equipotency basis suggested that bupivacaine was as safe and reliable as tetracaine for lower abdominal, lower extremity, and perineal procedures. Further trials are justified.

VII. Control of the level of anesthesia

A. A differential pattern of block (see **I**) appears with spinal anesthesia: **The segmental level of motor paresis** is two to three segments below the skin analgesia level, while that for **autonomic function** is blocked two to six segments cephalad to the sensory zone. The level required for the block depends on the surgical need: If a soft tissue lesion at T_{11} requires treatment, skin analgesia to $T_{9\text{-}10}$ will give a satisfactory anesthesia. If a herniorrhaphy ($T_{11\text{-}12}$) is planned with motor paresis required at that level, sensory anesthesia to $T_{7\text{-}8}$ becomes necessary.

B. For clinical purposes, **spinal anesthesia levels** are described as follows:

1. **Saddle block anesthesia.** The skin zone of sensory anesthesia involves the lower lumbar and the sacral segments.
2. **Low spinal anesthesia.** The level of skin anesthesia is at the umbilicus (T_{10}) and includes the lower thoracic, lumbar, and sacral segments.
3. **Midspinal anesthesia.** The sensory level of block is at the costal margin (T_6), and the anesthesia zone includes the lower thoracic, lumbar, and sacral segments.
4. **High spinal anesthesia.** The sensory level is at the nipple line (T_4), and the anesthesia zone includes thoracic segments $T_{4\text{-}12}$ and the lumbar and sacral segments.
5. **The higher the spinal,** the higher the vasomotor and motor block, and the more likely are both hypotension and respiratory inadequacy.

C. Levels of anesthesia. The following factors are important in determining the ultimate levels:

1. **Volume of solution.** The greater the volume, the greater the spread of the original bolus of drug. The resulting level also will be proportionately higher.
2. **Concentration of the solution.** The concentration of the local anesthetic is sufficient to block all components of the mixed nerve within the zone of injection (cauda equina). After dilution with CSF, the concentration eventually falls sufficiently to produce the differential blocks. In general, the level of anesthesia will increase in proportion to the strength of the concentration.
3. **Barbotage** is the use of repeated aspiration and injection of the local anesthetic solution and spinal fluid. Since vigorous barbotage will produce a higher analgesic level, it is preferable to aspirate only 0.1 ml of CSF before injection of the local anesthetic and 0.1 ml after injection, to ensure that the needle is still within the subarachnoid space during drug deposition.
4. **Speed of injection.** A slow injection leads to a minimal spread of the bolus of drug, producing a low spinal anesthesia, while rapid injection leads to turbulent currents within the CSF and a higher level of anesthesia. The recommended rate of injection is 1 ml in 3 sec.
5. **A Valsalva-like action** occurs from tensing of the chest and abdominal wall when an unaided patient moves to the supine position after injection of the drug. This leads to a rise in CSF pressure and a higher spinal anesthesia. Relaxation and panting by the patient are encouraged, along with utilizing sufficient personnel to help turn the patient so that the fear and sensation of falling, which prompt the straining, will not occur.
6. **The site of injection** plays a minor role. The vertebral column has several curvatures in the supine position (Fig. 15-4).
   a. **Injection at $L_{4\text{-}5}$** helps keep the mass of drug within the sacral concavity to maintain a desired saddle block.
   b. **Injection at $L_{2\text{-}3}$ or $L_{3\text{-}4}$** allows the drug to rise easily to the thoracic segments, producing higher levels of anesthesia.
7. **Specific gravity of the solution and the position of the patient.** The specific gravity of normal CSF is 1.003–1.006. **Hyperbaric solutions** vary from 1.023–1.035 and seek a dependent position. **Hypobaric solutions** have a specific gravity of 1.001–1.002 and tend to float. Thus if a high spinal anesthesia is desired, a head-down position is used with a hyperbaric solution and a head-up position with a hypobaric solution. For saddle block anesthesia, a head-up position favors anesthetizing only the sacral areas with a hyperbaric

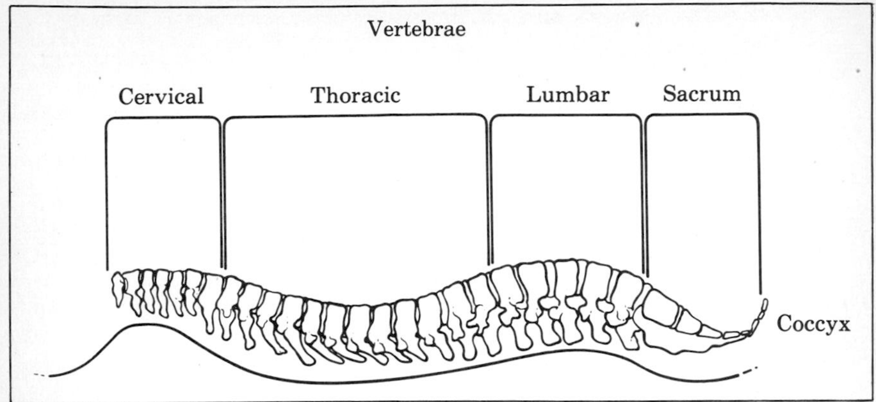

Fig. 15-4. The curvatures of the vertebral column. Note the characteristic thoracic concavity with the lowest point at $T_{6\text{-}7}$ and the lumbar lordosis with the apex at L_3.

solution, while a head-down position does the same with a hypobaric solution.

8. **Increased intraabdominal pressure,** by increasing the vertebral venous volume, effectively decreases CSF volume. Thus the lesser amount of CSF diluent would lead to higher levels of anesthesia. In clinical practice, a smaller dose is utilized in such a condition.

9. **Height of the patient.** The CSF volume varies with the length of the spinal cord. Thus a tall patient requires more drug to achieve a high level, while a short patient requires less drug than usual to achieve the desired level.

D. **Despite the many variables** that affect the anesthetic level, safe and consistently satisfactory conditions are obtainable with spinal anesthesia.

1. **Standardization of technique** allows for consistency. The amount of barbotage, the rate of injection, the drug concentration and specific gravity, and prevention of Valsalva-like maneuver on moving are easy to control.

2. **Only two factors** are allowed to vary: (1) the volume of the drug-containing solution, and (2) manipulation of the patient's position.

3. **In clinical practice,** a hyperbaric solution of 0.4% tetracaine is utilized. With 1 ml injected, a sensory level of T_{12}-L_1 is obtained. A volume of 2 ml will achieve a level to T_{10}, 3 ml produces a block to T_6, and 4 ml reaches T_4. An additional 0.25 ml of volume is added for patients taller than 6 ft, while 0.25–0.5 ml is subtracted for short patients (less than 5 ft), for patients with increased abdominal pressure (pregnancy), and when epinephrine is used.

4. **The patient is returned to the supine position** for 2–3 min after injection, during which time repeated testing of the skin analgesia level is done by pinprick. If the hypoesthetic level remains too low, manipulation to a 5- to 10-degree head-down position for several minutes will aid the spread of drug in the subarachnoid space and produce a higher anesthesia level.

VIII. Acute problems

A. Circulatory problems

1. **Cardiovascular changes** are due to the degree of sympathetic denervation and not to any systemic effect from the subarachnoid deposition of local

anesthetic or vasoconstrictor. In general, hypotension is more likely to occur in proportion to the height of spinal anesthesia. The segmental level of sympathetic block is two or more dermatomes cephalad to the zone of skin anesthesia. Thus a high spinal anesthesia (T_4 or higher) may be associated with a total block of the sympathetic nervous system. In healthy, well-hydrated volunteers, circulatory changes associated with high spinal anesthesia are mild, varying less than 15% from control values. **Parameters studied show:**

a. **A decrease in total peripheral resistance.**

   (1) **Arterial and arteriolar vasodilation** occurs in the zone of the block because of a decrease in sympathetic vasoconstrictor tone. Intrinsic autonomous tone, still retained by smooth muscle, can be diminished further by local or systemic hypoxia, acidosis, or alpha-adrenergic blocking drugs (chlorpromazine, droperidol, or phentolamine).

   (2) **Within the segments above the block,** compensatory vasoconstriction occurs, producing a cold skin with empty veins. Good clinical practice requires the start of an IV line prior to the block, because it will be more difficult to start later.

   (3) **Venous dilatation** leads to a marked increase in vascular capacity and a decrease in venous pressure and return.

b. **Decrease in systolic and mean arterial pressures.** These changes may be mild. Even so, they may significantly diminish flow to the brain or heart of a patient at risk. An early sign of **medullary ischemia** is nausea or vomiting.

   (1) **Systolic pressure** must not be allowed to fall more than 15 torr below the patient's lowest preoperative pressure.

   (2) **Maintenance of BP** is by:

      (a) Fluid infusions.

      (b) Vasoconstrictors.

      (c) Mild Trendelenburg (head-down 3 to 5 degrees) position, which helps venous return. Once assumed, the position is maintained until 30 min after dissipation of sensory block. Autonomic block will outlast sensory anesthesia.

c. **Decrease in heart rate** results from:

   (1) **Decrease in cardiac filling,** affecting the myocardial chronotropic stretch receptors.

   (2) **Anesthetic blockade** of the sympathetic cardiac accelerator fibers (T_{1-4}).

   (3) **Phenylephrine,** if used, increases vagal (baroreceptor) tone. The use of atropine (a vagal blocker) may increase the heart rate and possibly the BP.

d. **Stroke volume increase.** Myocardial contractility is not directly affected by spinal anesthesia.

   (1) **Indirectly,** spinal anesthesia decreases myocardial contractility because it affects preload, afterload, and rate and causes sympathetic adrenal suppression.

   (2) **The heart can pump** whatever volume returns to it. If venous return can be augmented by hydration or by the Trendelenburg position, preload effects can be maintained. The bradycardia permits more time for ventricular filling, with an increase in stroke volume (preload effect).

e. **Cardiac output increases** in normovolemic situations, while it decreases in hypovolemia. It is the product of stroke volume and heart rate and reflects their changes.

f. **In summary,** the heart attempts to compensate for changes in peripheral resistance to minimize BP changes. It is only indirectly affected by high spinal anesthesia.

2. **Regional flow changes associated with spinal anesthesia**

a. **The cerebral bed** retains its autoregulatory capability and allows for adequate flow in the face of a pressure drop unless intravascular obstructions are present.

b. **Coronary flow** is maximal during diastole. With a drop in BP, flow usually decreases. However, the rate–pressure index (heart rate × arterial pressure) is a major factor determining myocardial oxygen consumption and ultimately blood flow. Since the myocardium's oxygen need may decrease more than coronary flow, the heart will be relatively overperfused.

c. The percentage decrease in **renal blood flow** and glomerular filtration rate will diminish less than the mean arterial pressure.

d. **Hepatic flow** will diminish to a greater extent than the mean arterial pressure.

3. **Support of the BP** is most important if problems are to be averted. This is accomplished by the head-down position (3–5 degree Trendelenburg), along with the following two measures:

a. **Hydration.** The rapid infusion of 500–700 ml of electrolyte solution prior to middle and high spinal anesthesia will prevent significant hypotension in many patients. However, diuresis is promoted, and the urinary bladder will fill. Since bladder control is among the last functions to return, it is highly probable that either overdistention or catheterization will result. Either can lead to postoperative problems.

b. **Vasoconstrictors**

(1) **Phenylephrine,** 2–3 mg IM (usual route) and 0.25–0.50 mg IV (emergency route). Titration method: 10–20 mg/500 ml of 5% D/W IV.

(a) The onset of action is within 1 min IV and 5 min IM.

(b) The duration of action is 5 min IV and 25 min IM. The titration method permits continuous support for prolonged periods.

(c) Phenylephrine is a direct-acting alpha-adrenergic stimulant with slight positive inotropic actions.

(d) Bradycardia is common during its use.

(e) No tachyphylaxis is seen.

(f) Phenylephrine is the most useful vasopressor for the treatment of postspinal hypotension, except in obstetrics.

(2) **Ephedrine**

(a) The dose is 25–50 mg IM and 15–20 mg IV.

(b) The onset of action is within 2–4 min IV and 10–20 min IM.

(c) The duration of action is 1 hr.

(d) Ephedrine is an indirect-acting sympathomimetic drug with alpha- and beta-adrenergic effects. It may be less useful in patients on guanethidine or reserpine therapy because these drugs deplete norepinephrine stores.

(e) Tachycardia and occasional ectopic atrial and ventricular rhythms occur.

(f) Tachyphylaxis (with repeated doses, the response may be decreased).

(g) It does not reduce uterine blood flow and thus spares the placenta. This is a major advantage when treating hypotension in the obstetric patient.

4. **Use of vasopressors.** Prophylactic use is recommended in surgical patients. The selected drug is injected IM into the deltoid muscle or into the paraspinous muscles 2–3 min before subarachnoid injection of the local anesthetic. BP will be maintained for 25–30 min. This permits free use of patient-position manipulations to ensure a proper level of anesthesia.

5. **On cessation of the vasopressor** the BP may remain stable or may fall. If BP remains stable, no further treatment is necessary. **If BP falls** more than 15 torr below the lowest preoperative pressure recorded and this is not due to blood loss, a vasoconstrictor is indicated for the duration of the spinal anesthesia.

6. **When the duration of spinal anesthesia** is less than 2–2½ hr, an IM schedule is used, with repeat injections as required (usually every 30 min). If prolonged block is anticipated (up to 4–5 hr), the IV vasopressor is titrated.

7. Prophylactic use of vasopressors **in obstetric patients for vaginal delivery** is not recommended. The anesthesia level required is low, and a significant BP drop should occur in only a small number of patients. If it occurs, treatment is indicated, and ephedrine is administered. Vasoconstrictors and oxytocics may interact, resulting in a severe headache lasting up to several days.

B. Respiratory problems

1. General comments

a. **Blood gas exchange** is satisfactory under high spinal anesthesia if there is no underlying pulmonary disease. However, existing problems will worsen in proportion to how high the spinal anesthesia is given.

b. **Mean inspiratory capacity** falls only 8% with a motor block to T_4 (high spinal anesthesia), and only 19% after a total thoracic motor block. This emphasizes the preponderant role of **the diaphragm** in inspiration and explains why resting ventilation is unaffected by a high level of spinal anesthesia.

c. In contrast, **the mean expiratory reserve volume** diminishes with increasing motor block. There is a 15% volume decrease at a motor-block level of T_9 (midspinal anesthesia), a 40% decrease at T_5 (high spinal anesthesia), and volume rapidly falls to a 100% reduction with a total thoracic block, reducing the expiratory force to 50% of the control level. Coughing ability is impaired, and early airway closure, atelectasis, and hypoxia are promoted.

d. The patient should receive **oxygen** during middle to high spinal anesthesia. Patients with obstructive lung disease (such as emphysema, bronchitis, or asthma) are at risk with high spinal anesthesia because it prevents the active expiration essential for adequate ventilation.

2. **Respiratory difficulties** with spinal anesthesia are suggested by the onset of the following symptoms:

a. **Apnea**

(1) Commonly, apnea is due to **marked hypotension** with medullary ischemia. Treatment of the hypotension with vasoconstrictors or fluids

allows resumption of respiration. The patient must be ventilated until this occurs.

(2) Rarely, apnea is due to **high motor block of the phrenic nerve roots** (C_{3-5}). Treatment requires controlled intermittent positive-pressure breathing, often with tracheal intubation.

b. **A persistent dry cough** during spinal anesthesia may mean that the expiratory reserve is diminished, that expiratory flow rates are impaired, and that coughing cannot clear the airway effectively.

c. **Difficulty in phonation** indicates that the functional residual capacity is significantly reduced, affecting the air volume available for the flow of speech.

d. **Nausea or vomiting** occurs as a result of cerebral hypoxia. Oxygen administration is an effective antiemetic if respiratory inadequacy is the causative factor.

C. **Nausea and vomiting** are common during spinal anesthesia, occurring in 25% of cases. They are caused by:

1. **Hypotension,** a major cause of nausea during the course of spinal anesthesia. If hypotension is treated, nausea or vomiting will stop.

2. **Hypoxia** from respiratory inadequacy is the second most common cause. Oxygen therapy will treat this problem effectively.

3. **Marked anxiety** may be a cause. Verbal support and sedatives are helpful.

4. **Use of narcotics.** Gastrointestinal disturbances are a common side effect of narcotic usage. The use of the narcotic antagonist naloxone, 0.2–0.4 mg IV, may be an effective antidote. The use of narcotics for premedication is not recommended with spinal anesthesia.

5. **Parasympathetic overactivity.** Spinal block affects the sympathetic control of the gastrointestinal tract, allowing the vagus nerve to act without restraint. Constricted intestines, as well as abnormal peristaltic patterns, result from the enhanced tone. An additional dose of atropine 0.4 mg IV may restore a better balance and eliminate the symptoms.

6. **Traction reflexes.** The intestines respond to relatively few stimuli. These include manipulation of the gastrointestinal tract, which occurs whenever the surgeon explores an abdomen or packs off an intraperitoneal field. The afferent limb is by means of the vagus nerve. Preselection of patients with stoic personalities, gentleness by the surgeon, appropriate verbal support during the short maneuver, and even short-term sedation are means to prevent or treat gastrointestinal disturbances in the patient.

IX. Delayed problems following spinal anesthesia

A. Headache

1. **A postlumbar puncture** is identified by being aggravated in the erect position; it diminishes on recumbency. Its location is frontal in 50% of patients, occipital in 25%, and generalized in the remainder. The headache will appear within 3 days in 90% of patients. It has been reported as late as 12 days after lumbar puncture.

a. Headache lasts 4 days or less in 80% of cases and is disabling in 50% of cases.

b. It does not seem to be related to the duration of recumbency after lumbar puncture, to difficulty in the tap, or to whether paresthesias or a bloody tap occurs.

2. **Etiology**

   a. **The dural opening** may permit CSF leakage for 1–2 weeks. A net loss of 20 ml of CSF must take place for a headache to occur.

   b. **The proposed mechanism** states that when the patient assumes the **erect position,** the spinal fluid buffering the brain moves toward the dependent spinal cord. Thus the brain is not supported by sufficient fluid and is displaced. Traction of pain-sensitive structures produces the discomfort. **When the recumbent position** is resumed, spinal fluid flows back toward the cranium, supporting the brain, and the pain stops.

3. **Prevention factors**

   a. Use a fine needle (22- , 24- , or 26-gauge) for a small dural opening. Headache occurred in 10.7% of patients with the use of a 22-gauge needle and in 5% after the use of a 25-gauge needle. The incidence of headache related to needle size was the same in surgical patients and in patients with chronic pain having diagnostic spinal anesthesia.

   b. Insert the needle bevel, so that it is parallel to the longitudinal fibers of the dural sac. This parts, but does not sever, the dura, thus making a smaller opening.

   c. **Maintain adequate hydration** and encourage the patient to drink 3 L of fluid daily, in addition to permitted food, for at least 3 days. This tends to allow CSF secretion to keep up with the loss.

4. **Treatment**

   a. **The recumbent position** alleviates the discomfort and is maintained for 24 hr. By reducing CSF pressures, it lessens CSF leakage.

   b. **Active hydration.** Force fluids—up to 4 L PO daily, as well as 3 L IV—to encourage CSF production.

   c. **An abdominal binder** is useful, especially in postpartum patients. The increased intraabdominal pressure increases flow through the vertebral veins, which produces compression of the other contents of the vertebral canal. This helps coaption of the edges of the hole and promotes healing.

   d. **Avoid narcotics** that cause constipation. A stool softener will prevent straining, which increases the CSF pressure, thereby separating the dural opening and increasing the fluid loss.

   e. **Pitressin injection** (contains ADH) is not recommended because it can produce coronary vasospasm.

   f. **Lumbar or caudal epidural saline** is not recommended since it is too much work for what is considered a placebo response. If it helps, it does so by producing a transient increase in epidural pressure, simulating a binder action.

   g. **An epidural blood patch** is recommended. It is done by injecting up to 10 ml of freshly drawn autologous blood into a needle placed in the epidural space adjoining the hole. This will effectively alleviate the discomfort in 95% of patients with only one treatment. The blood clot seals the dural opening, preventing further leak, and, with maintenance of spinal fluid volume, eliminates the headache. Blood patch treatment does not obliterate the epidural space or prevent future successful epidural anesthesia.

5. **Problems associated with a headache** are quite rare.

   a. **Temporary paralysis of the cranial nerves** has been reported, with the exception of cranial nerves IX and X.

b. **The abducens (VIth cranial) nerve** is affected in over 90% of the rare patients who show cranial nerve paralysis and occurs 3–21 days after spinal puncture. The incidence is less than 0.1% in patients with postspinal headache. **Symptoms** reported are diplopia, photophobia, and blurred vision. The abducens nerve is particularly vulnerable to variations in CSF dynamics because of its long passage across the base of the skull, including the edge of the petrosal portion of the temporal bone. Spontaneous recovery may occur in days to months.

c. **Tinnitus and deafness** may occur in association with postspinal headache due to the concomitant fall in intralabyrinthine pressure.

d. It was suggested in a recent case report that headache may be a sign of serious sequelae and that treatment of headache should not be withheld. Apparently the sagging of the brain due to CSF loss can be associated with the rupture of small cerebral vessels, resulting in subdural hematoma with fatal herniation in patients without underlying intracranial disease.

B. **Backache** may be a problem following lumbar puncture for spinal anesthesia, as well as following general anesthesia. Many hospital factors contribute to backache. These are as follows:

1. **The hospital mattress** may be too soft and nonsupportive of the back.

2. **The patient may lie unsupported** on a stretcher, operating room table, or bed.

3. There may be **abrupt, traumatic transfers** from a stretcher, operating room table, or bed.

4. The patient may need to assume a position necessary for surgery that is stressful to the back muscles **(lithotomy).**

5. **The lumbar puncture needle** may injure the anulus that protects the intervertebral disc. However, this is rare and is attributable to gross inexperience. More commonly, the needle path itself is the source of pain, tenderness, and spasm. A well-placed puncture must pierce soft tissue and ligaments, and it often abrades the periosteum and pierces muscle and vessels when inaccurately directed. Injury to all these structures leads to local inflammation.

6. **Patients may attribute recurrence of back pain** and the sciatic radiation of pain to the sensitive needle site. Spinal anesthesia should be avoided whenever back problems exist unless other important reasons dictate its use. For all candidates for spinal anesthesia, careful history taking and neurologic examination before anesthesia are essential, along with support in a contoured back-relaxing position during and after surgery.

C. **Urine retention.** Problems of voiding are associated with spinal anesthesia. The causes are multiple and include the following:

1. **Bladder control** is the last function to return after anesthesia.

2. **Rapid fluid infusions** to minimize blood pressure changes may lead to early bladder filling.

3. Because of muscle spasm or pain, **operations on the perineum,** urogenital structures, and lower abdominal wall affect voiding ability.

4. **Catheterization** can produce chronic intermittent urinary tract infection. It is recommended that patients who are to have spinal anesthesia void just before coming to the operating room and receive slow infusions postoperatively until spontaneous voiding occurs. BP is supported by vasoconstrictors. If catheterization is necessary for surgery, there are no restrictions to infusion therapy other than the cardiac status of the patient.

D. **Permanent neurologic complications** associated with spinal anesthesia are extremely rare. Some factors of importance in maintaining a very low incidence of serious injuries are as follows:

1. **Heat sterilization** of all glass ampules used in spinal anesthesia eliminates the need for cold sterilization with alcohol and phenol, which formerly entered ampules through minute cracks in the glass and were injected into the subarachnoid space, causing injury.
2. **Disposable syringes and needles** eliminate the occasional institutional labor problem in cleansing when detergents, old blood, pyrogens, and bacteria contaminate reusable equipment.
3. **Spinal anesthesia** should be avoided in patients with **systemic diseases that have neurologic sequelae.** A partial list includes pernicious anemia, syphilis, porphyria, and acute or chronic viral disease. Spinal anesthesia is avoided in generalized sepsis or in hypotensive states.
4. **Aseptic technique** is used in performing lumbar puncture.
5. **Anesthesiologists must require** a neurologic history and physical examination of each patient before using spinal anesthesia.
6. The **CSF must be inspected** for color and free flow before injection.

E. **Chronic adhesive arachnoiditis**

1. **Some nerve injury** can occur following spinal anesthesia as a result of injection of foreign material. The most feared injury pattern is chronic adhesive arachnoiditis. This is a **proliferative arachnoid reaction** leading to fibrosis, distortion, and obliteration of the subarachnoid space. Numerous fibrous, cyst-like compartments are formed. This reaction is associated with an arteritis in which the media of the vessel is replaced with collagen and there is hypertrophy of the intima. This produces ischemia, resulting in cord softening and fibrosis.
2. **The primary injury** is still debated; it may appear soon after surgery or months later, with an insidious progression, and may be a patchy process or confluent.
3. The region of **the lumbar-sacral cord enlargement** is most frequently involved. Problems here affect bowel and bladder function with decreased perianal sensation and varied motor problems of the lower extremities. This has been termed the **cauda equina syndrome.**
4. **The electromyogram** has been useful in establishing whether a neurologic problem after spinal anesthesia is an unrelated, long-standing problem or is related to the anesthesia by time and pattern. Essentially, fibrillation potentials appear in denervated muscle after 2–3 weeks. The potentials do not appear in primary muscle problems or in upper motor neuron difficulties. Thus, if associated with spinal anesthesia, they cannot be present earlier than 2 weeks after the injury, and they will be confined to muscles innervated by the lumbar-sacral cord. Using the electromyogram, the most common nerve injuries seen after spinal anesthesia (to the peroneal and lateral femoral cutaneous nerves) were proved to be due to pressure injury and not to the spinal anesthesia.

Bibliography

Berkowitz, S., and Gold, M. I. Spinal anesthesia for surgery in patients with previous lumbar laminectomy. *Anesth. Analg.* (Cleve.) 59:881, 1980.

Benzon, H. T., Linde, H. W., Molloy, R. E., et al. Postdural puncture headache in patients with chronic pain. *Anesth. Analg.* (Cleve.) 59:772, 1980.

Chambers, W. A., Littlewood, D. G., Logan, M. R., et al. Effect of added epinephrine on spinal anesthesia with lidocaine. *Anesth. Analg.* (Cleve.) 60:417, 1981.

Eerola, M., Kaukinen, L., and Kaukinen, S. Fatal brain lesion following spinal anesthesia. Report of a case. *Acta Anaesthesiol. Scand.* 25:115, 1981.

Hatfalvi, B. I. The dynamics of post-spinal headache. *Headache* 17:64, 1977.

Moore, D. C. Spinal anesthesia. Bupivacaine compared with tetracaine. *Anesth. Analg.* (Cleve.) 59:743, 1980.

16 Lumbar Epidural and Caudal Anesthesia

I. Lumbar epidural (peridural, extradural) anesthesia

A. Lumbar epidural anesthesia is accomplished by injecting the local anesthetic solution into the epidural space of the lumbar area of the vertebral canal. Entrance to the epidural space is usually made at or below the level of the second lumbar vertebra.

1. Indications

a. Major abdominal operations.

b. Vaginal obstetric deliveries. In addition, intermittent (continuous) dose epidural anesthesia is employed to relieve the pain of all stages of labor.

c. Cesarean section.

d. Hysterectomy.

e. Anorectal and perirectal surgery.

f. Urologic procedures.

g. Lower extremity surgery.

h. Diagnosis and therapy of chronic pain related to circulatory or neoplastic diseases.

2. Contraindications

a. Severe hemorrhage or shock.

b. Local infection at the site of proposed puncture.

c. Septicemia.

d. Preexisting neurologic diseases.

e. Disturbances in blood morphology and/or anticoagulant therapy. If peridural anesthesia is administered during anticoagulant therapy, and blood vessels are pierced, consequent bleeding into the peridural space may result in neurologic complications.

f. Extremes of age.

g. Chronic backache or preoperative headache.

h. Hypotension or marked hypertension.

i. Arthritis or spinal deformity.

j. A patient who is psychotic or uncooperative.

B. Epidural anesthesia compared with spinal anesthesia

1. Advantages of spinal anesthesia

a. Less local anesthetic drug is needed.

b. Less time is needed to achieve an adequate block.

c. The level of anesthesia is more predictable.

d. Less technical skill is required.

2. **Advantages of epidural anesthesia**

a. Epidural anesthesia allows segmental anesthesia.

b. Postoperative headache does not occur.

c. Hypotension is less likely.

d. There are fewer adverse psychological objections on the part of the patient.

e. Because it achieves lessened motor effect, it may be used for both extrathoracic and extraperitoneal surgery in patients with severe respiratory impairment.

f. Epidural anesthesia can be maintained for 1–2 days into the postoperative period as a useful method for relief of pain.

3. **Disadvantages of epidural anesthesia as compared with spinal anesthesia**

a. Epidural anesthesia is technically more difficult to perform than subarachnoid injection.

b. Since the epidural space is very vascular and larger quantities of drugs are used, **systemic reactions** to absorbed drug can occur.

c. It is possible to pentrate the dura inadvertently and not realize it. If a large amount of anesthetic solution is injected into the subarachnoid space, a **high or total spinal anesthesia** may be produced; this will lead to respiratory arrest, loss of consciousness, and complete sympathetic block. Immediate respiratory and circulatory support is indicated.

d. Five to 10 times as much drug is needed to achieve a given level of anesthesia.

C. **Advantages of epidural anesthesia as compared to general anesthesia**

1. Respiration is less affected; it is a very useful technique in patients with asthma, bronchitis, or emphysema.

2. Analgesia, adequate motor relaxation, and contracted bowels are achieved.

3. Epidural anesthesia can be administered to patients who are not suitable candidates for muscle relaxants (e.g., those with myasthenia gravis).

D. **Anatomy of the epidural space**

1. **The spinal cord** is located within the spinal (vertebral) canal and is enveloped by the meninges, the **dura** being outermost. The spinal cord seldom extends below the L_1, but on occasion it extends to the upper level of the **second lumbar (L_2) vertebra.**

2. **The dura** is attached to the margins of the foramen magnum; this prevents the passage of anesthetic drugs from the peridural space into the cranial cavity. **The dura sac ends** at the lower border of the **second sacral (S_2) vertebra,** a point corresponding to approximately 1 cm below and medial to the level of the posterior superior iliac spines.

3. **The epidural space is located** between the spinal dura centrally, and the ligamentum flavum and the periosteum lining the spinal canal peripherally. **It extends** from the base of the skull (foramen magnum), where the periosteum of the skull and the dura fuse, to the coccyx (sacrococcygeal membrane). **Its diameter** is 0.5 cm, and it is widest in the midline posteriorly in the lumbar region.

4. On the average, **the distance** between the skin and the peridural space is 4–5 cm.

5. The epidural space contains loose areolar connective tissue and fat, arterial and venous networks, lymphatics, and the spinal nerve roots.

a. The veins, without valves and constituting the rich vertebral venous plexuses, connect the pelvic veins and the intracranial veins. Thus local anesthetic solutions or air injected into these venous plexuses may **ascend straight to the brain.**

b. The veins become distended when the patient strains or coughs (during bouts of increased intrathoracic pressure).

6. The size of the epidural space varies with alterations in the volume of the dural sac.

a. The main causes are changes in the CSF volume and distention of the peridural veins.

b. This variation in size of the epidural space may influence **the level** of the epidural anesthesia produced by a given amount of the local anesthetic solution.

c. The intervertebral foramina are more permeable in the young than in the old; therefore a given volume of solution tends to cause a higher block in the geriatric patient than in a young patient.

E. Drugs. See Table 16-1.

1. Lidocaine or mepivacaine

a. The dose of lidocaine (Xylocaine) or mepivacaine (Carbocaine) is 15–30 ml of a 1–2% solution with or without epinephrine 1:200,000.

b. The **onset** of anesthesia is established within 10–20 min, and the anesthesia **lasts** 1½ hr.

2. Bupivacaine

a. The dose of bupivacaine (Marcaine) is 15–30 ml of a 0.25–0.75% solution with or without epinephrine 1:200,000.

b. The **onset** of anesthesia is established within 10–20 min, and anesthesia **lasts** 3½–5 hr. The duration of anesthesia in intraabdominal surgery is 3½–5 hr with a 0.75% solution of bupivacaine.

3. Epinephrine

a. The addition of epinephrine 1:200,000 is recommended both to prolong the duration of anesthesia and to slow the absorption of the drug.

Table 16-1. Doses of Local Anesthetics for **Epidural (Peridural) Anesthesia** (Lumbar or Caudal Area), Single-Dose Technique

Drug	Concentration	Duration	Maximal Dose
Procaine (Novocain)	1–2%	1 hr	1000 mg
Lidocaine (Xylocaine)	1–2%	1½ hr	500 mg
Mepivacaine (Carbocaine)	1–2%	1½ hr	500 mg
Tetracaine (Pontocaine)	0.1–0.25%	2–3 hr	75 mg
Bupivacaine (Marcaine)	0.25–0.75%	3½–5 hr	225 mg
Etidocaine (Duranest)	0.5–1%	4–6 hr	300 mg

b. **A 1:200,000 concentration** of epinephrine solution in the epidural space should not be exceeded. A stronger solution, such as 1:100,000 will not prolong the duration of anesthesia greatly but may predispose the patient to the systemic actions of epinephrine, e.g., hypertension or arrhythmias.

c. **Phenylephrine should not be used** in the epidural space because it may cause severe hypertension.

4. **Site of effects**

a. The epidural local anesthetic solutions enter the CSF to some extent.

b. The local solutions anesthetize **the spinal nerve roots** as they traverse the peridural space and **the sympathetic fibers** traveling with the anterior roots.

F. Methods of identification of the epidural space

1. **The loss-of-resistance method** is most often used. The principle of this method is the fact that, because the advancing point of the needle is within the ligamentum flavum, there is a marked resistance to injection. When the point of the needle enters the epidural space, the marked resistance disappears completely.

a. **The simplest technique** is to exert pressure manually on the plunger of a glass syringe containing saline or air as the needle advances millimeter by millimeter through the ligamentum flavum.

b. **A spring-loaded syringe** or **small, air-filled balloon** attached to the advancing needle also may be used to demonstrate this loss of resistance.

2. **In the hanging-drop method,** a drop of saline or local anesthetic is placed into the hub of the needle following penetration of the ligamentum flavum. When the needle is advanced carefully into the peridural space, the drop of saline is sucked into it because of negative pressure in the peridural space.

G. Factors influencing the spread of the anesthetic solution into the epidural space are as follows:

1. **The volume and concentration** of the local anesthetic solution and **the level of the tap** determine the extent of segmental anesthesia. Four segments on both sides of the point of injection are affected by the epidural injection of 10–15 ml of anesthetic solution.

2. **Epinephrine** in a 1:200,000 concentration increases the duration of anesthesia.

3. **There is less influence** on the final response attributable to the speed of injection or the patient's position with epidural anesthesia than with spinal anesthesia. The specific gravity of the local anesthetic solution plays no role.

H. Effects of epidural anesthesia

1. **Neurologic effects**

a. The preganglionic autonomic fibers can be anesthetized with low concentrations of anesthetic solutions. Thus a **temporary sympathectomy** can be achieved, which is useful in causalgia of the lower extremities.

b. **Overdoses** of local anesthetic drugs may cause hallucinations and convulsions.

2. **The cardiovascular effects** depend on both the actions of the local anesthetic drug and whether epinephrine is added to the local anesthetic solution.

3. **Respiratory effects** are minimal.

I. Equipment. Many hospitals now have **disposable equipment.** The tray for sterile continuous epidural anesthesia contains:

1 25-gauge, 2-cm needle for the skin wheal.

1 22-gauge, 3.8-cm needle for infiltration.

1 1-ml tuberculin syringe for measuring epinephrine.

1 2.5-ml syringe for administration of the local anesthetic.

1 3-ml glass syringe.

1 10-ml glass syringe.

1 measuring cup for mixing solutions.

1 18-gauge, 3.8-cm withdrawal needle.

1 18-gauge, 9-cm, thin-walled Tuohy needle with a Huber point (directionally curved bevel).

1 marked radiopaque plastic epidural catheter with stainless steel stylet. The catheter has markings at 11, 12, 13, 14, 15, and 16 cm from the end.

1 23-gauge, 1 cm-adapter.

1 5-ml ampule of normal saline for wetting the plunger and barrel of the 5-ml syringe.

1 1-ml ampule of epinephrine solution 1:1000 (1mg/ml).

2 20-ml ampules of 1.5–2% lidocaine. The local anesthetic may be included on the tray or be made available to the anesthesiologist when the epidural anesthesia is administered.

J. Techniques

1. **Lumbar epidural anesthesia** can be performed by a single-dose method or by a **fractional technique** using a catheter placed into the epidural space.
2. **Continuous epidural anesthesia technique**
   a. Instead of a single-dose injection of solution, **repeated injections** are made through a plastic catheter inserted into the epidural space.
   b. The patient is placed in **the lateral decubitus (side) position** with full flexion of the spine. **A line is drawn between the iliac crests;** this line crosses either the spinous process of the L_4 vertebra or the interspace between the spinous processes of the L_4 and L_5 vertebrae (L_4 interspace).
   c. **The proper lumbar** spinal interspace is selected, and the area is prepared antiseptically.
   d. **In the midline** of the lumbar region, the skin and ligaments are infiltrated with a local anesthetic. **An 18-gauge needle** is placed through the skin wheal to make a hole in the skin, and **the 18-gauge, 9-cm Tuohy needle with a Huber point** (directionally curved bevel) is inserted into the peridural space.
   e. **The epidural puncture** should be made at the L_2 through L_4 interspace. The anterior-posterior diameter of the epidural space is greatest (0.5 cm) in this area.
   f. **The Tuohy needle** should be inserted through the hole in the skin wheal with the opening of the **curved bevel pointing cephalad.**
   g. **Identification** of the peridural space is made by the loss-of-resistance or hanging-drop method (see **F**).
   h. **Careful aspiration tests** are made. If no blood or CSF is aspirated during this entire procedure, the anesthesiologist may continue with the anesthesia.

(1) **If blood is obtained,** insert the stylet into the needle and wait for 2–3 min. If bleeding recurs, the needle is removed and inserted into another interspace.

(2) **If the dura is punctured** and CSF is obtained, the anesthesiologist should use spinal anesthesia, or abandon the regional route and use general anesthesia, or proceed to another interspace if epidural anesthesia is really indicated.

i. **A catheter** is inserted through the needle, and the tip is wedged at the needle point. The markings on the catheter indicate the distance from the tip.

j. **The wire stylet** in the plastic catheter is withdrawn 1–2 mm, and the catheter is advanced. When the catheter has passed the needle point into the epidural space, then, very carefully, the Tuohy needle is removed from the patient's back over the catheter and stylet. This is followed by withdrawal of the wire stylet.

k. The catheter should be introduced **not more than 1–2 cm** into the epidural space, or else it may either coil and interfere with spread of the local anesthetic solution or traumatize vessels or nerves.

l. **Withdrawal of the catheter should be avoided** while the introducing needle is still in place. The tip of the catheter can be sheared off if this precaution is not observed.

m. Following removal of the Tuohy needle and stylet, **a needle adapter** is connected in the free end of the catheter. This is followed by attachment of the catheter to the skin along the midline of the back and around the shoulder to permit repeated injections.

n. At this point, **further tests** are made to rule out the presence of CSF or blood.

o. **A 3-ml test dose** of the local anesthetic solution is injected, and **the patient is observed** for 5 min to rule out subarachnoid block (inability to move the feet). Then an appropriate amount of the solution is injected slowly at a rate of 1 ml/sec, with the total amount not to exceed 20 ml. The patient is then turned onto the back with a slight head-down tilt.

p. **Additional refill injections** are administered to maintain an adequate level of anesthesia. The refill doses depend on the agent used.

q. **A form of tolerance** known as **tachyphylaxis** is observed with all anesthetic drugs when they are injected during continuous epidural anesthesia.

r. **Caution** must be observed with regard to (1) asepsis and (2) avoidance of trauma.

s. On completion of surgery, **the catheter is removed slowly,** or it may be left in the peridural space 1–2 days postoperatively to provide analgesia and/or sympathetic block. The removed catheter should be examined to make sure **it is the same length** as when it was inserted.

K. Precautionary measures

1. Spinal (subarachnoid) or epidural anesthesia must never be administered without facilities at hand for **endotracheal intubation** and **artificial ventilation.** The anesthesiologist must have available a fully equipped anesthesia machine to administer general anesthesia and/or to treat circulatory and respiratory complications.

2. **If the dura is punctured,** the technique is repeated in another interspace, or spinal or general anesthesia is administered.

L. Complications

1. **Accidental puncture of the dura** may be followed by:

   a. **High or total spinal anesthesia** following injection of a full dose with more than 7 ml. **Immediate** respiratory and circulatory support is necessary.

   b. **Postspinal postural headache,** secondary to CSF leakage.

2. There may be **general systemic reactions** (see Chap. 14, sec. **IV**) from rapid absorption of the local anesthetic and epinephrine. The patient may complain of a bitter taste in the mouth, severe headache, ringing in the ears, and the presence of irritability and twitching. **Convulsions** may occur. Hypotension and loss of consciousness may occur, requiring specific treatment.

   a. An **overdose of epinephrine** may produce general systemic effects (tachycardia, pallor, palpitations, hypertension, and tremors) and local ischemic effects on the spinal cord.

   b. **Toxic reactions due to epinephrine** are particularly dangerous in patients with a history of arteriosclerotic heart disease.

3. The anesthesiologist **may fail to obtain anesthesia** because of misplacement of the needle or catheter. However, occasionally, even with correct epidural insertion, unilateral or unequal anesthesia may result. Such an inadequate block should be covered by general anesthesia.

4. Occasionally the catheter may leave the epidural space through an intervertebral foramen. Pulling back the catheter and reinjecting more drug may then produce adequate anesthesia.

5. **Additional problems**

   a. Epidural anesthesia causes constricted bowels, yet surgical manipulation and traction of the gastrointestinal tract may cause visceral pain, nausea, vomiting, or hypotension.

   b. Deep sedation permits surgery to continue but may result in ventilatory obstruction or in aspiration of vomitus.

II. Caudal anesthesia

A. Caudal anesthesia is accomplished by introducing the local anesthetic solution through the sacral hiatus into the epidural space of the sacral (caudal) canal (Fig. 16-1).

1. **Indications**

   a. **Obstetric patients,** for vaginal deliveries.

   b. **Surgery** related to the sacral area (anorectal and vaginal procedures).

2. **Contraindications.** See section **I.A.2.**

B. Anatomy

1. **The sacrum** is a triangular bone formed by the fusion of five sacral vertebrae. It articulates above with the fifth lumbar vertebra and below with the coccyx and is interposed between the two iliac bones of the pelvis.

2. **The sacral canal** is situated within the sacrum and is limited posteriorly by the periosteum, covering the four fused sacral spinous processes with the four sacral foramina located laterally. Through these posterior sacral foramina pass the posterior primary divisions of the sacral nerves.

3. **The sacral hiatus.** The spinous process of S_5 is not fused, thus creating the two sacral cornua with an opening between them known as the sacral hiatus, which is covered by the sacrococcygeal ligament.

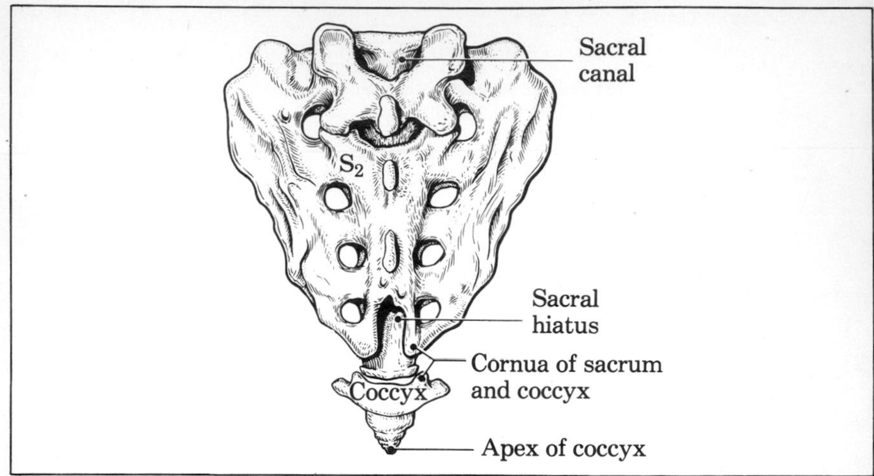

Fig. 16-1. The posterior view of the sacrum and coccyx.

4. **The epidural space** within the sacral canal contains the nerves from the **cauda equina,** which leave the sacral canal through the anterior and posterior sacral foramina. The **dura sac ends** at the lower border of the S_2 foramina (Fig. 16-2).

5. In caudal epidural anesthesia, the nerves involved are the **lumbosacral plexus** (T_{12}, $L_{1\text{-}5}$, $S_{1\text{-}3}$) and the coccygeal plexus (formed by the S_4 and S_5 nerves and the coccygeal nerve).

6. **The contents** within the epidural space are similar to what has been described for the higher levels (see sec. **I.D.5**).

C. Drugs. See Section **I.E.**

D. Techniques

1. The patient is placed in the **prone position** on the table, which is slightly flexed upward. The legs are separated, with the heels rotated outward. **In the pregnant patient,** for vaginal delivery, the lateral decubitus position with the uppermost thigh acutely flexed is more comfortable.

2. **Bony landmarks**

   a. **The posterior superior iliac spines,** with S_2 foramina 1 cm below and medial to the spines.

   b. **The tip of the coccyx.**

   c. **The sacral hiatus** between the sacral cornua, about 4 cm above the tip of the coccyx. The sacral hiatus can be located by the distinct V depression it occupies.

3. **A gauze sponge** is placed in the anal cleft to prevent burns of the anus and genitalia from the antiseptic solution (alcohol tincture burns; povidone-iodine [Betadine] does not burn), and the sacral region is prepared antiseptically. With a 25-gauge needle, the skin and underlying ligaments are injected with a local anesthetic.

4. **A 22-gauge, 3.8-cm needle** is inserted perpendicular to the skin, injecting as the needle advances through the sacrococcygeal ligament at the midline at an angle of 90 degrees. When the needle reaches the floor of the canal, the

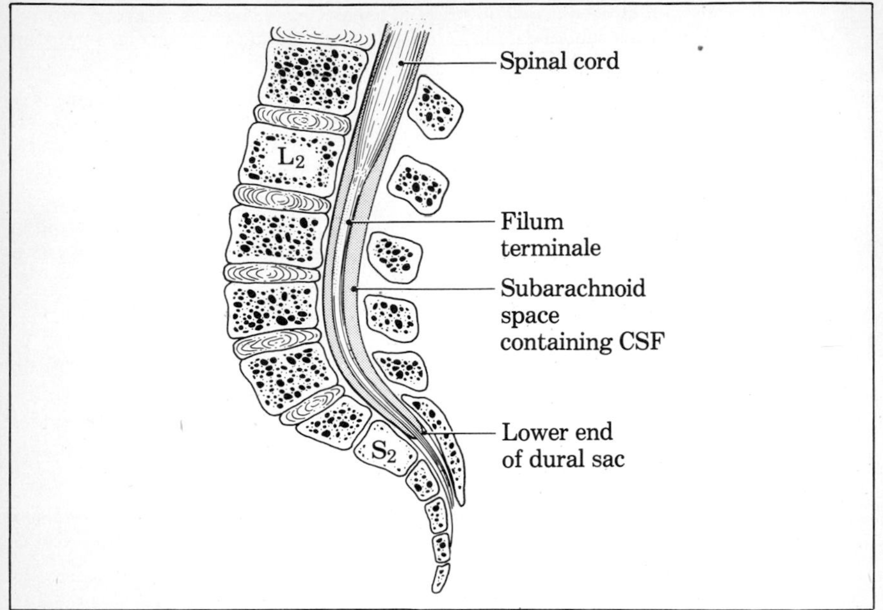

Fig. 16-2. The spinal cord ends at the L_2 vertebra. The subarachnoid space and the contained CSF end at the S_2 vertebra.

angle of inclination is decreased, and the needle is rotated so that the bevel faces anteriorly. Then it is advanced 2 cm into the sacral canal.

5. **The point of the needle** should not reach the S_2 level where the dural sac ends. Aspiration for blood or CSF is attempted in four quadrants, because occasionally (in less than 1% of cases) the dural sac ends below the S_2 level.
   a. **If blood is aspirated,** the needle is repositioned. If, after this, blood is still aspirated, a spinal block or lumbar epidural is instituted, or general anesthesia is administered.
   b. **If CSF is aspirated,** the anesthesiologist should use spinal anesthesia or abandon the regional technique and administer general anesthesia.
6. If no blood or CSF is aspirated, **5–10 ml of air is injected** rapidly, testing whether the needle is located subcutaneously. **In the pregnant patient,** a rectal examination is performed to rule out accidental penetration of the fetal head, the rectum, or the retrorectal space.
7. **Caudal anesthesia with the single-dose technique**
   a. **A test dose** of 3–5 ml of the anesthetic solution is administered. If there is no evidence of spinal anesthesia within 5 min, the full dose of 15–20 ml of 2% lidocaine with epinephrine 1:200,000 is injected.
   b. A **2% solution of lidocaine** provides good muscular relaxation. With **epinephrine** 1:200,000, anesthesia may last up to 2 hr. No epinephrine is needed for short procedures up to 1 hr.
   c. **Headache** or discomfort in the thighs may follow the injection.
8. **Continuous caudal anesthesia**
   a. **The plastic catheter method** is similar to that described for lumbar epidural anesthesia (see sec. **I.J.2.**). A 19-gauge, 5-cm or 6.3-cm continu-

ous caudal needle with a stylet is used. The catheter is placed about 3–5 cm into the caudal canal. Following withdrawal of the needle, aspiration for CSF or blood is attempted with a syringe.

b. **A test dose** of 3–5 ml of the anesthetic solution is injected. If there is no evidence of spinal anesthesia within 5 min, the catheter is attached to the skin, the patient is positioned, and the first dose of 15–20 ml of 2% lidocaine with epinephrine 1:200,000 is injected.

c. **Reinforcing doses** should be given on a timed basis; for example, lidocaine should be administered hourly. Both the volume and concentration of the reinforcing dose should be decreased to approximately two-thirds of the original effective dose.

E. Disadvantages

1. It is difficult to obtain high levels of anesthesia.
2. **Systemic reactions** are possible.
3. Due to anatomic anomalies or incorrect methods, there is a **5–10%** rate of failure.
4. Infection is possible.

F. Precautionary measures. The anesthesia machine and equipment for endotracheal intubation and cardiopulmonary support should be at hand from the start of any caudal anesthesia.

G. Complications are similar to those of lumbar epidural anesthesia (see sec. **I.L**). They include:

1. **Accidental puncture** of the dura.
2. **General systemic reactions** to local anesthetics and epinephrine.
3. Rarely, **infection** develops at the site of the caudal anesthesia injection.

Bibliography

Apostolou, G. A., Zarmakoupis, P. K., and Mastrokostopoulos, G. T. Spread of epidural anesthesia and the lateral position. *Anesth. Analg.* (Cleve.) 60:584, 1981.

Behar, M., Olshwang, D., Magora, F., et al. Epidural morphine in treatment of pain. *Lancet* 1:527, 1979.

Boas, R. A. Sympathetic blocks in clinical practice. *Int. Anesthesiol. Clin.* 16:159, 1978.

Carrie, L. E. S., and Mohan, J. Horner's syndrome following obstetric extradural block. *Br. J. Anaesth.* 48:611, 1976.

Cooper, G. M., Holdcroft, A., Hall, G. M., et al. Epidural analgesia and the metabolic response to surgery. *Can. Anaesth. Soc. J.* 26:381, 1979.

Evans, J. M., Gauci, C. A., and Watkins, G. Horner's syndrome as complication of lumbar extradural block. *Anaesthesia* 30:774, 1975.

Grundy, E. M., Samanurthy, S., Patel, K. P., et al. Extradural analgesia revisited. A statistical study. *Br. J. Anaesth.* 50:805, 1978.

Hodgkinson, R., and Husain, F. J. Obesity, gravity, and spread of epidural anesthesia. *Anesth. Analg.* (Cleve.) 60:421, 1981.

Kane, R. E. Neurologic deficits following epidural or spinal anesthesia. Anesth. Analg. (Cleve.) 60:150, 1981.

Maitra, A. M., et al. Continuous epidural analgesia for cesarean section in a patient with morbid obesity. *Anesth. Analg.* (Cleve.) 58:348, 1979.

Mohan, J., and Potter, J. M. Pupillary constriction and ptosis following caudal epidural analgesia. *Anaesthesia* 30:769, 1975.

Moore, D. C., Bush, W. H., and Burnoff, L. L. Celiac plexus block. A roentgenographic, anatomic study of techniques and spread of solution in patients and corpses. Anesth. Analg. (Cleve.) 60:369, 1981.

Sharrock, N. E. Epidural anesthetic dose responses in patients aged 20–80 years old. *Anesthesiology* 49:425, 1979.

Sharrock, N. E. The influence of height in young and old patients. *Anesthesiology* 51:5225, 1979.

Stanton-Hicks, M. Cardiovascular effects of extradural anaesthesia. *Br. J. Anaesth.* 47:253, 1975.

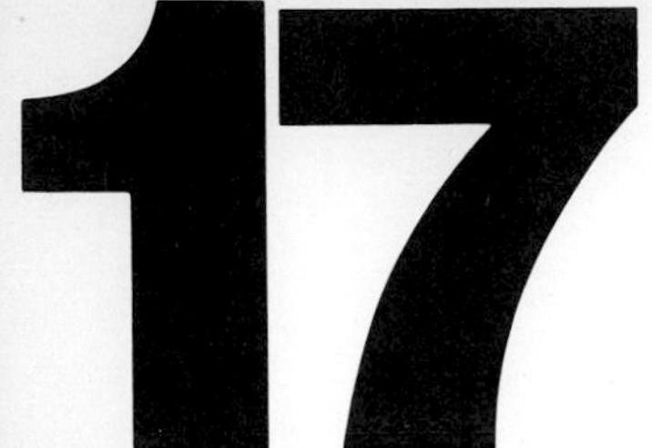

Regional Nerve Block Anesthesia

I. General considerations

A. Preanesthesia medication. See Chapter 3.

B. Monitoring. See Chapter 6.

C. Local anesthetics and reactions to local anesthetic drugs. See Chapter 14.

D. The most valuable drug we have today for regional block procedures, particularly in teaching institutions, is **bupivacaine (Marcaine)** (Table 17-1). It is a safe drug, and the doses given should result in no systemic toxic reactions unless injected intravascularly.

E. Basic rules

1. Start an IV infusion with a plastic catheter.
2. Monitor the patient's BP and the electrical activity of the heart.
3. Make sure that a laryngoscope, endotracheal tube, and resuscitation equipment are available.
4. Use sterile technique.
5. Aspirate before injection of the local anesthetic solution to ensure that neither a blood vessel nor the subarachnoid space has been entered.
6. **Diazepam,** as a preanesthetic or a postreaction drug, can decrease the incidence and severity of systemic toxic reactions occurring secondary to direct vascular injection or total overdose of the local anesthetic solution. If diazepam is to prevent or ameliorate systemic toxic reactions, it must be given IV about the same time as the block is being performed. Furthermore, it must be given in doses greater than 10 mg.

II. Paravertebral nerve blocks

A. Cervical plexus block

1. **Indications.** Surgery on the neck and occipital part of the scalp.
2. **Anatomy.** The cervical plexus is formed by the anterior rami of the first four cervical nerves. It lies opposite the upper four cervical vertebrae and in front of the levator scapulae muscle and the middle scalene muscle.
   a. The cervical plexus is divided into superficial and deep plexuses. **The superficial cervical plexus,** which innervates the skin and the superficial structures, emerges along the posterior margin of the midportion of the sternomastoid muscle. **The deep plexus** supplies the muscles and other deep structures of the neck.
   b. **The first cervical nerve** has no sensory component.
   c. **The phrenic nerve** arises from the 4th cervical nerve and receives minute branches from the 3rd and 5th cervical nerves.

Table 17-1. Adult Doses of Bupivacaine (Marcaine)

Block	Concentration[a]	Volume (ml)	Total (mg)	Epinephrine (mg)[b]
Cervical plexus				
Unilateral	0.25	40	100	0.2
	0.5	40	200	0.2
Bilateral	0.25	80	200	0.25
Brachial plexus				
Axillary	0.25	50	125	0.25
	0.5	50	250	0.25
Interscalene	0.25	50	125	0.25
	0.5	50	250	0.25
Supraclavicular	0.25	50	125	0.25
	0.5	50	250	0.25
Stellate ganglion	0.25	10	25	0.05
	0.5	10	50	0.05

[a]If a rapid onset is needed and complete motor block must be ensured, whenever possible, the stronger concentration should be employed.
[b]Optimal final concentration of epinephrine is 1:200,000 (0.25 mg in 50 ml). Seldom should 0.25 mg of epinephrine be exceeded. Therefore, when more than 50 ml of the local anesthetic solution is employed, the concentration of epinephrine is less than that considered optimal.

3. **Technique**
   a. **The patient lies supine,** with the face turned to the side opposite that being anesthetized and with arms at the sides.
   b. **A straight line** is drawn between **the mastoid process** and **the anterior tubercle of the transverse process of the C_6 vertebra** (Chassaignac's tubercle), which is the most prominent of the cervical transverse processes and which is located at the same levels as the thyroid cartilage. This line gives the plane in which the cervical transverse processes are located.
   c. **The transverse process of the C_2 vertebra** is located 1.5 cm below the tip of the mastoid process and 0.5 cm posterior to the line drawn.
   d. The transverse processes of **C_3 and C_4** lie along the line, caudad to C_2 and 1.5 cm from each other.
   e. **Under the palpating fingers,** skin wheals are raised, and 23-gauge, 3.8-cm needles are inserted perpendicular to the skin and slightly caudad and pushed downward until they rest on the transverse process of the second, third, and fourth cervical vertebrae. The transverse processes lie 1.5–3 cm under the skin.
   f. **Through each needle,** after careful aspiration, 7 ml of the anesthetic solution is injected. As the needle is withdrawn, an additional 3 ml is injected.
   g. **Paresthesias** are not sought.
   h. **The superficial cervical plexus** is anesthetized with 10 ml of the anesthetic solution injected at the posterior border of the sternomastoid muscle.
4. **Complications.** These include intravascular, epidural, or subarachnoid injection, cervical sympathetic block with Horner's syndrome (blepharoptosis,

enophthalmos, and miosis), phrenic nerve paralysis, recurrent laryngeal nerve paralysis, and hematoma.

B. Other paravertebral nerve blocks include intercostal nerve block and paravertebral somatic nerve block.

III. Nerve blocks of the upper extremity

A. Anatomy

1. The upper extremity is innervated by **the brachial plexus,** which is formed by the anterior rami of spinal nerves $C_{5\text{-}8}$ and T_1. These nerves converge toward the upper surface of the first rib, where they emerge together (with the subclavian artery) between the anterior and middle scalene muscles and pass under the midportion of the clavicle to the apex of the axilla.
2. **In the axilla,** the brachial plexus forms three cords, which provide the nerve supply to the upper limb: **the radial, median, ulnar, musculocutaneous, and axillary nerves.**
3. The sensory nerves of the **hand** are the radial, median, and ulnar nerves.
4. The sensory nerves of the **forearm** are the radial, median, and musculocutaneous nerves.

B. Nerve blocks of the arm

1. Supraclavicular block of the brachial plexus

a. **Indications.** Surgery or manipulations on the shoulder joint, arm, forearm, and hand.

b. **Anatomy.** In the neck, the brachial plexus with the subclavian artery lies between the anterior and middle scalene muscles.

c. **Technique**

(1) The patient lies supine, with the face turned to the side opposite that being anesthetized and arms at the sides.

(2) **The clavicular head** of the sternomastoid muscle is identified, and the anterior scalene muscle is palpated. The brachial plexus makes its exit at the lateral border of the **anterior scalene muscle.** This point lies at the **middle of the clavicle** and 1–2 cm from the clavicular head of the sternomastoid muscle.

(3) **The subclavian artery** is located by palpation; it emerges with the brachial plexus lateral to the anterior scalene muscles (midpoint of the clavicle).

(4) Through a raised intradermal wheal, a 23-gauge, 3.8-cm needle, connected by tubing to a syringe containing local anesthetic solution, is inserted **1 cm above the midpoint of the clavicle** (just lateral to the subclavian artery) and is advanced slowly backward, inward, and downward toward **the first rib.** If the patient coughs, the needle is removed, since the cough is a sign that the pleura may have been stimulated or penetrated.

(5) The index finger of the anesthesiologist's opposite hand feels for and protects the subclavian artery. **If paresthesias** to the forearm and fingers are elicited 40–50 ml of 1% lidocaine with epinephrine 1:200,000 is administered after aspiration. Injection of the anesthetic solution without obtaining paresthesias increases the probability of failure of the block.

(6) **If the first rib is contacted** and paresthesias are obtained, the needle is traversing the length, rather than the breadth, of the first rib, and 40–50 ml of the anesthetic solution is injected after aspiration.

(7) **Tourniquet pain**

(a) **The intercostobrachial nerve (T_2)** innervates the medial and inner surfaces of the arm and is not a part of the brachial plexus. **When a pneumatic tourniquet** is used, the intercostobrachial (T_2) and the medial brachial cutaneous (T_1 and T_2) nerves should be anesthetized. For prevention of tourniquet pain, anesthesia is carried out by half-ring subcutaneous infiltration with 10 ml of the local anesthetic solution in the axilla.

(b) Many times **nerve fibers of the autonomic nervous system** that accompany the blood vessels to the arm are not blocked by the brachial plexus block. In addition, not every nerve fiber in the brachial plexus, especially the large ones, is anesthetized. Following 45 min inflation of the tourniquet, ischemia may cause these unanesthetized nerves to transmit pain stimuli. This tourniquet pain may be relieved by (1) IV doses of analgesics, (2) releasing and reapplying the tourniquet, or (3) a half-ring of local infiltration distal to the axilla when the block is performed.

d. **Complications**

(1) **Pneumothorax** occurs in 1 to 3% of the cases. Symptoms are chest pain, dyspnea, and coughing. **Diagnosis** is made by physical examination and chest x-ray. **Therapy** is not needed if the pneumothorax is less than 20%; when therapy is indicated, aspiration of air from the pleural cavity is done by intercostal, underwater closed-chest drainage. Examination by x-ray should be carried out until the lung is completely expanded.

(2) **Other possible complications** include intravascular injection, subarachnoid injection, phrenic nerve paralysis, recurrent laryngeal nerve block, Horner's syndrome (stellate ganglion block), hematoma, and neuropathy.

2. **Interscalene block of the brachial plexus**

a. **Indications.** Surgery or manipulations on the shoulder joint, arm, forearm, and hand.

b. **Anatomy.** The nerves of the brachial and cervical plexuses emerge from their grooved transverse processes and enter **the interscalene space** formed by the fascia covering the anterior and middle scalene muscles. The greater part of this space is above the subclavian artery and the cupula of the pleura.

(1) The interscalene block has the advantage that the anesthetic solution is administered close to the origin of the nerves of the brachial plexus.

(2) The musculocutaneous and axillary nerves, which come off high in the arm, are anesthetized.

c. **Technique**

(1) The patient lies supine, with the face turned to the side opposite that being anesthetized and arms at the sides. To allow identification of **the clavicular head** of the sternomastoid muscle, the patient raises the head. The anesthesiologist places a finger behind the muscle and locates the **anterior scalene muscle;** when the finger is moved laterally on this muscle, it falls into **the interscalene groove,** between the anterior and middle scalene muscles.

(2) **The interscalene groove** is palpated, and the level of **the C_6 vertebra** is identified by extension of a line from the **cricoid cartilage** to the interscalene groove. The line passes over the anterior tubercle of the C_6 transverse process (Chassaignac's tubercle).

(3) **As the index and middle fingers** impinge on this groove while astride the line drawn from the cricoid cartilage, a 23-gauge, 3.8-cm needle, connected by a small-bore disposable IV tubing to a syringe containing local anesthetic solution, is inserted perpendicular to the skin through a skin wheal into the groove (caudad, dorsad, and mesiad).

(4) **Another useful landmark** for the introduction of the needle is the **external jugular vein,** which crosses the groove at this point.

(5) The needle is advanced until **paresthesias** are obtained and/or contact is made with the C_6 transverse process. If the needle makes contact with the C_6 transverse process without producing paresthesias, it is moved laterally until paresthesias are obtained.

(6) **With paresthesias,** and following a careful aspiration, 30–40 ml of 1% lidocaine, 1–2% procaine, 1% mepivacaine, or 0.5% bupivacaine is administered. All local anesthetic solutions should contain 1:200,000 epinephrine.

(7) **The volume** of anesthetic solution injected is important, since, with large volumes, both cervical and brachial plexuses are anesthetized.

(8) **If a pneumatic tourniquet is used,** the intercostobrachial (T_2) nerve should be anesthetized by half-ring subcutaneous local infiltration with 10 ml, in the axilla where axillary artery pulsations are felt.

d. Complications

(1) Neuropathies.

(2) The needle may enter the vertebral artery or the subarachnoid space.

3. Axillary block of the brachial plexus

a. Indications are surgery or manipulations of the arm, forearm, and hand. **Contraindications** are local infection or inflammation of the axillary nodes.

b. Anatomy

(1) **In the axilla,** the brachial plexus, axillary artery, and axillary vein are enclosed in a neurovascular compartment. Solution injected into the axillary sheath is limited and can spread only up or down, parallel to the neurovascular bundle.

(2) At the third part of the axillary artery, the cords of the brachial plexus form the three major nerves of the upper limb: **The radial nerve** lies behind the axillary artery, **the median nerve** is located in front and above it, and **the ulnar nerve** lies in front and below it.

(3) **The musculocutaneous nerve,** which innervates the lateral side of the forearm, arises from the brachial plexus at the lower border of the pectoralis minor muscle. **The intercostobrachial nerve,** which innervates the skin of the upper half of the medial and posterior side of the arm, arises from the second intercostal nerve (T_2). During axillary block, these two nerves may not be blocked.

c. Technique

(1) The patient lies supine, with the arm abducted to 90 degrees, the forearm flexed, and the hand placed under the head. **A tourniquet** (Penrose drain) is applied tightly on the arm distal to the point of injection; this will prevent spread of the anesthetic solution peripherally. It is removed 5–10 min following completion of the block.

(2) **The axillary artery** is palpated as high as possible and is fixed against the humerus by the anesthesiologist's index finger. A skin wheal is raised, and a 23-gauge, 2.5-cm needle, connected by tubing to a sy-

ringe containing local anesthetic solution, is inserted until pulsations of the axillary artery are transmitted to the needle. This is most often preceded by a palpable click as the needle penetrates the deep fascia forming the axillary sheath.

(3) **Correct placement of the needle** within the neurovascular bundle is verified by (1) **paresthesias** radiating down the arm to the fingers, or (2) **aspiration of blood** into the syringe.

(4) **If paresthesias** are obtained, 30–40 ml of 1% lidocaine with epinephrine 1:200,000 is administered following aspiration.

(5) **If blood** is aspirated, the needle is withdrawn until the aspiration of blood stops, and then the anesthetic solution is administered. The small size of the needle decreases the possibility of hematoma.

(6) **The musculocutaneous nerve** need not be blocked if the injection for the axillary block is high in the axilla.

(7) **The intercostobrachial nerve (T_2)** is anesthetized by subcutaneous injection of 3 ml of anesthetic solution over the axillary artery.

(8) **If a pneumatic tourniquet** is applied or surgery on the arm at or above the elbow is to be carried out, a subcutaneous ring of local anesthesia, using 10 ml around the inner half of the arm, is necessary to anesthetize the medial brachial cutaneous nerve and the intercostobrachial nerve.

d. **Complications** include intravascular injection, broken needles, injury to the nerves, and hematoma. There is no risk of pneumothorax.

IV. Nerve blocks of the arm at the elbow and wrist

A. Radial nerve block

1. **Indications.** Surgery or manipulations of the arm and hand that are limited to the innervation of the radial nerve.

2. **Anatomy.** The radial nerve is a branch of the brachial plexus and is derived from $C_{5\text{-}8}$ and T_1 nerves. It runs on the medial side of the humerus with the brachial artery in front. At the lateral condyle of the humerus, the radial nerve is divided into branches that innervate parts of the forearm, upper arm, and hand.

3. **Technique**

a. **Radial nerve block at the elbow.** The radial nerve is anesthetized as it descends in the lateral aspect of the humerus. The lateral condyle of the humerus is palpated, and 7.5 cm above it a skin wheal is raised on the lateral aspect of the arm. A 22-gauge, 5-cm needle is inserted until contact is made with the bone. In the presence of paresthesias, the needle is withdrawn 1 cm and, following aspiration, 1% lidocaine 3 ml with epinephrine 1:200,000 is administered. This procedure is repeated 3 to 4 times, to cover an area 2 cm above and below the first injection site. A total of 20 ml of the anesthetic solution is injected.

b. **Radial nerve block at the wrist.** The radial nerve is anesthetized by subcutaneous infiltration at the dorsolateral aspect of the wrist. A 22-gauge, 5-cm needle is introduced through a skin wheal, and in the presence of paresthesias and following aspiration, 10 ml of 1% lidocaine is injected in ring fashion, beginning lateral to the radial artery and extending to the radial half of the back of the wrist, at the level of the styloid process of the ulnar bone. A total of 20 ml of the anesthetic solution is injected.

4. **Complications** include intravascular injections; hematoma of the joint.

B. Median nerve block

1. **Indications.** Surgery or manipulations of the arm and hand that are limited to the innervation of the median nerve.

2. **Anatomy.** The median nerve is a branch of the brachial plexus and is derived from $C_{6\text{-}8}$ and T_1 nerves. At the elbow, it is located very close and medial to the brachial artery. At the wrist, it lies behind and to the radial side of the tendon of the palmaris longus muscle.

3. **Technique**

   a. **Median nerve block at the elbow.** The median nerve is anesthetized at the cubital fossa and at the level of the medial condyle of the humerus, where it is located medial to the brachial artery. Through a skin wheal, a 22-gauge, 5-cm needle is introduced medial to the brachial artery. Following verification of paresthesias and subsequent aspiration, 20 ml of 1% lidocaine with epinephrine 1:200,000 is administered.

   b. **Median nerve block at the wrist.** The median nerve is anesthetized at the superficial and ventral aspect of the wrist and under or lateral to the palmaris longus tendon. Through a skin wheal, a 25-gauge, 2-cm needle is introduced lateral to the palmaris longus tendon at the level of the proximal crease of the wrist. When paresthesias are obtained and aspiration is done, 10 ml of 1% lidocaine with epinephrine 1:200,000 is injected.

4. **Complications** include intravascular injections and intracapsular bleeding.

C. Ulnar nerve block

1. **Indications.** Surgery or manipulations of the arm and hand that are limited to the little finger and fifth metacarpal bone.

2. **Anatomy.** The ulnar nerve is a branch of the brachial plexus and is derived from $C_{7\text{-}8}$ and T_1 nerves. Located at the medial side of the upper arm, it becomes superficial in the groove between the medial condyle of the humerus and the olecranon process of the ulnar bone. Above the wrist, it is divided into dorsal and palmar branches.

3. **Technique**

   a. **Ulnar nerve block at the elbow.** The ulnar nerve is anesthetized at the elbow at the site where it runs in the groove between the medial condyle of the humerus and the olecranon process of the ulnar bone. Through a skin wheal, a 22-gauge, 5-cm needle is introduced in the direction of the nerve and parallel with it. Following verification of paresthesias and aspiration, 10 ml of 1% lidocaine with epinephrine 1:200,000 is injected.

   b. **Ulnar nerve block at the wrist.** The ulnar nerve is divided into dorsal and palmar branches 5 cm proximal to the wrist. **The palmar branch** is located on the ventral aspect of the wrist, lateral to the tendon of the flexor carpi ulnaris muscle, where it can be anesthetized at the level of the styloid process of the ulnar bone. Through a skin wheal, a 25-gauge, 2-cm needle is inserted close to the ulnar artery and, following verification of paresthesias and aspiration, 5–10 ml of 1% lidocaine with epinephrine 1:200,000 is injected as a subcutaneous ring of anesthesia of the ulnar aspect of the wrist. **The dorsal branch** of the ulnar nerve is blocked by subcutaneous injections following the line drawn through the styloid process from the ulnar side of the flexor carpi ulnaris tendon to the middle of the back of the wrist.

4. **Complications** include intravascular and intracapsular injections.

D. Hand and digital block

1. **A nerve block of the hand** is of the field and infiltrative variety, so the anesthetic solution is injected through the dorsum of the hand rather than

through the skin of the palm. Both excessive distention of tissues and epinephrine should be avoided, since both may compromise circulation to the fingers. Local anesthetic solution injected is 1% lidocaine, 5–10 ml **without epinephrine.**

2. **The fingers** are anesthetized by local infiltration of both sides at the base of the finger. The finger block is superior to ring block of a finger because it provides complete anesthesia and causes less ischemia and consequently less necrosis. Local anesthetic solution infiltrated is 5 ml of 1% lidocaine **without epinephrine.**

V. Nerve blocks of the lower extremity

A. Anatomy. The nerve supply of the lower extremity consists of the lumbar and sacral plexuses. The femoral, obturator, and lateral femoral cutaneous nerves arise from the lumbar plexus, and the sciatic nerve arises from the sacral plexus.

B. The following nerve blocks are performed for surgery on the lower extremity:

1. Sciatic nerve block.
2. Femoral nerve block.
3. Obturator nerve block.
4. Lateral femoral cutaneous nerve block.
5. Peroneal nerve block.
6. Tibial nerve block.
7. Ankle block.
8. Toe block, which is similar to finger block.

VI. Sympathetic nerve blocks

A. Stellate ganglion block

1. **Indications.** Diagnosis and/or therapy of peripheral vascular disease, sympathetic dystrophy, and arterial embolism of the upper extremity.

2. **Anatomy.** The stellate ganglion is formed by fusion of the inferior cervical and first thoracic sympathetic ganglia. It is located on the transverse process of the C_7 vertebra and the neck of the first rib. The following structures are close to the stellate ganglion: carotid sheath, vertebral artery, vertebra, subclavian artery, recurrent laryngeal nerve, spinal nerves, and cupula of the pleura.

3. **Block of the stellate ganglion** interrupts the sympathetic nerve supply and visceral afferent nerves to the head, upper extremity, and thorax.

4. **Technique**

a. Median paratracheal approach

(1) The patient lies supine with a small pillow under the shoulders for hyperextension of the neck. At the level of the **cricoid cartilage,** the anesthesiologist, using two fingers, displaces the sternomastoid muscle laterally.

(2) Through a skin wheal, **a 23-gauge, 4-cm needle** is introduced perpendicular and lateral to the cricoid cartilage. The needle is forwarded 2.5–4 cm until contact with bone is made and then is withdrawn 0.5 cm. Following careful aspiration, 10–20 ml of the anesthetic solution is administered.

(3) **Symptoms and signs** of successful block include (a) Horner's syndrome (blepharoptosis, miosis, and enophthalmos), (b) increased tem-

perature of the face and arm, (c) increased lacrimation, (d) anhydrosis of the arm and face, and (e) stuffiness of the nose. These effects are limited to the anesthetized side.

b. **Other techniques** used are the anterior approach and the posterior approach.

5. **Complications** include intravascular injections, subarachnoid injection; pneumothorax, phrenic nerve paralysis, recurrent laryngeal nerve paralysis, and hematoma. Bilateral blocks should be avoided.

B. **Other sympathetic nerve blocks** include paravertebral lumbar block and celiac plexus block.

VII. Intravenous regional anesthesia

A. Local anesthetic drugs occasionally are **injected IV** in spite of the low margin of safety and short duration of effect that characterize this procedure. Lidocaine is the drug most often used.

B. **Indications.** Surgery and manipulations of 1¾ hr duration or less on the upper and lower limbs from the lower pneumatic tourniquet distally. This technique is recommended particularly for soft tissue surgery, such as ganglionectomy and surgery for Dupuytren's contractures.

C. Technique

1. **A vein** on the upper or lower extremity is entered with a 20-gauge plastic catheter through a skin wheal and is kept patent by injection of lactated Ringer's solution.

2. The upper or lower extremity is elevated. **Exsanguination** is accomplished by firm wrapping of the limb with **the Esmarch bandage** from the digits or toes proximally or by a pneumatic splint.

3. **A double pneumatic tourniquet** is placed on the upper or lower limb, and **the most proximal tourniquet is inflated** to a pressure of 275 torr (for the upper extremity) or to 550 torr (for the lower extremity).

4. The Esmarch bandage is removed, and **the venous system is infused** with 50 ml of 0.5% lidocaine with no epinephrine (for the upper limb) or 100 ml (for the lower limb). Total anesthesia of the extremity follows within 10 min. The anesthetic solution should not contain preservative or epinephrine. Surgery is performed in a bloodless area of an analgesic extremity.

5. **During surgery,** the patient may complain of discomfort under the inflated proximal tourniquet (tourniquet pain). If this happens, **the distal cuff is inflated,** since it is overlying tissues that are now analgesic, and **the proximal cuff is deflated.**

6. **Anesthesia lasts** as long as the extremity remains ischemic. Sensory and motor function return within 10 min following deflation of the pneumatic tourniquet.

7. **When surgery is completed,** the tourniquet is deflated slowly over a period of 2–3 min to prevent a massive loading of the local anesthetic solution into the systemic circulation. The deflation must not be carried out until the incision has been sutured and a pressure dressing applied, because the congestion will cause bleeding in the wound.

D. Disadvantages

1. The technique can be used only up to 1¾ hr.

2. **Discomfort** is produced by application of the Esmarch bandage over sensitive wounds, lesions, or fractures.

3. A satisfactory **anesthesia may not result** if the limb is not adequately exsanguinated.
4. **Sudden release** of the cuff is a hazard that may necessitate brachial plexus block or general anesthesia.

Bibliography

Enright, A. C., Smith, C. G., and Wyant, G. M. Comparison of bupivacaine and lidocaine for intravenous regional analgesia. *Can. Anaesth. Soc. J.* 27:553, 1980.

McClure, J. H., and Scott, D. B. Comparison of bupivacaine hydrochloride and carbonated bupivacaine in brachial plexus block by the interscalene technique. *Br. J. Anaesth.* 53:523, 1981.

Skretting, P. Hypotension after intercostal nerve block during thoracotomy under general anesthesia. *Br. J. Anaesth.* 53:527, 1981.

Snow, J. C., Kripke, B. J., Sakellarides, H., et al. Broken disposable needle during an axillary approach to block the brachial plexus. *Anesth. Analg.* (Cleve.) 53:89, 1974.

Teddy, P. J., Fabinyi, G. C. A., Kerr, J. H., et al. Bupivacaine infiltration after lumbar laminectomy. Local infiltration in the control of early postoperative lumbar laminectomy pain. *Anaesthesia* 36:380, 1981.

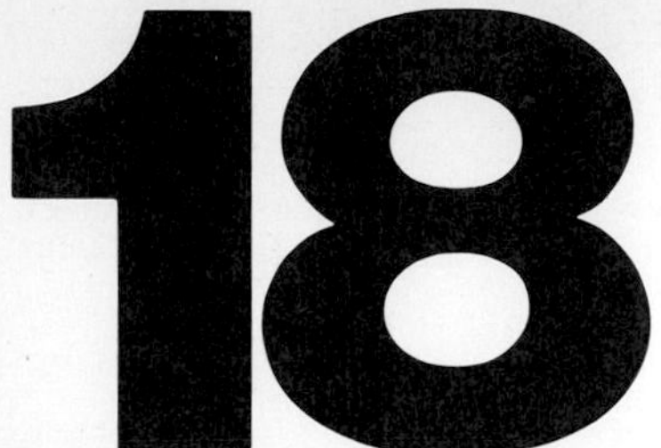

Vasopressors and Adrenergic Blocking Agents

I. General considerations

A. The variety of hemodynamic effects of the vasopressor or adrenergic agents has been attributed to their differential actions on two categories of sympathetic receptors, alpha and beta receptors.

1. Alpha receptors. Stimulation of alpha adrenergic receptors causes peripheral vasoconstriction (skin, mucosa, intestine, and kidney), mydriasis, and myometrial contraction.

2. Beta receptors. Stimulation of the beta adrenergic receptors causes smooth muscle relaxation, vasodilation (heart, skeletal muscle), bronchial relaxation, myocardial stimulation (increased rate, contractility, and excitability, and facilitation of atrioventricular conduction), hyperglycemia, and CNS excitation. Recently the beta-adrenergic receptors have been subdivided into $beta_1$ and $beta_2$.

a. Stimulation of **$beta_1$ receptors** causes, in addition to bronchodilation, tachycardia, palpitation, hypertension, insomnia, tremor, and increased cardiac contractility. Typical representatives of this group of stimulants are isoproterenol, epinephrine, and ephedrine.

b. Stimulation of **$beta_2$ receptors** causes vasodilation and bronchodilation.

B. Most adrenergic agents act on both alpha and beta receptors but differ in their degree of effectiveness in stimulating these two categories of receptors.

C. All so-called vasopressors are **adrenergic drugs.** These include the **catecholamines** (epinephrine, norepinephrine, isoproterenol, and dopamine) as well as the **noncatecholamines** (metamphetamine, ephedrine, mephentermine, metaraminol, phenylephrine, and methoxamine).

D. Monoamine oxidase inhibitors may potentiate the hypertensive effects of the sympathomimetic amines.

E. The hypotension occurring in the obstetric patient during labor or delivery—usually following spinal or epidural anesthesia—can decrease uterine blood flow enough to cause fetal hypoxia.

1. Vasopressor therapy can be dangerous to the fetus because the uterine blood vessels appear to have only alpha receptors and can react to vasopressors only by constricting.

2. Prior to drug treatment, an effort should be made to increase the BP by changing the mother's position, displacing the uterus to the left, and administering fluids. If these efforts fail, and the signs of cerebral or coronary ischemia develop in the mother, a vasopressor should be given. **Ephedrine** is often preferred.

F. The alpha-adrenergic blocking drugs include phenoxybenzamine (Dibenzyline), phentolamine (Regitine), and droperidol (Inapsine). **The beta-adrenergic blocking drugs** include propranolol (Inderal).

II. Epinephrine

A. Description

1. Epinephrine (Adrenalin) is a naturally occurring catecholamine that constitutes 85% of the catecholamines in the adrenal medulla. It is the most widely used sympathetic drug in anesthesia.
2. It is released endogenously from the adrenal medulla by a variety of stimuli, including fear, anger, anoxia, hypercapnia, and hypotension.

B. Actions

1. Epinephrine is a sympathomimetic agent and the physiologic transmitter of the adrenal medulla. It activates an adrenergic receptive mechanism on effector cells and imitates the action of the sympathetic nervous system.
2. It acts on both alpha-, $beta_1$-, and $beta_2$-adrenergic receptors of the entire sympathetic nervous system, and it is the most potent alpha receptor activator.
3. **Epinephrine stimulates the heart** and the CNS and increases the heart rate, cardiac output, and cardiac irritability; ventricular arrhythmias may follow its administration. It dilates coronary arteries and bronchi and constricts veins. Epinephrine is a potent vasopressor agent that increases systolic BP and decreases diastolic BP. Total peripheral resistance is decreased with moderate to small doses.
4. Epinephrine is an effective vasoconstrictor when infiltrated into the skin and subcutaneous tissues.
5. The effects of epinephrine and the contractile force of the heart are decreased as **acidosis** is increased.
6. **Kidney.** Epinephrine markedly decreases renal blood flow and urinary output.

C. Indications. Epinephrine is used:

1. When a vasoconstrictor is needed in local anesthetic solutions.
   a. To retard absorption and decrease toxicity systemically.
   b. To prolong the action of local, regional, spinal, epidural, and caudal anesthesia.
2. When a bronchodilator is needed.
3. For treatment of hypersensitivity or allergic reactions to drugs, particularly in anaphylactic shock, for which it is the drug of choice.
4. For hemostasis.
5. When very potent stimulation is needed to restore cardiac rhythm in an arrested heart.

D. Contraindications

1. Patients with angina pectoris, hypertension, mitral valve disease, heart failure, thyrotoxicosis, or diabetes and in pregnant patients.
2. Use with local anesthetics for surgery of certain areas (e.g., fingers, toes, penis, or external ear) because of the danger of vasoconstriction that would produce sloughing of tissues.
3. During halothane anesthesia, epinephrine should be given very cautiously. Halothane sensitizes the myocardial conduction system to the action of epinephrine.

E. Adverse reactions

1. Epinephrine may cause headache, restlessness, anxiety, weakness, pallor, vertigo, tremor, precordial pain, palpitation, and respiratory distress.

2. **Overdose** or inadvertent IV administration of epinephrine may cause convulsions, cerebral hemorrhage, and ventricular disturbances.

3. As a catecholamine, epinephrine may induce serious ventricular arrhythmias in patients undergoing general anesthesia with certain anesthetics—particularly in the presence of anoxia and hypercapnia.

F. Usual dosage

1. A 1-ml ampule of 1:1000 solution contains 1 mg of epinephrine.

2. The usual dose is 0.1 mg IV and 0.2–0.3 mg IM or SQ. Start with a small dose and increase it if required. If on rare occasions the drug is given IV, it should be diluted sufficiently and injected slowly. As an IV drip (4 mg in 250 ml 5% D/W or normal saline) the average dose is 0.1 microgram/kg/min.

3. With local anesthetic solutions, epinephrine 1:200,000 (1 mg/200 ml) is the usual concentration employed.

4. For intraspinal use, the usual dose is 0.2 mg added to the spinal anesthetic mixture; by limiting absorption, this technique may extend the period of anesthesia by 50%.

5. For cardiac resuscitation (see Chap. 8, secs. **V.E,H,J**), a dose of 0.5 mg is diluted to 10 ml with sodium chloride and can be injected IV or intracardially to restore myocardial contractility. The IV dose of 0.5 mg may be repeated every 5–15 min if necessary. The rapid biodegradation of the drug dictates frequent readministration.

III. Norepinephrine

A. Description. Norepinephrine (Levophed) (also called levarterenol) is a naturally occurring catecholamine that differs from epinephrine because of the absence of a methyl group on the nitrogen atom. It is released in small quantities from the adrenal medulla. A large fraction of the circulating norepinephrine arises from sympathetic nerve endings.

B. Actions

1. Norepinephrine is a strong peripheral vasoconstrictor (alpha-adrenergic action) and potent inotropic stimulator of the heart and dilator of coronary arteries (beta-adrenergic action). Both these actions result in increased systolic and diastolic BP and coronary artery blood flow.

2. **Kidney.** Norepinephrine decreases renal blood flow and urinary output.

C. Indications. Norepinephrine has little application in anesthesia. It is used:

1. For the restoration of BP in controlling certain acute hypotensive states.

2. For treatment following pheochromocytoma removal.

3. As an adjunct in the therapy of cardiac arrest and profound hypotension.

D. Contraindications

1. Patients who are hypotensive from blood volume deficits.

2. During halothane anesthesia, it should be given very cautiously.

E. Adverse reactions

1. Headache, angina, hypertension, and arrhythmias.

2. **Tissue necrosis and sloughing** at the site of injection. This has occurred following extravasation during IV infusion. Therapy of extravasation includes local infiltration with phentolamine.

F. Usual dosage

1. A 4-ml ampule of solution contains 4 mg of norepinephrine.

2. Whenever possible, norepinephrine should be administered into a large vein, especially an antecubital vein or a central venous pressure line, so that the risk of necrosis of the overlying skin from prolonged vasoconstriction is very slight.

3. Norepinephrine should be given **only IV and diluted** as follows: 1 ampule containing 4 mg in 4 ml (0.1% solution) to 250 ml of 5% D/W with slow drip; the average dose is 0.1 microgram/kg/min. It is administered at a rate sufficient to maintain the systolic BP no higher than 20–30 torr below normal. The onset of action is rapid, and the duration is short.

IV. Isoproterenol

A. Description. Isoproterenol (Isuprel) is a synthetic sympathomimetic amine that is related structurally to epinephrine.

B. Actions

1. Isoproterenol acts exclusively on $beta_1$- and $beta_2$-adrenergic receptors. It is devoid of alpha effects.

2. It stimulates the heart, dilates blood vessels (primarily those in skeletal muscles), and relaxes bronchial and alimentary smooth muscles.

3. It increases the cardiac output by increasing the strength of cardiac contraction, heart rate, and venous return. It lowers peripheral vascular resistance, so diastolic BP falls.

4. **Kidney.** Isoproterenol has no significant effect on blood flow or urinary output.

C. Indications. Isoproterenol is used:

1. As a valuable vasopressor agent when the desired action is an increase in heart rate.

2. In a patient in shock (hypoperfusion syndrome).

3. As an effective bronchodilator.

4. To maintain increased heart rate in patients who have undergone cardiac surgery and in patients with heart block.

5. In cardiac arrest.

D. Isoproterenol is contraindicated:

1. In patients with tachycardia caused by digitalis intoxication.

2. During general anesthesia with anesthetics that sensitize the heart to catecholamines.

E. Adverse reactions

1. Isoproterenol may cause headache, flushing, tachycardia, precordial distress, palpitation, tremors, vertigo, and arrhythmias.

2. Isoproterenol and epinephrine should not be administered simultaneously, since both drugs are direct cardiac stimulants and their combined effects may induce serious arrhythmias.

3. Isoproterenol must be used with caution because it can assist in the development of escape rhythms and rapidly produce premature ventricular contractions. Hypokalemia potentiates these arrhythmias.

F. Usual dosage

1. Each milliliter of the 1:5000 solution contains 0.2 mg.
2. A 5-ml ampule (1 mg) is diluted in 250 ml of 5% D/W. Start at 6 microdrops per minute and increase in multiples of 6 microdrops per minute. The average dose is 0.025 microgram/kg/min.

V. Phenylephrine

A. Description. Phenylephrine (Neo-Synephrine) is a synthetic vasoconstrictor and vasopressor drug related chemically to epinephrine and ephedrine.

B. Actions

1. Phenylephrine acts almost exclusively on alpha receptors.
2. It is a direct-acting sympathomimetic amine that stimulates receptors directly but for a longer time than epinephrine. Its chief effect is to cause vasoconstriction by direct action on the walls of the vessels. It stimulates the force of contraction of the ventricular muscle, but the dose needed to elicit this effect is larger than the ordinary dose that will elevate the BP.
3. When applied topically or infiltrated into the tissues, phenylephrine produces vasoconstriction that lasts longer than that produced by epinephrine and ephedrine.
4. Its action on the heart contrasts sharply with that of epinephrine and ephedrine in that it slows the heart rate and increases the stroke output, inducing no disturbance in the cardiac rhythm. It dilates and increases the blood flow in the coronary arteries.
5. Phenylephrine increases systolic and diastolic BP by peripheral constriction of arterioles. **Bradycardia** results from reflex response mediated via pressoreceptors that can be inhibited by atropine. Occasional ventricular arrhythmias occur if the drug is administered in large doses.
6. Phenylephrine dilates the pupils, relieves nasal congestion, and does not stimulate the cerebral cortex.
7. **Kidney.** Phenylephrine decreases renal blood flow and urinary output.

C. Indications. Phenylephrine is used:

1. For control of acute hypotension during general anesthesia.
2. For treatment of postspinal hypotension (except in obstetrics) and to prolong spinal anesthesia.
3. For treatment of orthostatic hypotension.
4. For treatment of vascular failure in shock, shock-like states, and drug-induced hypotension.
5. As a topical vasoconstrictor in the nose (0.25% solution).
6. Phenylephrine can be used with halogenated anesthetics.

D. Contraindications

1. Patients with hypertension or ventricular tachycardia.
2. Patients receiving monoamine oxidase inhibitors.

E. Adverse reactions

1. Bradycardia due to reflex vagal effects.
2. Headache.
3. Ventricular extrasystoles and ventricular tachycardia.

F. Usual dosage

1. A 1-ml ampule of solution contains 10 mg of 1% phenylephrine.
2. Phenylephrine is commonly injected SQ, IM, or slowly IV or is infused in dilute solution as a continuous IV drip.
3. The dose is 2–3 mg IM or 0.25–0.5 mg IV.
4. The onset of action is within 1 min IV or within 5 min IM, and the duration of action is 5 min IV or 25 min IM.
5. Phenylephrine is a powerful agent that is best given by the drip method. The continuous IV solution is prepared by dilution of 10 mg of phenylephrine in 250 ml of 5% D/W and is administered at a rate of 1–50 micrograms/min.

VI. Mephentermine

A. Description. Mephentermine (Wyamine) is a synthetic adrenergic drug that is pharmacologically similar to ephedrine.

B. Actions

1. Mephentermine acts directly and indirectly and is both an alpha and a beta stimulator.
2. It stimulates the heart; increases venous tone, cardiac output, and coronary blood flow; and elevates systolic and diastolic BP. It does not produce ventricular arrhythmias.
3. Mephentermine stimulates the CNS and may induce euphoria.
4. **Kidney.** Renal blood flow and urinary output are increased.

C. Indications. Mephentermine is used:

1. For maintenance of BP during spinal or epidural anesthesia or following ganglionic block.
2. For control of acute hypotension during general anesthesia (if stimulation of the heart is not contraindicated).
3. Mephentermine may be used with halogenated anesthetics.

D. Contraindications

1. Severe essential hypertension.
2. Chronic heart disease.

E. Adverse reactions

1. Anxiety due to CNS stimulation.
2. Palpitation, headache, vertigo, and ventricular tachycardia.

F. Usual dosage

1. A 1-ml ampule contains 15 mg and is administered IM, SQ, or IV.
2. The dose is 5–15 mg IV or 10–30 mg IM. The action following IV injection is immediate and lasts for 30–45 min. After IM injection, the onset of action begins within 10–15 min and lasts for 1–2 hr.

3. The continuous IV infusion consists of 500 mg (0.1% solution) diluted in 500 ml of 5% D/W and is given at a rate that will maintain the systolic BP at about 90–100 torr.

VII. Ephedrine

A. Description. Ephedrine is available as a natural and as a synthetic adrenergic drug. Clinically, it is allied to epinephrine.

B. Actions

1. Ephedrine is a direct alpha-, beta$_1$-, and beta$_2$-adrenergic stimulator and owes part of its peripheral action to the release of norepinephrine.
2. It is a potent sympathetic stimulant that raises systolic and diastolic BP, stimulates the myocardium, constricts arterioles, relaxes smooth bronchial and intestinal muscles, dilates the pupils, and stimulates the cerebral cortex and medulla. The effect on the bronchial muscle is less prominent but more sustained than with epinephrine.
3. Ephedrine dilates the coronary arteries and increases heart rate and cardiac output.
4. Tachyphylaxis occurs (with repeated doses, the response may be decreased).
5. It does not reduce uterine blood flow and thus spares the placenta. This is a major advantage when treating hypotension in the obstetric patient.
6. **Kidney.** Its effect is similar to that of epinephrine but less intense.

C. Indications. Ephedrine is used:

1. For maintenance of normotension during spinal or epidural anesthesia.
2. For control of acute hypotension following ganglionic block or during general anesthesia (if cardiac stimulation is not contraindicated) and to treat orthostatic hypotension.
3. In severe attacks of bronchial asthma, when the administration of epinephrine is not warranted.
4. For **obstetrics,** in which it is the ideal agent because of its minimal deleterious effects on the fetus.

D. Contraindications

1. Severe essential hypertension.
2. Chronic heart disease.

E. Adverse reactions

1. Palpitation, ventricular tachycardia, headache, vertigo, and insomnia may occur.
2. Urine retention may result in men with prostatic hypertrophy.
3. Ephedrine plus oxytocin may cause postpartum hypertension.
4. Ephedrine may be less useful in patients on therapy with guanethidine or reserpine, because these drugs deplete norepinephrine stores.

F. Usual dosage

1. A 1-ml ampule contains 50 mg.
2. Ephedrine is given IM, SQ, and IV. The IM or SQ dose is 25–50 mg, determined by the response of the patient.
3. The IV initial dose is 10–25 mg, accompanied by 25–50 mg IM for a prolonged effect. If an adequate IV response is not obtained, the IV injection may be repeated in 5–10 min.

4. The onset of the IV effect occurs within 2–4 min; the onset of IM action, within 10–20 min. The duration of action is 1 hr.

VIII. Methamphetamine

A. Description. Methamphetamine (Methedrine) is a synthetic adrenergic drug that is similar in its clinical effects to ephedrine and amphetamine.

B. Actions

1. Methamphetamine is a sympathomimetic amine that stimulates alpha, $beta_1$, and $beta_2$ receptors; it acts in the same manner as ephedrine, buts its action lasts longer.
2. Methamphetamine stimulates the heart and CNS and increases the heart rate, force of contraction, and output. It constricts peripheral blood vessels, elevates BP, and dilates the coronary arteries and bronchi. It may cause bradycardia through a vagal effect, but this can be abolished by atropine.
3. It is a powerful cerebral stimulant with potential for abuse.
4. **Kidney.** It increases renal blood flow and urinary output.

C. Indication. While its use has been discontinued in many hospitals for social (not pharmacologic) reasons, methamphetamine is used as a pressor agent during spinal anesthesia.

D. Methamphetamine is contraindicated in patients with thyrotoxicosis and heart disease.

E. Adverse reactions are the same as those induced by ephedrine, but the reactions are more marked.

F. Usual dosage

1. The dose is 5–10 mg IV, accompanied by 10–20 mg IM for prolonged action.
2. The onset of the IV effect occurs within 1–2 min; the onset of IM action occurs within 3–5 min. The duration of action is 2 hr.

IX. Metaraminol

A. Description. Metaraminol (Aramine) is a potent synthetic sympathomimetic amine that is more potent than ephedrine but with similar sites and mechanism of action.

B. Actions

1. Metaraminol is an alpha stimulator with slight $beta_1$-stimulating effects. It produces marked vasoconstriction. Its effect is partly the result of direct action on the vessel walls and partly due to the liberation of norepinephrine from stores in nerve endings or chromaffin cells.
2. Metaraminol stimulates the heart without producing arrhythmias. It increases cardiac output and coronary blood flow as well as systolic and diastolic BP (due to peripheral vasoconstriction). It is accompanied by reflex bradycardia that can be abolished by the use of atropine.
3. Unlike ephedrine, it does not stimulate the cortex.
4. Tachyphylaxis occurs (with repeated doses, the response may be decreased).
5. **Kidney.** Renal vasoconstriction is not pronounced.

C. Indications. Metaraminol is used:

1. As an adjunct in the treatment of hypotension due to hemorrhage, reactions to medications, surgical complications, and shock associated with brain damage from trauma or tumor.
2. To prevent and treat the acute hypotensive state that occurs with spinal anesthesia.

D. Contraindications

1. Halothane anesthesia.
2. Metaraminol should be used very cautiously in patients with heart or thyroid disease, hypertension, or diabetes.

E. Adverse reactions

1. Sympathomimetic amines, including metaraminol, may cause tachycardia or arrhythmias, particularly in patients with myocardial infarction.
2. Abscess formation, tissue necrosis, or sloughing may follow the use of metaraminol. The large veins of the antecubital fossa should be preferred to veins in the dorsum of the hand.

F. Usual dosage

1. Each milliliter of solution (1%) contains 10 mg; solution comes in 1-ml and 10-ml containers. Metaraminol is a potent vasopressor that can be given IM or IV.
2. The dose is 2–5 mg IM and 0.5–2 mg IV. The pressor effect begins in 1–2 min after IV infusion and within about 10 min after IM injection. The effects last from about 20–60 min.
3. Metaraminol is best administered in a continuous IV infusion by adding 100 mg in 500 ml of 5% D/W at a rate sufficient to maintain the systolic BP at about 90–100 torr.

X. Methoxamine

A. Description. Methoxamine (Vasoxyl) is a synthetic sympathomimetic drug that is similar to phenylephrine.

B. Actions

1. Methoxamine is an adrenergic drug that stimulates the alpha receptors almost exclusively. It has no beta activity. It acts peripherally, on the vessels, and does not stimulate the heart.
2. It increases BP by peripheral vasoconstriction. Bradycardia results from compensatory reflexes. There is no effect on the cardiac output. It increases peripheral resistance and central venous pressure.
3. It does not produce arrhythmias and does not stimulate the higher centers.
4. There is evidence that methoxamine enriches blood flow to non-vital organs, such as muscle, at the expense of vital organs, e.g., the heart.
5. **Kidney.** Due to vasoconstriction, the renal blood flow and urine output are decreased, but the desire to empty the bladder is stimulated.

C. Indications. Methoxamine is used:

1. To maintain arterial pressure following spinal or epidural anesthesia and to control severe hypotension following ganglionic block.
2. To control acute hypotension during general anesthesia when cardiac stimulation is contraindicated.

D. Contraindications

1. As a combination with local anesthetics to prolong their action at local sites.
2. Methoxamine should be used carefully in patients with hypertension, heart disease, or hyperthyroidism.

E. Adverse reactions

1. Marked hypertension (associated with severe headache, pilomotor response, and vomiting), tremor, or myocardial depression.

2. Reflex bradycardia via the carotid sinus and vagus nerve. This can be abolished by the use of atropine.

3. Increased left ventricular workload and diminished venous return.

4. Tingling of the extremities, pilomotor stimulation, and desire to urinate.

F. Usual dosage

1. Each milliliter of solution (1%) contains 10 mg; the solution comes in 1-ml and 10-ml containers. Methoxamine, a potent vasopressor, is administered IM and IV.

2. The IM dose is 5–10 mg. The IV dose is 2–5 mg and should be reserved for emergencies in which a strong immediate pressor response is imperative.

3. The onset of action begins within 15 min IM and within 2 min IV. The duration of action is about 1 hr.

XI. Dopamine

A. Description. Dopamine (Intropin) is a potent, naturally occurring biochemical catecholamine precursor to the formation of epinephrine in the intragranular pool at the adrenergic nerve endings.

B. Actions

1. Dopamine exerts an inotropic effect on the myocardium, resulting in an increased cardiac output.

2. It usually increases systolic BP, with either no effect on or a slight increase in diastolic BP.

3. **Kidney.** Dopamine has been reported to dilate the renal vasculature presumptively by activation of a dopaminergic receptor. This action is accompanied by increases in glomerular filtration rate, renal blood flow, and sodium excretion. An increase in urine output produced by dopamine usually is not associated with a decrease in osmolality of the urine.

C. Indications. Dopamine is used for the correction of hemodynamic imbalances present in shock syndrome due to myocardial infarction, trauma, endotoxin septicemia, open heart surgery, renal failure, or chronic cardiac decompensation, as in congestive heart failure.

D. Contraindications

1. Pheochromocytoma.

2. Uncorrected tachyarrhythmias or ventricular fibrillation.

E. Adverse reactions. The most common adverse reactions observed in clinical evaluation of dopamine include ectopic beats, nausea, vomiting, tachycardia, anginal pain, palpitation, dyspnea, headache, hypotension (especially at lower infusion rates), and vasoconstriction.

F. Usual dosage

1. Each milliliter of solution (4%) contains 40 mg; the solution comes in 5-ml containers.

2. Dopamine is administered in a continuous IV infusion by adding the contents of one 5-ml ampule (containing 200 mg) to 250 or 500 ml of 5% D/W.

3. Do not add dopamine injection to 5% sodium bicarbonate or other alkaline IV solutions because the drug is inactivated in an alkaline solution.

4. Close monitoring of urine flow, cardiac output, and BP is necessary during dopamine infusion, as it is with any adrenergic agent.

XII. Propranolol

A. Description. Propranolol (Inderal) is an adrenergic beta-receptor blocking drug.

B. Actions

1. **Propranolol has strong beta-blocking activity.** Its effects depend on the degree of sympathetic activity. When sympathetic activity is high, propranolol will reduce the cardiac rate, prolong atrioventricular conduction, and increase the P–R interval while reducing myocardial contractility—negative inotropic action.
2. It blocks the beta-adrenergic receptors in the heart, bronchioles, uterus, and vascular bed.
3. It exerts a depressant effect on the cardiac muscle similar to that of quinidine.
4. Its myocardial depressant effect dictates that treatment with propranolol should be discontinued at least 24 hr before a patient is exposed to general anesthesia, unless the discontinuation would lead to aggravation of an arrhythmia or an ischemic sign.

C. Indications. Propranolol is used:

1. In the presence of certain arrhythmias, hypertrophic subaortic stenosis, pheochromocytoma, angina pectoris, and certain hypertensive states.
2. In controlling supraventricular arrhythmias in patients with thyrotoxicosis. It appears to be especially useful here.
3. In ventricular tachycardia.

D. Contraindications

1. Bronchial asthma.
2. Sinus bradycardia and heart block greater than first degree.
3. Right ventricular failure secondary to pulmonary hypertension.
4. Congestive heart failure.
5. Patients receiving adrenergic-augmenting psychotropic drugs, including monoamine oxidase inhibitors.

E. Adverse reactions

1. Propranolol can produce multiple nonspecific adverse effects, such as nausea, vomiting, dizziness, and insomnia. It also can produce more serious adverse effects, such as fever, visual disturbances, hypotension, and bradycardia.
2. Bronchospasm may develop in patients with chronic obstructive lung disease.
3. Propranolol is liable to precipitate and intensify heart failure.
4. Several deaths have been reported during the use of propranolol.

F. Usual dosage

1. A 1-ml ampule contains 1 mg. Tablets contain 10 mg and 40 mg.
2. The dose is 0.5–1 mg IV, up to a maximum of 2 mg. The injection should be carried out with careful monitoring of the ECG. Larger doses may result in vagal overactivity unless atropine is also given.
3. Blockade usually develops within 30 min following oral ingestion of propranolol and is maintained for approximately 3–8 hr. Almost no blocking effect is evident after 12–24 hr.

4. When propranolol is administered IV, the onset of effect occurs within 2 min, and peak action is reached in 3–5 min. The total duration of action is 2–4 hr.

Bibliography

Cooper, G. M., Paterson, F. L., Mashiter, K., et al. Beta-adrenergic blockade and the metabolic response to surgery. *Br. J. Anaesth.* 52:1231, 1980.

Dollery, C. T., Paterson, J. W., and Conolly, M. E. Clinical pharmacology of beta-receptor-blocking drugs. *Clin. Pharmacol. Ther.* 10:765, 1969.

Holland, O. B., and Kaplan, N. M. Propranolol in the treatment of hypertension. *N. Engl. J. Med.* 294:930, 1976.

Smith, N. T., and Corbascio, A. N. The use and misuse of pressor agents. *Anesthesiology* 33:58, 1970.

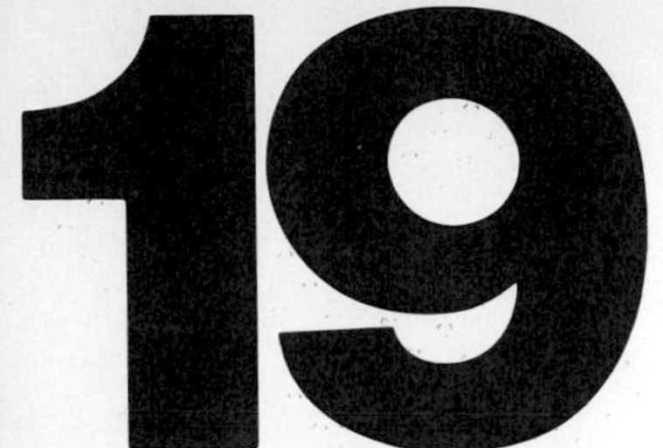

Hypotensive Techniques and Induced Hypothermia

I. Controlled hypotension

A. It is incumbent on those who intend to utilize the potent and potentially dangerous techniques and drugs required in controlled hypotension to be thoroughly conversant with the pharmacology and physiology involved. **The agents and their dosages must be carefully selected** following a comprehensive review of the entire case, including the patient's age and physical and mental status; the surgical procedure contemplated; and the skill and experience of the surgeon, anesthesiologist, and operating room, recovery room, and intensive care unit personnel.

1. Before selecting the method of controlled hypotension, one must be sure the advantages outweigh the disadvantages following a thorough review of all the facts.
2. When indicated and carefully conducted, controlled hypotension can be an effective, safe technique that provides good operating conditions for some operations.

B. Advantages

1. The method minimizes blood loss and the need for blood transfusion.
2. It decreases oozing.
3. Decreased amounts of anesthetics are necessary.

C. Indications

1. Head and neck surgery.
2. Neurosurgical operations: for aneurysm, meningioma, and excision of vascular tumors.
3. Cancer operations in which bleeding may be difficult to control.
4. Pelvic procedures, such as pelvic exenteration with node dissection.
5. Vascular surgery, such as portacaval shunt.
6. Orthopedic surgery: for disarticulation procedures and correction of scoliosis.

D. Contraindications

1. Heart failure.
2. Arteriosclerosis.
3. Hypertension (severe).
4. Cerebrovascular disease.
5. Impaired renal or hepatic function.
6. Marked anemia and/or decreased blood volume.
7. Respiratory insufficiency.

8. Narrow-angle glaucoma, when ganglionic blocking drugs are not used because of pupillary dilation.
9. An anesthesiologist who is not familiar with the technique, a slow operating room team and/or surgeon(s), and/or postoperative care personnel with little or no experience.

E. Requirements

1. Advantages must outweigh risks.
2. Proper selection of patients.
3. Proper positioning of the patient.
4. Careful monitoring.
   a. Arterial BP monitoring, preferably with an indwelling radial artery cannula, to monitor the BP continuously.
   b. Central venous pressure monitoring.
   c. Use of the electrocardioscope.
   d. Gravimetric monitoring (weighing of sponges) and close observation of the amount of blood in the suction bottle (be aware of fluids used for irrigation of the surgical area).
   e. Temperature monitoring.
   f. Determination of arterial blood gases and hemoglobin and hematocrit should be done as indicated during the procedure.
5. Adequate ventilation and oxygenation.
6. Replacement of blood loss.
7. Normal preoperative blood volume.
8. Minimal duration of the hypotensive period.
9. An experienced anesthesiologist and a skillful surgeon.
10. Excellent postoperative care and supervision in the recovery room or intensive care unit.
    a. Ascertain that the blood loss has been replaced.
    b. The patient should be awake, responding, and ventilating well and have good color.
    c. Oxygen should be administered by mask or nasal cannula.

F. Drugs and methods

1. **Trimethaphan** (Arfonad) produces hypotension by ganglionic block, direct vasodilation (reduction in peripheral resistance), and histamine release.
   a. Trimethaphan is short acting; reversal of hypotension takes place in 10–30 min.
   b. Trimethaphan should be avoided in patients with allergies or increased intracranial pressure.
   c. The drug provides graded, rapidly reversible falls in BP.
   d. The mechanism for its short action is probably the rapid excretion of 30% of the drug in the urine.
   e. The level of BP must be correlated with the vascular ooze, then maintained. Try not to let the BP get below 80–90 torr, if at all possible, to diminish postoperative complications. In an ASA class 1 patient, a fall to 70 torr may be permissible.

f. Disadvantages

(1) Tachyphylaxis.

(2) Occasional onset of tachycardia.

g. Dose. A 0.1% solution (1 mg/ml or 500 mg/500 ml in 5% D/W) as an IV drip infusion.

2. Nitroprusside

a. Nitroprusside (Nipride) is a potent, rapid-acting hypotensive drug administered by IV infusion.

b. Its effects are achieved by peripheral vasodilation and decreased peripheral resistance.

c. Its mechanism is direct action on blood vessel walls, independent of the autonomic innervation.

d. Shortly after administration the drug is slowed down or discontinued, and the BP begins to rise; it returns to the preoperative level within 1–10 min.

e. Tachyphylaxis is rare.

f. The prepared stock solution is sodium nitroprusside dihydrate, 50 mg. From the stock solution, a final preparation of nitroprusside in 500 or 1000 ml of 5% D/W is made up in strengths of 0.01% to 0.002%, depending on the age and physical status of the patient.

g. Degradation of nitroprusside occurs in the presence of light and/or low pH, and yields sodium ferrocyanide and cyanide. Thus cyanide poisoning is a possibility.

(1) The presence of these compounds can be detected by a change in color of the solution from normal brown-pink to an abnormal dark brown or blue; either of these colors indicates the preparation is chemically unfit for use.

(2) This photosensitive breakdown can be prevented by either storing nitroprusside in amber-colored vials or wrapping opaque foil around the containers.

h. Nitroprusside should be administered by an infusion pump or by microdrip regulator, and BP should be recorded directly via a radial artery cannula.

i. Although nitroprusside is a good hypotensive agent—rapidly reversible and predictable in its action—it can have an adverse metabolic effect if administered in a dose over 3 mg per kilogram of body weight. In high doses, severe hypotension and/or methemoglobinemia have been reported.

j. The average dose of nitroprusside is 3 micrograms/kg/min (range of 0.5–8 micrograms/kg/min). One vial (50 mg) of nitroprusside is diluted in 500 ml of 5% D/W; each milliliter contains 100 micrograms.

3. Nitroglycerin

a. Nitroglycerin can be used IV to reduce BP.

b. It has a short plasma half-life, is easy to control, and has no direct toxic effects or toxic metabolites.

c. Nitroglycerin dilates vessels directly by reacting with vascular smooth muscles and acts predominantly on capacitance vessels, resulting in decreased venous return.

d. Nitroglycerin may not induce hypotension in young patients, especially during narcotic-supplemented nitrous oxide–oxygen anesthesia. These patients may require other agents or techniques for significant BP reduction.

e. Nitroglycerin is supplied in 20-ml glass ampules containing 10 mg of nitroglycerin, or 500 micrograms/ml. Nitroglycerin solution as obtained from the manufacturer is relatively stable when it is exposed to light and can be kept up to 3 years without refrigeration.

f. The drug is absorbed by plastic bags and should be infused from glass bottles. An infusion pump is best for infusion at a beginning rate of 1 microgram/kg/min, with increases to achieve the desired BP level.

4. Halothane, enflurane, and isoflurane may be used alone or with hypotensive agents to produce controlled hypotension. However, the anesthesiologist should be alert to the possibility of overdosage in the effort to decrease the systolic BP.

G. Physiologic effects on vital organs

1. Brain

a. Cerebral metabolism may not be at the usual levels during the hypotensive period if the BP is very low and the patient is in the head-up position.

b. When the BP is reduced below 60 torr, additional cerebral vasodilation is not possible; therefore lower levels of BP may be accompanied by a reduction in cerebral blood flow.

c. Oxygen consumption does not change significantly.

d. Mental function may be altered to a minor degree in the postoperative period; however, this is usually transient.

2. Heart and blood vessels

a. Coronary perfusion remains adequate.

b. There is no permanent myocardial damage, although there may be some transient myocardial ischemia in elderly patients or those with hypertension if the BP is allowed to fall below 60 torr. In these patients, a systolic pressure of at least 80 torr should be maintained at all times.

c. Cardiac output changes vary with the agent or technique utilized.

(1) Trimethaphan causes slight changes in cardiac output.

(2) With pentolinium (Ansolysen), changes in cardiac output are rate-dependent.

(3) High spinal block and deep general anesthesia yield a significant decrease in cardiac output.

(4) Nitroprusside causes no change in cardiac output if BP is maintained above 80 torr and all other conditions are stable.

3. Liver

a. Due to the physiology and anatomy of the liver's blood supply, it is subject to a higher critical level of hypotension.

b. The liver has two sources of blood: (1) the hepatic artery supplies 20% of the total hepatic blood supply, at high oxygen tension (95% saturated), and (2) the portal vein supplies 80% of the hepatic blood supply, at 74% oxygen saturation.

c. When the systolic BP falls below 60 torr, the liver becomes cyanotic and turgid.

d. When the liver is subjected to anoxia, (1) it cannot form urea from ammonium salts or amino acids, and (2) it also cannot inactivate vasodepressor substances.

4. Lungs

a. Physiologic dead space is increased.

b. Vital capacity is increased.

5. Kidney

a. Urine formation. Renal filtration is reduced with a fall in systolic BP. Below 60 torr, urine formation ceases; however, this does not mean that kidney damage has occurred.

b. Renal blood flow. Initially depressed, it then returns to preoperative levels. It is maintained, as the systolic BP falls, through a compensatory vasodilation. This mechanism will start to fail when BP goes below 60 torr.

H. Complications. Induced hypotension can be the cause of morbidity and mortality.

1. The most common complications

a. Cerebral thrombosis and hypoxia.

b. Reactionary hemorrhage.

c. Renal failure, oliguria, and anuria.

d. Coronary thrombosis, cardiac failure, and cardiac arrest.

e. Thromboembolic phenomena.

f. Delayed awakening.

g. Persistent hypotension.

2. The incidence of these complications has been decreasing as anesthesiologists gain experience with this technique.

I. Use of vasopressors: two points of view

1. Some hold that the BP should be allowed to return to preoperative levels prior to wound closure, so that bleeders may be ligated or cauterized.

2. Another point of view is that administration of a vasopressor is contrary to the express purpose of induced hypotension. Clots form in the dilated vessels. When reversal of the hypotension is proceeding, the veins contract on the formed clots. The vasopressor might dislodge the clot and cause bleeding.

II. Induced hypothermia (total body)

A. The main purpose of induced hypothermia is to give the surgeon increased time to operate in which the circulation to vital organs is temporarily occluded.

B. Surface cooling by use of the tub technique

1. For the adult patient, **premedication** includes 8 mg of morphine and 0.4 mg of atropine IM 1 hr before induction of anesthesia.

2. Preoxygenation consists of administration of 100% oxygen for several minutes.

3. ECG leads are applied. (Use of the EEG monitor is optional.)

4. Thiopental, 4 mg/kg is injected, and succinylcholine, 1.5 mg/kg is administered IV to facilitate intubation. Then 0.5–1% halothane or 1% enflurane is given with a mixture of 50% N_2O and 50% O_2.

5. **Tympanic, rectal, and/or esophageal** thermistors are placed to monitor body temperature.
6. Tubocurarine 0.2 mg/kg or pancuronium 0.1 mg/kg is administered to control **shivering** and is supplemented as necessary.
7. **When the vital signs are stable,** the patient is immersed in cold water, keeping the chin and hands above the water level. When the vital signs again stabilize, ice cubes are added to the water. Cooling usually takes 30–60 min. The patient is kept in the ice water until body temperature has dropped to about 40% of the desired value, since after the patient is removed from the tub and transferred to the operating table, the temperature continues to drop (drift), frequently by 3° to 4° C. Thus, if the desired temperature is 28° C, the patient is removed from the ice water when the temperature is 32° C.
8. Another technique involves the use of a **hypothermia blanket.** A modified antifreeze solution is run through the coils of the unit to a preset temperature. The blanket should be precooled before the patient is placed on it and should be lined with protective cloth sheeting to prevent skin damage at pressure sites. The patient is anesthetized on the stretcher and then moved to the blanket.
9. **As the body temperature drops,** the concentration of anesthetics is gradually reduced until their administration is stopped with the body temperature at 28° to 30° C. From this point on, no further administration of anesthetics is necessary, but controlled hyperventilation with oxygen continues for the duration of surgery. The pupils are ordinarily dilated during the hypothermic period.
10. The patient is removed from the ice water, thoroughly dried with bath towels, and placed on water-filled mattresses for rewarming. If the patient moves spontaneously while being rewarmed, a mixture of 50% N_2O and 50% O_2 is usually sufficient to keep him quiet.
11. **The methods of rewarming** vary. During rewarming, reflexes and spontaneous movements reappear at about 31° C and consciousness returns at 32° to 34° C.
12. **Extubation** is carried out when respirations are adequate.
13. The tympanic or rectal **temperature is monitored** for at least 24 hr postoperatively to ensure that the temperature is maintained at about 36.5° C. Also, the patient is observed carefully during this period for any signs of shock or reactive hyperthermia.

C. Physiologic considerations

1. Effects on metabolism

a. When blood is cooled, the oxygen dissociation curve shifts to the left.

b. The rate of oxygen consumption falls as the body temperature falls (but tissue oxygen need does not fall in a direct ratio).

c. Essential oxidative enzymes are not inactivated by hypothermia.

2. Effects on respiration

a. As body temperature falls, the solubility of carbon dioxide in the blood increases.

b. There is little change in blood sodium, potassium, or chloride during and after cooling.

3. Effects on the heart

a. The heart rate, coronary flow, and oxygen uptake of the heart are decreased by 50% when the body temperature is 25° C.

b. The cardiac output falls if shivering is prevented.

c. ECG features: The QRS complex lengthens, the P–R interval is prolonged, and there is elevation of the early part of the S–T segment (the precursor of ventricular fibrillation).

D. General circulatory changes

1. The blood flow through the brain, kidney, and splanchnic areas decreases as body temperature decreases.
2. The mean arterial pressure is decreased by 5% for each degree centigrade below 37° C.

E. Nervous system

1. Cerebral oxygen consumption falls at 25° C; the oxygen uptake of the brain decreases to 33% of that at 37° C.
2. The rate of reduction in blood flow in the brain decreases by 7% for each degree centigrade below 37° C.
3. The cerebrospinal fluid pressure falls.
4. Cortical function is decreased, so there is retrograde amnesia for events happening under hypothermia.
5. During circulatory arrest, the 3-min period at 37° C before gross irreparable damage will occur is extended at 25° C to 15 min.

F. Renal function

1. Hypothermia protects the kidney from adverse effects when the blood supply is occluded during surgery.
2. The glomerular filtration rate and renal blood flow are reduced by 30% at 25° C.

G. General considerations

1. **The use of dextrose solutions** during hypothermia carries a risk, because dextrose is metabolized very slowly during hypothermia and therefore accumulates in the extracellular fluid and, by its osmotic effect, draws water from the cells. The extra water dilutes the extracellular fluid and thus serum electrolytes.
2. **The serum potassium** tends to be low when the pH is high (alkalosis). The extracellular potassium rises whenever there is tissue anoxia.
3. **During rewarming,** dextrose solutions should be administered because dextrose levels will then tend to fall.

H. Liver

1. If circulatory arrest occurs in such a manner that there is increased central venous pressure and marked hepatic venous congestion, there may be severe structural damage to the liver, causing loss of hepatic function and marked postoperative metabolic acidosis.
2. **Morphine** is slow to be conjugated and detoxified in the liver.
3. The metabolism of **barbiturates** is impaired.
4. It is possible that norepinephrine and/or tubocurarine could remain undestroyed in areas of vascular stasis and, on rewarming, be released into the general circulation.
5. **Changes in the clotting mechanism**

   a. The bleeding time is increased.

   b. Clot retraction is poor.

I. Anesthetic drugs

1. **The effects of thiopental** are potentiated and prolonged during hypothermia. Thiopental has a direct depressant effect on the myocardium, so its use should be restricted to the induction of anesthesia.

2. **Inhalation agents**

   a. **Hypothermia potentiates** the effects of the anesthetic drugs and delays their excretion. Therefore, as hypothermia progresses, smaller amounts of anesthetic agents are required.

   b. **Halothane** is a potent vasodilator.

3. **Muscle relaxants**

   a. The effects of tubocurarine are decreased during the cooling period. Caution should be exercised during rewarming, when the action of the nondepolarizing muscle relaxants may become manifest.

   b. Muscle stiffness may be present at 33° C; it may remain until rewarming.

   c. The metabolism and excretion of tubocurarine and its reversal by neostigmine are not altered.

J. Drugs influencing cardiovascular activity

1. The decreased heart rate during hypothermia could be augmented by preoperative administration of **digitalis.** Therapy consists of injection of small doses of atropine.

2. **Quinidine** has been used for prevention of ventricular fibrillation.

3. The action of **atropine** is gradually decreased as cooling progresses.

4. **Neostigmine** maintains its action during hypothermia.

5. **Epinephrine** retains its activity in the cooled patient, at least to 25° C. **Norepinephrine** is less active in the hypothermic patient and may remain partially inert until rewarming, when it can cause a marked degree of hypertension.

K. Acid-base balance

1. The buffering capacity of the blood is reduced during hypothermia.

2. Alveolar ventilation and the kidney's ability to regulate acid-base disturbances are decreased.

3. The heart is sensitive to low blood pH, which can increase both its irritability and its tendency to ventricular fibrillation; therefore the patient should be hyperventilated to raise the blood pH.

4. The oxygen hemoglobin curve is shifted to the left; therefore the hemoglobin has more affinity for oxygen.

5. On rewarming, there is some metabolic acidosis (mostly lactic acidemia).

L. Hypothermia by use of the heat exchanger

1. **Advantages**

   a. The rate and depth of temperature drop are controlled.

   b. Cooling to the temperature desired is rapid in the heart-lung circuit.

   c. The cooling is not started until the chest is opened and the cardiac condition is confirmed; thus the total period of hypothermia is reduced.

2. **Disadvantages.** The requirements of cannulation of major blood vessels and, usually, an open chest preclude its use in neurosurgery and abdominal surgery.

3. **Principles of bloodstream cooling.** Some form of heat exchange is necessary, together with a coil of plastic tubing, 10–15 ft long, through which the blood circulates.

4. **The methods** of inducing bloodstream cooling include arteriovenous cooling, venovenous cooling, and cooling with the heart-lung machine (cooling coil or heat exchanger).

M. Hypothermia applied to neurosurgical patients

1. **General effects**

   a. The metabolic and oxygen requirements are decreased.

   b. The BP usually falls with induction of anesthesia; then, as cooling starts, a rise in BP is followed by a gradual fall as the body temperature decreases.

2. **Brain**

   a. The intracranial pressure and brain volume are decreased.

   b. The brain's metabolism rate is lowered.

   c. The blood circulation should be restored if there is an increase in delta activity on the EEG.

   d. Occlusion of the middle cerebral artery should be limited to 15 min at 30° C.

   e. The edema due to brain trauma is lessened.

   f. There may be less bleeding during brain surgery.

3. **Indications**

   a. Aneurysmectomy.

   b. Carotid artery surgery in the neck.

   c. Surgery for vascular tumors, such as meningiomas.

N. Induced hypothermia. This technique **may be useful** in the management of (1) severe head injuries, especially brainstem injuries with high fever, coma, tachycardia, tachypnea, and rigidity, (2) acute cerebral vascular accident, and (3) ruptured intracranial aneurysm.

O. Complications of prolonged hypothermia

1. Prolonged hypothermia may mask infection and signs of cerebral compression.

2. There may be pressure necrosis of the skin.

P. Local refrigeration analgesia. This method can be useful for handling severely traumatized limbs that require amputation.

1. The tissues are chilled for about 1 hr; then a tourniquet is applied. The tourniquet must be tight enough so that the tissues distal to the tourniquet are blanched rather than congested.

2. The limb is placed in cracked ice and cooled for 2–3 hr, depending on whether it is an arm or a leg. The limb is placed so that the melting ice will drain away from the bed.

3. The patient is placed on the operating table and the limb is dried. The analgesic effects will last for 1 hr.

4. When the larger vessels have been tied, the tourniquet is released, and adequate hemostasis is obtained.

5. Ulceration of tissues will not occur if actual freezing and excessive pressures are avoided.

6. **Disadvantages.** The labor and time involved in preparing the patient for surgery.

Bibliography

Enderby, G. E. H. (ed.). Symposium on deliberate hypotension. *Postgrad. Med. J.* 50:555, 1974.

Fahmy, N. R., and Laver, M. B. Hemodynamic response to ganglionic blockade with pentolinium during N_2O-halothane anesthesia in man. *Anesthesiology* 44:6, 1976.

Khambatta, H. J., Stone, J. G., and Khan, E. Propranolol alters renin release during nitroprusside-induced hypotension and prevents hypertension on discontinuation of nitroprusside. *Anesth. Analg.* (Cleve.) 60:569, 1981.

Leigh, J. M., and Millar, R. A. (eds.). Symposium on deliberate hypotension in anaesthesia. *Br. J. Anaesth.* 47:743, 1975.

Leighton, K. M., Bruce, C., and MacLeod, B. A. Sodium nitroprusside-induced hypotension and renal blood flow. *Can. Anaesth. Soc. J.* 24:637, 1977.

Rao, T. L. K., Jacobs, K., Salem, M. R., et al. Deliberate hypotension and anesthetic requirements of halothane. *Anesth. Analg.* (Cleve.) 60:513, 1981.

Salem, M. R., Wong, A. Y., Bennett, E. J., et al. Deliberate hypothermia in infants and children. *Anesth. Analg.* (Cleve.) 53:975, 1974.

Skene, D. S., Sullivan, S. F., and Patterson, R. W. Pulmonary shunting and lung volumes during hypotension induced with trimethaphan. *Br. J. Anaesth.* 50:339, 1978.

Snow, J. C., Sideropoulos, H. P., Kripke, B. J., et al. Autonomic hyperreflexia during cystoscopy in patients with high spinal cord injuries. *Paraplegia* 15:327, 1977.

Thompson, G. E., Miller, R. D., Stevens, W. C., et al. Hypotensive anesthesia for total hip arthroplasty. A study of blood loss and organ function (brain, heart, liver and kidney). *Anesthesiology* 48:91, 1978.

Tinker, J. H., and Michenfelder, J. D. Sodium nitroprusside. Pharmacology, toxicology and therapeutics. *Anesthesiology* 45:340, 1976.

Verner, I. R. Sodium nitroprusside. Theory and practice. *Postgrad. Med. J.* 50:576, 1974.

Vesey, C. J., Cole, P. V. Linnell, J. C., et al. Some metabolic effects of sodium nitroprusside in man. *Br. Med. J.* 2:140, 1974.

Wildsmith, J. A. W., Drummond, G. B., and MacRae, W. R. Metabolic effects of induced hypotension with trimethaphan and sodium nitroprusside. *Br. J. Anaesth.* 51:875, 1979.

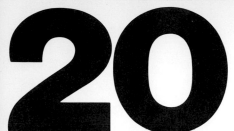

Intravenous Fluid Therapy

I. Objectives of fluid therapy

A. IV fluids are used to restore or maintain the **interior environment** within physiologic limits. It is the anesthesiologist's responsibility to assess the preoperative and intraoperative fluid losses and to plan replacement of crystalloid, colloid, and blood elements that become deficient while the patient is under his care.

B. There are no readily available simple, accurate means to make this assessment. **Multiple observations** of the patient's body functions and general appearance are needed to provide, at best, an educated guess as to the patient's needs.

II. Preoperative assessment

A. History

1. **A careful history of the present illness** should include changes in weight, body functions, and intake and output during the illness.

2. **Medications.** Determine whether the patient has been taking any medications that would alter renal function, such as diuretics, or is a chronic user of antacids or laxatives that alter bowel absorption. Certain antibiotics, such as neomycin, also alter bowel absorption and the formation of precursors to vitamin K. The use of drugs that affect coagulation should be determined before surgery, and steps should be taken to correct clotting times. The patient's use of medications that affect metabolism, water and electrolyte balance, and the elements of blood production should be known and their effects anticipated.

B. Physical examination

1. Central nervous system

a. **Abnormalities in water and electrolytes** can alter the sensorium and muscle strength.

b. Patients on IV fluids for more than 24 hr with no sodium may begin to show signs of **hyponatremia,** such as lethargy and mental confusion.

c. The CNS symptoms in hyponatremia, water intoxication, hypokalemia, and diabetic hyperglycemia may be similar. **Differentiation** is made by the history and laboratory findings.

2. Vital signs

a. Blood pressure

(1) Unless the volume deficit is sudden, there may be no change in BP. Narrowing of the pulse pressure may indicate slowly occurring fluid deficits.

(2) BP is maintained by peripheral vasoconstriction; the skin may appear mottled because of the body's attempt to preserve flow to vital organs.

(3) A drop in BP indicates rapid volume loss.

b. **Heart rate.** Tachycardia is very common in hypovolemic patients.

c. **Heart sounds**

(1) In hypovolemia, heart sounds change even before changes in BP.

(2) Especially under anesthesia, the heart sounds become muffled, more distant.

d. **Temperature**

(1) Temperature variations are the result of many factors, including ambient temperature, a disease process, and circulatory function.

(2) Pure hypovolemia will cause an elevation in temperature secondary to the peripheral vasoconstriction.

e. **Respiration.** Rate and depth will vary with the cause of the fluid and electrolyte disturbances.

3. **Skin**

a. In the acutely hypovolemic patient, the skin may appear mottled and feel cool to the touch. The core temperature may be elevated.

b. Water and colloid changes will cause alterations in the skin turgor.

c. Overhydration or low colloids will cause dependent edema.

d. Hypovolemia secondary to water loss without electrolyte deficits will produce thirst, furrows in the tongue, and folds in the skin if there is moderate dehydration, and sunken eyes in severe dehydration. When dehydration is severe, the patient is usually in shock.

C. **Laboratory tests**

1. **Serial sodium, potassium,** chloride, blood urea nitrogen, and creatinine determination will aid in the diagnosis of hypovolemia or hypervolemia.

2. **Hematocrit changes** will reflect changes in both blood volume and extracellular volume.

3. **Urinalysis**

a. **Specific gravity values** will provide information about the kidney's ability or need to concentrate urine. High concentration and low urine output, when previously kidney function was normal, is evidence of hypovolemia.

b. **Sugar in the urine** may be present in diabetic patients, in patients receiving glucose solutions IV at rapid rates, or, especially, in **elderly** patients receiving IV glucose. The elderly patient's kidney may have a lowered glucose threshold and spill sugar at lower blood levels than the normal 175 mg/100 ml. Glucose may act as an osmotic diuretic, contributing to water loss without electrolyte loss.

4. **ECG**

a. The ECG reflects serum levels of **potassium and calcium.**

b. **Changes in potassium concentrations are:**

(1) **Hyperkalemia**

(a) The P wave flattens down.

(b) The QRS complex widens.

(c) The T wave becomes peaked.

(2) **Hypokalemia**

(a) The T wave becomes flat or inverted.

(b) There is a U wave.

c. **Changes in calcium alterations**

(1) **In hypercalcemia,** the Q–T interval shortens.

(2) **In hypocalcemia,** the Q–T interval becomes prolonged.

5. **Blood volume determination**

a. Blood volume determination requires an isotope tracer technique or dye dilution, using methods that tag the albumin fraction of the red cell.

b. The methods are reasonably accurate within 10% of actual volumes as measured by more precise techniques of research laboratories.

c. The determinations are useful only if there is no active bleeding at the time the measurements are made.

6. **Serum proteins,** when less than 5 gm/100 ml, will lead to peripheral edema, which must be distinguished from congestive heart failure and hypervolemia secondary to excess water.

III. Normal values and minimum daily requirements

A. Blood

1. Blood volume 75–80 ml/kg.
2. Hematocrit Male 42–50%.
Female 40–48%.

B. Normal blood values

1. Sodium 136–145 mEq/L.
2. Potassium 3.5–5 mEq/L.
3. Calcium 8.5–10.5 mg/100 ml.
4. Chloride 100–106 mEq/L.
5. Blood urea nitrogen 8–25 mg/100 ml.
6. Creatinine 0.7–1.5 mg/100 ml.
7. Serum proteins 6–8 g/100 ml.
   a. Albumin 4–5 g/100 ml.
   b. Globulin 2–3 g/100 ml.
8. Glucose (fasting) 70–100 mg/100 ml.

C. **Daily maintenance requirements** for the normal 70-kg adult are:

1. Water 3000 ml.
2. Sodium 77–102 mEq (4.5–6 g NaCl).
3. Potassium 52–78 mEq (4–6 g KCl).
4. Calories 25 cal/kg (at bed rest).

IV. Calculating deficits

A. **Measured differences between intake, output, and daily requirements** will aid in determining whether there is a preoperative deficit.

B. **If intakes and outputs are not available,** subtract from the preillness and current weight difference, 0.5 kg/day catabolic losses per day of fasting; the difference obtained may be regarded as a water deficit. In the normal adult subject, 60% of the body mass is water. Therefore weight loss after subtracting for catabolism gives a reasonable guide for fluid losses.

C. **To calculate electrolyte needs,** only a rough approximation is possible because there is currently no method to measure total body electrolytes; serum levels may not reflect true losses.

1. **If electrolyte values are low,** to calculate replacement, the following formula is helpful: normal value minus the patient's value times the patient's weight in kilograms times 60% equals the number of milliequivalents the patient is behind.

   Example: Patient's sodium 120 mEq
   Body weight 50 kg
   Normal sodium 140 mEq
   (140 − 120 × 50 × 0.6 = 600 mEq deficit)

2. **If the patient has a higher value,** this reflects water loss.
3. **Potassium levels** do not reflect the state of potassium stored in the body. Severe depletion may be present with low-normal serum potassium levels.

V. Common causes of fluid and electrolyte imbalances

A. Volume depletion (water and sodium)

1. Gastrointestinal losses

- **a.** Diarrhea.
- **b.** Vomiting.
- **c.** Bowel fistulas (colostomy, ileostomy).
- **d.** Gastric or small-bowel drainage (T-tubes).

2. Renal losses

- **a.** Diuretics.
- **b.** Osmotic diuresis.
- **c.** Chronic renal failure.
- **d.** Adrenal insufficiency.
- **e.** Postobstructive nephropathy.
- **f.** Diuretic phase of acute tubular necrosis.

3. Skin losses

- **a.** Burns.
- **b.** Sweating.

4. Third-space losses

- **a.** Ascites.
- **b.** Free fluid in the bowel.
- **c.** Interstitial edema.

B. Causes of potassium deficiency

1. Renal

a. Diuretics

- **(1)** Mercurials.
- **(2)** Ethacrynic acid.
- **(3)** Thiazides.
- **(4)** Furosemide.
- **(5)** Carbonic anhydrase inhibitors.

b. Renal disease

c. Adrenal steroids

- **(1)** Adrenal steroid therapy.

(2) Cushing's syndrome.

(3) Aldosteronism.

2. **Extrarenal**

a. Vomiting.

b. Gastric drainage.

c. Diarrhea.

C. **Water and electrolyte losses in gastrointestinal secretions**

Origin	Na^+	K^+ (in mEq per 1000 ml)	Cl^-	Water (ml/24 hr)
Stomach	60	9	84	2500
Small bowel (suction)	110	5	104	3000
Ileostomy (recent)	130	11	116	100–4000
Ileostomy (adapted)	46	3	21	100–500
Cecostomy	52	8	43	100–3000
Bile	149	5	100	700–1000
Pancreatic juice	141	5	77	1000

D. **Skin losses**

1. Normal losses from the skin: water, 350 ml/day; sodium, 10–60 mEq/day.

2. Loss/day/°C fever: water, 500 ml (maximum 4000 ml/hr); sodium, maximum 300 mEq/hr.

VI. **Replacement therapy**

A. **The normal surgical patient** requires 2000 ml of fluid. This may be administered as a solution of 5% dextrose in 0.5% NaCl for half the maintenance fluid, with the remainder given as 5% D/W.

1. **Surgical patients** usually fast from midnight of the day scheduled for the surgery. Fluid requirements should be figured starting with the time of fasting in the patient for elective surgery who is otherwise in good health.

2. If there is sufficient raw surface exposed during the surgical procedure, or if the procedure is prolonged under general anesthetics, **fluid losses due to evaporation** from the surface and losses because of inhalation of the dry anesthetic gases should be calculated into the maintenance requirements. Antidiuretic hormone secretion is usually elevated during the surgical procedure and early postoperative period. Water should be given with this in mind.

3. **Various electrolyte solutions** are favored in different medical centers. In the healthy patient scheduled for elective surgery, the choice of fluid therapy during the intraoperative period may be any fluid that fulfills the maintenance requirements for water and sodium.

B. **Replacement of preexisting losses**

1. **The dehydrated and salt-deficient patient** presents a serious operative risk. Partial replacement of preexisting losses should be attempted whenever possible.

2. **Restoration of plasma volume** and improvement of renal function are primary objectives.

3. **In the patient with serious dehydration and salt depletion,** it may be necessary to give 5–10 ml/kg/hr for the first 1–2 hr of a replacement solution of 0.45% NaCl, 0.33% NaCl in water, or the salt solution in 5% D/W. Hydration will be adequate to begin surgery when the **urine output is about 50 ml/hr.**

Surgery should not be started without attempts to rehydrate unless the delay in commencing surgery will further increase the threat of death or loss of a limb. In such a situation, rehydration must be vigorous during surgery.

4. **Profound collapse** of the seriously dehydrated, salt-deficient patient may be anticipated when anesthesia is attempted.

5. **To gauge the patient's response to fluid therapy during anesthesia correctly,** a central venous pressure (CVP) line is required; a Swan-Ganz catheter can be used if it is available. The Swan-Ganz catheter is preferable because it allows monitoring of both right and left heart functions and cardiac output if a thermistor is incorporated. The CVP will indicate if the fluid load is exceeding the right heart's functional capacity. If 100 ml of fluid is administered rapidly and the CVP remains elevated longer than 5 min after cessation of fluid administration, the patient is approaching right heart failure, and additional fluids should be administered slowly.

6. **The patient should be catheterized,** and urine volume should be measured hourly.

7. If it is not possible to have a CVP line or a Swan-Ganz catheter, **an esophageal stethoscope** may be used to detect pulmonary edema. **Signs of pulmonary edema under anesthesia** may be the development of rales and rhonchi if these were not present previously. There may be an increased resistance to controlled ventilation as circulatory overload develops. Should fluid therapy be excessive, small doses of ethacrynic acid or furosemide may be given, but with caution, since they may provide a brisk diuresis of such magnitude as to bring the patient to the verge of circulatory collapse.

8. In addition to crystalloid replacement, about one-fourth of the fluid deficit can be given as colloid. **Albumin preparations** are useful. In their absence, **low molecular weight dextrans** may be used. Allergic reactions to the dextrans are uncommon, but the possibility must be kept in mind.

9. **Correction of hyperkalemia** may be accomplished by using **1 unit of regular insulin per 1 g of dextrose IV.** If time permits, potassium chelating agents may be administered rectally.

C. The acutely burned patient

1. **The anesthesiologist** may be involved in the acute resuscitation and subsequent care. Proper management during the first 48 hr may be lifesaving.

2. **Large volumes of fluids** are lost through burned surfaces. The fluid shift to the burned area occurs rapidly in the first 8 hr after the burn, peaking in the first 24–48 hr. It is desirable to replace the fluid at the same rate as it is lost to avoid oligemic shock and renal insufficiency. Fluid needs are calculated on the basis of the extent and depth of the burn and body weight.

3. **The rule of nines.** The extent of burn is expressed as a percentage of body surface. The body is divided into parts that correspond to 9% of the surface or multiples thereof.

Area	Adults	Infants or Young Children
Whole head	9%	18%
Each upper limb	9%	9%
Front of trunk	18%	18%
Back of trunk	18%	18%
Each lower limb	18%	14%
Perineum	1%	1%

4. **Two widely used formulas for replacement** in burn patients are the Evans and the Brook Army Hospital formulas.
   a. **Evans formula**
      (1) 50% colloids.
      (2) 50% lactated Ringer's solution.
   b. **Brook Army Hospital formula**
      (1) 75% of the calculated volume should be lactated Ringer's solution.
      (2) 25% colloids.
         (a) 10–15 ml/kg should be whole blood.
         (b) The remainder of the calculated colloids can be plasma or albumin.
         (c) Blood should be given after the first 8 hr of injury.
   c. In addition to the preceding solutions, the normal insensible fluid losses should be replaced by dextrose in water.
5. **Calculating the total fluids needed per day** is done by multiplying the preinjury weight of the patient in kilograms times the percentage of body burned times 2.

   Example: The patient weighs 70 kg and has a 20% burn: $70 \times 20 \times 2 = 2800$ ml of fluids required above normal daily requirements. The 2800 ml should be given according to one of the preceding formulas.
6. **The adequacy of replacement** may be determined by the urine output and hematocrit. It is desirable to have a urine output of at least 50 ml/hr and not more than 100 ml/hr. When output exceeds the latter figure, decrease the rate of fluid administration. **Hematocrit values** are a useful guide to plasma volume. A hematocrit of greater than 45% suggests a low plasma volume, which can be corrected by giving additional albumin or plasma.
7. **The "rules" of fluid therapy** are meant only to serve as guidelines. Hourly assessments of the burned patient must be made and fluid therapy adjusted to meet the patient's changing needs.
8. **Should acidosis develop,** about one-third of the lactated Ringer's solution should be replaced by 1-molar sodium lactate solution diluted with an equal volume of 5% D/W.

D. **Standard surgical procedures**

1. **Recommended fluid replacement** during routine surgery in healthy patients is 1.5 ml/kg/hr in adults, 3 ml/kg/hr in children, and 6 ml/kg/hr in infants.
2. **The simplest method of judging blood loss** that is reasonably accurate is **measuring blood lost into the suction bottles and weighing the surgical sponges.**
3. **Weigh all types of sponges** to be used during the procedure, measuring both dry and wet weights. A dietetic gram scale is ideal and inexpensive. **If a dry sponge is used,** weigh it after it has been thrown off the field. Subtract the dry weight from the used weight. The difference in grams is the amount of blood it contains, or the milliliters of blood lost. **If the surgeon uses wet sponges,** substitute the preoperative wet weight for the dry weight.
4. **If there is ascitic fluid,** colloids may be used to replace the lost volume; measure in a similar manner. The vigorousness of colloid replacement will depend on the patient's response to the sudden loss of fluid. A drop in pres-

sure or a sudden tachycardia will require infusion of albumin or fresh-frozen plasma if available.

5. **When irrigation fluids are used,** the scrub nurse should be asked to keep track of the amount and make the necessary calculations to exclude this from the measured protein and blood losses.
6. **Blood replacement in infants** should be milliliter for milliliter. Infants tolerate volume losses poorly. **Larger children and adults,** depending on their preoperative hematocrit, will need replacement of whole blood when 15–20% of their blood volume is lost.
   a. **Blood volume can be calculated** approximately by multiplying body weight in kilograms by 75.
   b. **A patient with a low hematocrit** for his or her age may need packed cells in addition to replacement of acute losses.
   c. **It is desirable** to have all existing blood deficits replaced at least 24 hr before surgery, rather than try to catch up on the day of surgery. This will allow time for cardiovascular adjustments under the most desirable conditions.

E. Massive transfusions

1. **Massive transfusion** may be defined as replacement of over half the patient's calculated blood volume in less than 24 hr.
2. **Blood loss** may be replaced with whole blood or with components of whole blood. **Blood components** are available as fresh-frozen preparations and washed red cells, and they have the advantage of tailoring the component replaced to the patient's specific needs.
3. **Citrate-phosphate-dextrose (CPD) bank blood** is the most commonly available form. Its disadvantage is the deterioration of the components with age, so using large amounts of whole bank blood may cause clotting deficiencies and significantly alter the oxygen-carrying capacity of the red cells.
4. **It is desirable to use 1 unit of fresh-frozen plasma** or fresh-frozen whole blood after 4–5 units of CPD blood. **Using blood components** reduces the incidence of transfusion reactions by eliminating the **white cell,** a common source of mild transfusion reactions.
5. **Fresh-frozen plasma** contains all the clotting elements except platelets. **Thrombocytopenia occurs after transfusion of 20–30 units of bank blood.** Platelet counts should be done after each 15 units replaced. **Fresh blood** had viable platelets in sufficient concentration for 5 hr. Only 2% of the platelets are viable after 48 hr.
6. **Clotting factors V and VIII** are decreased in ACD blood. Factor V is at 20% of normal concentration after 21 days. Factor VIII concentration is at 50% of normal after 21 days. For adequate clotting, the patient's blood levels of factor V should not be less than 5% of normal and blood levels of factor VIII, not less than 20% of normal.
   a. **Clotting factors** can be consumed by tissue trauma and acute coagulopathies.
   b. **The partial thromboplastin test** measures these factors and should be used as a monitor to determine the need for the replacement of factors V and VIII.
7. **The citrate in bank blood** can be metabolized at an infusion rate of 500 ml/5 min before calcium levels begin to fall. This rate decreases in shock and in the presence of liver disease. If calcium is to be administered to counteract

the citrate intoxication, it should not be given at a rate greater than 100 mg/5 min.

8. **Stored blood has high levels of potassium,** and should ECG changes occur secondary to serum elevation of potassium, they may be treated by using **1 unit of regular insulin per gram of dextrose in water** to lower the serum potassium by transferring it into the cell. An alternative method, if renal function is present, is to use **furosemide or ethacrynic acid** as directed in the package insert. There may be massive water loss and cardiovascular collapse secondary to sudden hypovolemia from the brisk diuresis that follows administration of these drugs. Fluids must be pushed to prevent this occurrence.
9. **Stored blood contains cellular debris,** and the lungs are the physiologic filter for this debris. To prevent shock lung syndrome, the blood should be filtered through **micropore membrane filters**. There are many suitable types on the market. The membrane filters on the traditional blood-transfusion set should not be used for more than 2 units of blood.
10. **Hypothermia** caused by rapid transfusion of massive amounts of cold stored blood in a short period of time may cause serious cardiac arrhythmias. To prevent this, **the transfused blood should be passed through a warmer.** A simple, inexpensive method is to **add a blood-warming coil** to the IV line. The coil is placed in a bucket and warm water is added as needed to keep the water temperature at 27°–38° C. The water temperature can be monitored by a thermometer.

F. **Patients with known kidney failure or those on dialysis** should be treated in consultation with their nephrologist. Patients with chronic renal failure will know their daily water allowance. Their fluid replacement should be adjusted to their usual needs, and their regimen added to only according to measured and calculated losses. **Do not add potassium to their fluids** unless directed to do so by their nephrologist.

Bibliography

Aronson, H. B., Horne, T., Blondheim, S. H., et al. Blood viscosity and the overnight fast. *Can. Anaesth. Soc. J.* 27:550, 1980.

Gabow, P. A., Anderson, R. J., and Schrier, R. W. Acute renal failure. *Cardiovasc. Med.* 2:1161, 1977.

Levinsky, N. G. Pathophysiology of acute renal failure. *N. Engl. J. Med.* 296:1453, 1977.

Merin, R. G. New implications of fasting. *Anesthesiology* 48:236, 1978.

Shires, G. T., and Canizaro, P. C. Fluid, Electrolyte, and Nutritional Management of the Surgical Patient. In S. I. Schwartz (Ed.), *Principles of Surgery*. New York: McGraw-Hill, 1974. Chap. 2.

Wilkinson, A. W. (Ed.). *Body Fluids in Surgery*. New York: Longman, 1974.

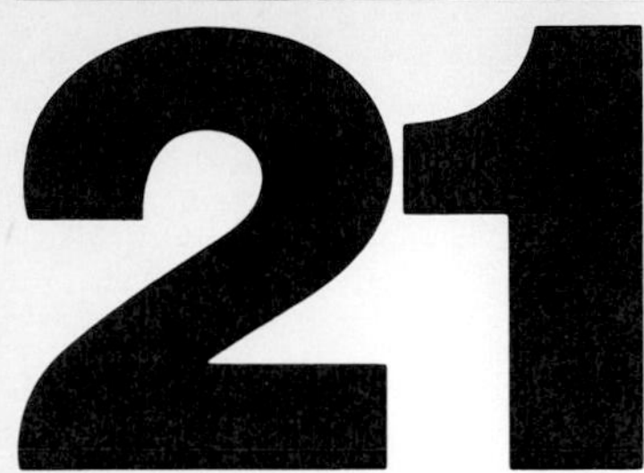

Blood Transfusions

I. General considerations

A. Stored, refrigerated blood (4° C) is administered to surgical patients to improve the oxygen-carrying capacity of the patient's blood and to maintain the circulating blood volume.

B. Following acute blood loss, blood volume can be maintained by adequate administration of **whole blood or plasma volume expanders,** such as albumin, dextran, and balanced electrolyte solutions.

1. **Albumin or plasma protein solutions** are as effective as blood for simple volume expansion. They are readily produced in quantity, and they do not transmit hepatitis or cause hemolytic transfusion reactions.
2. **Dextran** is available for blood volume expansion in two molecular weights, 40,000 and 70,000. It is associated with **reactions,** including clotting disorders and allergic reactions. In addition, blood for blood typing and cross matching should be obtained before dextran infusion, because dextran causes marked rouleau formation, which interferes with blood typing and cross matching.
3. **The quantity of electrolyte solutions** (such as physiologic saline and lactated Ringer's solution) required to maintain the intravascular volume is 3 to 4 times the volume of the blood lost.
4. Blood volume loss **cannot be made up by 5% D/W,** because it is dissipated rapidly into the urine and interstitial spaces. Infusion of large amounts of 5% D/W can lead to **water intoxication** (vomiting, hypothermia, convulsions, and coma leading to death).

C. For blood transfusions

1. An 18-gauge (or better, a 16-gauge) IV plastic catheter is satisfactory for blood transfusion. For rapid, massive transfusions, one or two 16-gauge plastic catheters are preferable.
2. **Banked blood** is stored at 4° C and should be warmed before transfusion to decrease the incidence of heart arrhythmias and prevent lowering of the patient's temperature.
3. **Medications should never be added** to the blood used in transfusions or to solutions in immediate contact with it.
4. **Fluids intended to precede or follow** blood transfusion in the infusion set should be isotonic **without calcium** (calcium will clot citrated blood).
   a. **Physiologic saline** (0.9%) and balanced electrolyte solutions are the only solutions that can precede or follow blood transfusion.
   b. **Dextrose 5% in water** will clump red blood cells and on prolonged contact will injure them.
5. **Blood left out of the refrigerator** for more than 30 min should not be used for transfusion.

II. The blood groups

A. The A, B, AB, and O groups. The blood from different individuals is classified in four principal groups on the basis of A and B antigen (agglutinogen) in their red cells. These groups are called A, B, AB, and O. The antibodies (agglutinins) in the serum are anti-B for group A, anti-A for group B, none for group AB, and anti-A and anti-B for group O.

1. **ABO grouping** is the most significant system used for blood transfusion. **The donor's antigen group** in the red cells and **the recipient's antibody group** in the serum are the important criteria.
2. **During transfusion,** the transfused red cells, which contain corresponding antigen for the patient's antibody group, may be rapidly destroyed, leading to serious complications.

B. The Rh factor

1. **The Rh factor is an inherited trait** based on a division of individuals into Rh-positive and Rh-negative categories, according to their reactions to an anti-Rh serum.
2. **First transfusion.** A patient with Rh-negative blood transfused with Rh-positive blood for the first time will not show any clinical response, but this first transfusion will cause a sensitizing effect. The antibody will be fully developed within 8 weeks.
3. **Second transfusion.** Once anti-Rh is produced, the titer begins to rise within 2 days following the second transfusion and may reach a peak within 7 days.
4. **The severity of the reaction** is increased with each succeeding transfusion of Rh-incompatible blood.
5. **Signs and symptoms**
   - **a.** Chills, fever, and transient hemoglobinemia.
   - **b.** Flushing of the face, distention of the neck veins, hypotension, and vascular depression.

C. Other blood groups. Blood groups other than ABO and Rh play smaller roles in hemolytic transfusion reactions. These are MN, P, Ss, Lutheran, Kell, Lewis, Duffy, Kidd, and Vel.

D. Blood typing and cross matching are performed to identify any antibodies in the recipient's serum that will react with blood group antigen in the donor's blood cells.

III. Normal blood values

pH 7.4

Blood volume 75–80 ml/kg

Hemoglobin Male 13–16 g/100 ml
Female 12–15 g/100 ml

Hematocrit Male 42–50%
Female 40–48%

Red blood cells 5,000,000/mm^3

White blood cells 8,000/mm^3

Platelets 200,000–350,000/mm^3

IV. Bank blood

A. Composition of bank blood

1. **One unit (500 ml)** of refrigerated (4° C) whole blood in citrate-phosphate-dextrose (CPD) solution contains 450 ml of human blood plus 63 ml of the anticoagulant CPD solution.

2. **CPD solution** is superior to acid-citrate-dextrose (ACD) solution for the preservation of bank blood. The CPD anticoagulant solution is both satisfactory and safe, and it offers significant advantages over the ACD solution.

3. **The following altered values** are seen in 14-day-old stored blood preserved in CPD and ACD solution:

Component	CPD	ACD
pH	6.9	6.7
Hemoglobin	21	35
Potassium (mEq/L)	20	29
2,3-DPG (microgram per gram of Hgb)	7 (40% of normal)	3.5 (10% of normal)
Viable RBC (%)	85	85

4. Blood transfused later than 28 days after its withdrawal from a donor undergoes a great decrease in the number of surviving RBCs. As a general rule, **blood should be infused within 21 days** of withdrawal.

5. **Advantages of CPD-preserved whole blood**
   a. Maintains a higher pH, a lower potassium level, and a higher 2,3-diphosphoglycerate (2,3-DPG) level in stored blood than in ACD-preserved blood.
   b. Maintains a better functional state and longer erythrocyte survival time.
   c. Maintains a higher level of 2,3-DPG when stored in the refrigerator, so there is better oxygenation of the tissues.

6. **All coagulation factors** except platelets and factors V (proaccelerin) and VIII (antihemophilic globulin) are present in stored blood.

B. Heparin

1. Blood is collected in heparin only for special use, such as in extracorporeal circulation.
2. Blood collected in heparin has a fast rate of glycolysis and deterioration. It may be administered safely for only 48 hr after collection.

C. Blood components. Whole blood can be separated into its components: packed red cells, fresh plasma, fresh-frozen plasma, platelet-rich plasma, platelet concentrate, cryoprecipitate, and reconstituted whole blood. The advantages of **packed red cells** include both an increase in oxygen-carrying capacity with a minimum of volume expansion and a reduction in sodium, free potassium, excess acids, and ammonia.

D. Other sources of blood

1. **Cadaver blood.** The erythrocytes in cadaver blood have a normal in vivo survival rate; however, the coagulation factors, platelets, and white cells are decreased. Another disadvantage is that usually the autopsy examination has to be completed before the blood can be used.
2. **Frozen glycerinated erythrocytes.** Blood may be frozen and stored for long periods at very low temperatures (−80° to −190° C). The process comprises adding glycerol to freshly collected blood after removing the plasma. The glycerination protects the erythrocytes during the freezing and thawing process.
3. **Autologous banked blood.**

V. Complications

A. Despite the accepted regimens of ABO and Rh testing and the development of increasingly sensitive methods of cross matching, a variety of transfusion reactions continue to occur, with a mortality of about 1 in 3000 recipients. The two main causes of death are serum hepatitis and hemolytic transfusion reactions.

1. In blood transfusions, the most serious complications arise from **human errors,** such as mistaken identity (of blood specimens, blood containers, or recipients). Blood typing and cross matching should be performed by two laboratory technicians working independently, and the administration of blood in the operating room and recovery room should be checked carefully and independently by both the anesthesiologist and another physician or the circulating registered nurse. This is especially important during anesthesia, when transfusion reactions are more difficult to recognize.

2. **Every blood transfusion** should be supervised carefully, and the first 100 ml of blood should be infused slowly to allow early detection of any reactions.

3. **Recognition of a reaction** early in the blood transfusion of an anesthetized patient depends directly on the alert observation of the anesthesiologist or nurse-anesthetist.

B. Immediate reactions

1. **Overloading the circulation** is an occasional complication of blood transfusion, especially in patients with heart disease and chronic anemia and in aged patients. It may occur if blood is given faster than the heart can accept it or is infused in excessive volumes.

   a. **The diagnosis** is established from the presence of left heart failure with acute pulmonary edema. The central venous pressure monitor is useful in the differential diagnosis of congestive heart failure and hypovolemia.

   b. **Therapy of acute pulmonary edema**

      (1) Oxygen is administered under intermittent positive pressure.

      (2) The patient is placed in a semisitting position.

      (3) Tourniquets are placed on the extremities without occlusion of the arterial pulse.

      (4) Calcium, isoproterenol, digitalis (ouabain), morphine, and furosemide are administered.

2. **Allergic reactions,** characterized by urticaria and pruritus, occur in mild form in 1% of transfused patients. Laryngeal edema and bronchial asthma are rare but serious reactions.

   a. The **diagnosis** is made from the skin manifestations.

   b. **Treatment**

      (1) The rate of blood transfusion is decreased (the transfusion is not stopped unless symptoms worsen and fail to respond to therapy).

      (2) Antihistaminics (diphenhydramine 50 mg IM or IV) and corticosteroids (dexamethasone, 8–16 mg IV) are given.

      (3) Patients with known histories of severe allergic reactions should receive prophylactic doses of antihistaminics and corticosteroids and be treated with packed, washed, plasma-free red cells.

      (4) Laryngeal edema and bronchial asthma are treated with epinephrine and corticosteroids.

3. **Hemolytic transfusion reactions**

   a. A hemolytic reaction is a **rare but serious complication,** occurring once in 20,000 transfusions. An intravascular hemolysis takes place; the incompatible donor's red cells are destroyed by antibodies of the recipient's plasma.

b. **As little as 25–50 ml** of the transfused blood may create a major reaction, or as much as 500 ml may be administered before the reaction can be diagnosed.

c. **A serious hemolytic reaction** from mismatched blood carries a mortality of 40% from as little as 200 ml of incompatible blood.

d. **Human error** is frequently involved in such accidents. Incorrect laboratory work and mislabeling or misreading of labels on blood bags or bottles are the usual sources of error.

e. **In the conscious recipient,** the clinical manifestations include chills, fever, flushing of the face, distention of the neck veins, headache, chest and flank pain, nausea, vomiting, tachypnea, tachycardia, hypotension, hemoglobinuria, oliguria, unexplained bleeding, and jaundice.

f. **In the anesthetized or unconscious recipient,** a hemolytic transfusion reaction is manifested by tachycardia, hemoglobinuria, hypotension, sudden increase in bleeding, and, later, jaundice and oliguria. The **diagnosis** is established by recognition of hemoglobinemia and hemoglobinuria.

g. **The major complications** of incompatible blood transfusion and **intravascular hemolysis** are vascular collapse and **acute renal failure,** with signs of oliguria, anuria, and uremia.

h. When a hemolytic reaction is suspected, **the blood transfusion should be discontinued immediately,** and the remaining donor blood, with a fresh sample of the recipient's blood and urine, should be sent to the blood bank for repeat compatibility testing.

i. **Urine samples** may become dark brown to black and may contain hemoglobin, red cells, and casts.

j. **Therapy**

(1) Generous administration of **IV fluids and diuretics,** in excess of 75 ml/hr, for maintenance of urine output.

(a) Mannitol 25%, 25 g IV, followed by an infusion of 40 mEq of sodium bicarbonate.

(b) Furosemide 80 mg IV or ethacrynic acid.

(2) **Hypotension** is treated with lactated Ringer's solution, albumin, and compatible blood. If blood volume is normal and hypotension persists, vasopressors are indicated.

(3) **Oxygen**

(4) In the presence of **anuria,** the patient is treated for acute renal failure. Peritoneal dialysis, hemodialysis, or massive hemodilution using cardiopulmonary bypass under moderate hypothermia (28° – 30° C) is performed when indicated.

4. **Air embolism**

a. **There is danger of air embolism** if blood is given under pressure applied to its surface within the container. This complication has been almost entirely eliminated since the introduction of the disposable plastic blood bag and its pneumatic cuff for rapid transfusion.

b. **Diagnosis** in the anesthetized or unconscious patient includes the mill-wheel murmur, ECG changes, and hypotension.

c. **Therapy** consists of placing the patient on the left side in the head-down position. This will help to trap the air bubbles in the right ventricle and keep them away from the pulmonary outflow tract.

C. Massive blood transfusions. See Chapter 20, section **VI.E.**

1. **In the operating room, massive transfusion** may be defined as the acute administration of more than half the patient's calculated blood volume.

2. **Monitoring.** Patients receiving massive blood transfusions (more than 15 units) require careful monitoring to allow diagnosis of inherent and acquired abnormalities.

   a. An **ECG** to detect changes in calcium or potassium concentration in circulating blood. Treat only when indicated.

   b. **Central venous pressure and urine output per hour.**

   c. **PO_2, Pco_2, and pH** every 5 units of transfused blood, to allow precise bicarbonate infusion.

3. Along with the immediate and late complications of blood transfusion, rapid infusion of large amounts of CPD-stored blood is associated with **the following additional hazards:**

   a. **Hypothermia**

      (1) **Transfusion within 30 min of 5 units of blood** at refrigerator temperatures may decrease body temperature by 4° C.

      (2) **At 33° C, hypothermia** results in metabolic acidosis and depressed cardiac output. Changes in body position or respiration may lead to cardiac arrest.

      (3) **Blood should be prewarmed** when infused very fast and in large quantities. Warming is accomplished by administering the blood through a very long blood-warming plastic coil immersed in water maintained at 37° C. Blood warmed in waterbath units undergoes fewer changes than blood warmed in other types of units.

   b. **Citrate toxicity** is a very rare complication that occurs primarily in patients with severe liver disease or in shock, whose ability to metabolize sodium citrate is decreased. Citrate has a calcium-binding property that results in low calcium levels.

   c. **Hyperpotassemia.** During storage of blood, the potassium content of the erythrocytes decreases, and that of the plasma increases. The plasma potassium may reach 20 mEq/L in 14-day-old CPD-stored blood. When the transfused red cells become reoxygenated, the potassium returns to them, thus decreasing the plasma potassium concentration to the normal level of 3.5–5 mEq/L. Hyperpotassemia very rarely occurs following massive transfusion, so routine prophylactic calcium infusion is not recommended.

   d. **Acidosis.** The pH of 14-day-old CPD- or ACD-banked blood is 6.7–6.9; this acidosis is the result of hypoxia of the red cells during storage. Following transfusion, the hydrogen radicals are returned to the red cells or buffered by the recipient's plasma.

   e. **Coagulopathies**

      (1) **Abnormal bleeding** may be associated with compatible blood transfusion, particularly when large quantities of blood are infused. This bleeding is due to thrombocytopenia and abnormalities of coagulation factors.

      (2) During surgery, a common cause of coagulation defect is **dilutional thrombocytopenia,** which occurs following massive administration of stored blood when the platelet count has reached 50,000–75,000/mm^3. **Therapy** includes administration of platelet concentrates or, if they are not available, freshly drawn blood less than 6 hr old.

(a) Platelet levels can be decreased from a normal 200,000–350,000/mm^3 to below 50,000/mm^3 before the coagulation mechanism is impaired.

(b) **The first 10 units of blood** infused to an adult can be any storage age within a 21-day limit. When using blood stored for more than 21 days, the ratio of 1 unit of freshly collected blood for every 5 units of stored blood should maintain an adequate platelet count.

(3) Following massive transfusion, the patient may be **deficient in factors V and VIII,** which can be restored by infusion of fresh-frozen plasma or fresh blood.

(4) **Disseminated intravascular coagulation** occurs when tissue materials that induce blood coagulation and platelet aggregation are infused into the blood circulation in great quantities. This complication combines thrombosis and bleeding and activates a secondary fibrinolysis. **Therapy** includes heparin. Epsilon-aminocaproic acid is needed for the rare patient with extensive secondary fibrinolysis.

f. **Pulmonary complications.** The stored blood contains clots and debris that increase with the time of storage. During massive transfusion in patients with severe trauma and hemorrhage, pulmonary insufficiency with vascular obstruction may result from the accumulation of undesirable and unfilterable debris in the lungs. These pulmonary microemboli can be prevented by transfusing blood that is as fresh as possible and by using membrane filters with a small pore size (20–40 microns) as compared with 170 microns, the pore size of standard blood filters.

D. Late complications

1. Serum hepatitis

a. **Posttransfusion hepatitis** is a serious complication. It may follow the transfusion of whole blood, plasma, or other products prepared from human blood, such as fibrinogen. **Serum albumin,** which is heated to 60° C for 10 hr during preparation, is thereby rendered noninfectious.

b. With the more refined current methods of **Australia antigen (HAA)** detection, 80% of all posttransfusion hepatitis occurrences can be prevented.

c. There is no proof of the effectiveness of **gamma globulin** in preventing the disease.

2. **Syphilis** may be transmitted by fresh blood from a donor with the disease, but storing the blood for more than 96 hr at 4° C inactivates the spirochetes.

3. **Malaria.** Donors with histories of malaria are rejected. Malaria parasites will survive storage for 3 weeks at 4° C.

4. **Brucellosis** is rarely transmitted by transfusion. For treatment, tetracycline or chloramphenicol is indicated.

Bibliography

Dornette, W. H. L. Jehovah's Witnesses and blood transfusion. *Anesth. Analg.* (Cleve.) 52:272, 1973.

Grindon, A. J. The use of packed red blood cells. *J.A.M.A.* 235:389, 1976.

Hilgard, P. Immunological reactions to blood and blood products. *Br. J. Anaesth.* 51:45, 1979.

Jesch, F., Webber, L. M., Dalton, J. W., et al. Oxygen dissociation after transfusion of blood stored in ACD or CPD solution. *J. Thorac. Cardiovasc. Surg.* 70:35, 1975.

Myrhe, B. A. Fatalities from blood transfusion. *J.A.M.A.* 244:1333, 1980.

Robertson, H. D., and Poll, H. C. Blood transfusions in elective operations: Comparison of whole blood versus packed red cells. *Ann. Surg.* 18:778, 1975.

Schmidt, P. J. Red cells for transfusion. *N. Engl. J. Med.* 299:1411, 1978.

Schmidt, P. J. Transfusion mortality. With special reference to surgical and intensive care facilities. *J. Fla. Med. Assoc.* 67:151, 1980.

Umlas, J. Washed, hyperpacked, frozen and shelf red blood cells. *Transfusion* 15:111, 1975.

Van der Walt, J. H., and Russell, W. J. Effect of heating on the osmotic fragility of stored blood. *Br. J. Anaesth.* 50:815, 1978.

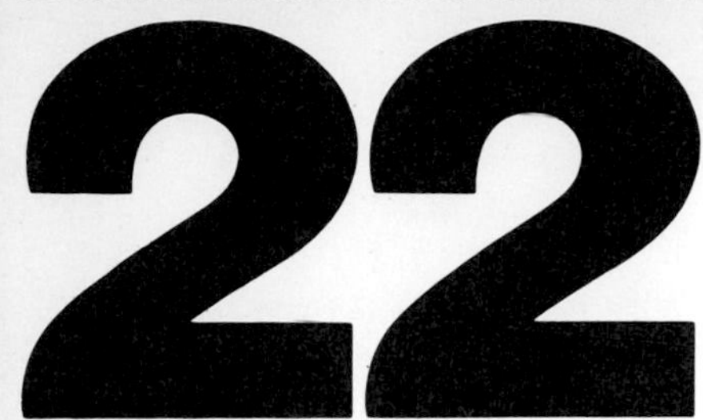

Liver and Anesthesia

I. Physiology

A. Function of the liver

1. Protein synthesis

a. Most of the plasma protein, except the immunoglobulins, is produced by the liver cell (hepatocyte).

b. The liver cell also produces certain carrier proteins and a variety of alpha and beta globulins.

c. In addition, the liver is the site of manufacture of important coagulant factors, such as factor II (prothrombin) and factors V, VII, IX, and X. Except for factor V, all these are dependent on vitamin K for their synthesis.

2. Carbohydrate metabolism

a. The liver is involved in the handling of absorbed monosaccharides (glucose, galactose, and fructose) and in their conversion to glucose and glucose 6-phosphate.

b. The healthy liver contains about 100 g of glycogen, which can be released into the circulation as free glucose (the conversion of glycogen to glucose is made by either phosphorylase or amyloglucosidase).

3. Fat metabolism

a. Neutral fat derived from the diet is oxidized in the liver, releasing adenosine triphosphate as well as producing glycerol and free fatty acids.

b. Free fatty acids are also stored in the liver after conversion to neutral fat. Approximately 5% of the weight of a normal liver is made up of neutral fat.

c. Another important hepatic function is the release of lipoproteins into the circulation. This is effected by the incorporation of protein coupled with neutral fat.

4. Metabolism of bile salt and cholesterol

a. The primary bile acids (cholic and chenodeoxycholic acids) are produced from cholesterol in the liver and excreted in the bile as conjugates.

b. Bile salts are essential for the absorption of dietary fats, cholesterol, and fat-soluble vitamins.

5. Drug metabolism

a. The endoplasmic reticulum is the site of primary drug metabolism. The processes involved are the conversion of lipid-soluble and potentially toxic compounds to harmless water-soluble derivatives, which are excreted in the bile.

b. The basic processes in hepatic drug metabolism are drug hydroxylation, demethylation, dealkylation, and other drug-specific breakdown processes, which are all functions of cytochrome P-450.

c. Conjugation with substances such as glucuronic acid sulfate renders a drug water-soluble for excretion; this function is also largely microsomal.

d. By stimulating the formation of excess cytochrome P-450, one drug can seriously affect the metabolism of others. Drugs that are good inducers of cytochrome P-450 include barbiturates, meprobamate, phenytoin, phenozone, and glutethimide.

e. Other factors that influence the rate of drug metabolism include age, sex, the presence of liver disease, and nutritional status.

B. The excretion of bilirubin. Bilirubin is a waste product of the breakdown of hemes. The principal source of bilirubin is hemoglobin. Linked to serum albumin, bilirubin is transported to the liver, is conjugated there with glucuronic acid, and then is actively excreted into the biliary canaliculi.

C. Hepatic storage. The liver is a major storage site for a variety of substances normally present; these include vitamin B_{12}, copper, iron, and glycogen.

II. Liver and anesthesia

A. In the last 15 years, there has been a renewed interest in **the effects of anesthesia and surgery on the liver,** mainly for two reasons: (1) the controversial matter of the alleged hepatotoxicity of halothane and (2) the discovery that volatile anesthetics are metabolized to a greater extent than had been previously believed.

1. **The biochemical methods** designed to determine the liver's condition, although valuable in differential diagnosis, are less helpful when it comes to screening a normal surgical patient.

2. Another problem is the **large anatomic and functional reserve of the liver,** which enables the organ to regenerate even after gross trauma.

3. **A small degree of liver impairment** may be significant but difficult to detect and, when detected, difficult to interpret. In any case, biochemical tests, radiology, isotope and immunologic studies, and liver biopsy do not necessarily predict or reveal the liver's response to the stress of anesthesia and surgery.

B. Direct hepatotoxic potential of anesthetic drugs. The problem is not merely to look at the direct hepatotoxic potential of anesthetic drugs (regional or general). Many other ill-defined stresses surround anesthesia and operations. Examples of these are hypoxia, hypocapnia and hypercapnia, hypotension, hemorrhage, hepatic hemodynamics, and hypersensitivity. It is also necessary to assess the influence of enzyme induction and protein binding, general health, drug-taking, and nutritional status.

C. The role of the liver in the breakdown of some anesthetics justifies differential consideration and selection of anesthesia in surgical patients with hepatic dysfunction.

1. **The choice of anesthetic drugs** and techniques requires knowledge of liver disease, the role of the liver in detoxification of drugs, and the effect of drugs on the liver.

2. **The anesthesiologist** must make his own preoperative assessment and consult with colleagues to determine the type of liver disease present, the degree of hepatocellular damage or functional disability, and whether other factors are present that may complicate the operation, particularly those that encourage bleeding.

D. Detoxification of drugs

1. When there is **evidence of liver damage,** the organ's ability to break down drugs is likely to be impaired, leading to abnormal patterns of excretion.

2. The actions of both **opiates and barbiturates** are prolonged in patients with severe liver disease. However, intravenous barbiturates depend for their duration of action on redistribution into other nonnervous tissues, so, provided repeated doses are not given, there should be no prolongation of their effect.

E. Cholinesterase

1. **Serum cholinesterase** (pseudocholinesterase) is synthesized in the liver. Its plasma concentration is reduced in patients with hepatocellular damage.

2. The action of **depolarizing muscle relaxants** (succinylcholine) is likely to be prolonged in such patients, but this should not be considered a contraindication for the drug because the possible prolongation of its effect is of short duration.

F. Plasma proteins

1. The first evidence of impaired protein synthesis is usually a fall in **plasma albumin level,** which will encourage formation of ascites and peripheral edema. By contrast, the level of globulins will tend to be raised.

2. **Protein levels** assume particular importance in anesthesia using **drugs that are protein-bound.** The amount of a drug available to exert a pharmacologic effect may be significantly altered if the liver's protein synthesis capability is defective. When protein-binding is decreased, the pharmacologically active fraction of the drug is increased and "unexpected" drug sensitivity may occur.

III. Choice of anesthetic techniques

A. Effects of anesthetic drugs on the liver

1. Where the integrity of liver function is concerned, **important factors** in an anesthetized patient are:

   a. The preoperative preparation (particularly restoration of clotting factors).

   b. Maintenance of an adequate oxygen delivery (avoiding hypoxia and hypotension).

   c. Accurate replacement of blood lost.

2. **The choice of drugs** should take into account both direct hepatotoxicity and effects on hepatic blood flow.

3. **Halothane** has proved relatively harmless to the liver. On the other hand, there are reports suggesting that halothane hepatitis is a real, even if extremely rare, occurrence. In view of this, halothane is probably best avoided during operations on the liver.

4. Of other agents, **methoxyflurane** has been shown to cause changes that suggest it is hepatotoxic. Liver damage has not been reported after clinical doses of **trichloroethylene** or **cyclopropane.**

5. **General anesthetic agents** may seriously influence **splanchnic** (and hence hepatic) **flow,** with untoward effects on the liver.

6. **Hypoxia, hypercapnia,** oligemia, induced hypotension, and vasoconstrictor agents all may cause splanchnic vasoconstriction and reduction in hepatic blood flow.

B. The choice of anesthetic

1. **The choice of drug(s).** The **skill** with which the anesthetic is administered is of more importance than the choice of the individual drug(s) employed.
   a. Generally, one should employ drugs that **are not hepatotoxic** and, whenever possible, that do not depend on the liver for their degradation.
   b. A conventional technique, using **nitrous oxide and relaxant drugs** with occasional analgesic supplements, is recommended.
2. **Preoperative medication** in a conscious patient may consist of 10 mg of diazepam given IM 1 hr before surgery and 0.5 mg of atropine given IV before induction of anesthesia.
3. **Induction of anesthesia** with an inhalation agent, a sleep dose of a barbiturate, or a nonbarbiturate agent IV is usually followed by succinylcholine injection, which permits a quick, safer endotracheal intubation, particularly in a patient whose stomach is not empty.
   a. The risk of **prolonged apnea** due to low plasma cholinesterase levels is not significant, especially in operations that last a considerable amount of time.
   b. **If succinylcholine is to be avoided,** a nondepolarizing muscle relaxant may be used to facilitate intubation.
4. **Anesthesia is maintained** with a muscle relaxant, nitrous oxide, and oxygen.
   a. **Tubocurarine** is protein-bound, so higher than average doses may be required.
   b. **Pancuronium** does not appear to be affected by liver disease and does not induce hypotension, so it is regarded as the relaxant agent of choice.
   c. When necessary, supplementation by intermittent small doses of an **analgesic** or a low concentration of an inhalation agent may be used.
5. **Mechanical ventilation,** producing a moderate respiratory alkalosis, ensures adequate oxygenation and helps to maintain a normal pH in the face of metabolic acidosis (see sec. **IV.A.2**). Mechanical ventilation causes **minimal disturbance** to the circulation and ensures a satisfactory distribution of cardiac output.
6. **Local or regional anesthesia** may be preferred in some patients, but in either case meticulous attention to details is essential. Early detection of changes by physiologic and biochemical monitoring is very important.

IV. Operations for liver transplantation

A. Patients receiving liver transplants present **special problems** to the anesthesiologist, both during the operation and in the postoperative period. The main problems are:

1. **Circulatory changes**
   a. There may be **heavy bleeding** from engorged anastomotic vessels in patients with portal hypertension and cirrhosis or in case of clotting deficiencies.
   b. When the inferior vena cava is clamped, venous return flow will be reduced by one-half, which will lead to a fall in cardiac output.
   c. The fall in blood pressure can be prevented by adequate blood transfusion. The arterial and venous pressures return to normal when the grafted liver is revascularized.

2. Acid-base changes

a. In such operations, the development of **metabolic acidosis** is due to different factors:

(1) The administration of massive blood transfusions (fresh blood is preferred).

(2) The clamping of the inferior vena cava. The stagnation of the blood will encourage anaerobic metabolism, with the production of organic acids.

(3) The donor liver itself, which contains perfusate that has equilibrated with the intracellular pH of about 6.9.

b. To deal with metabolic acidosis, **sodium bicarbonate** should be given.

c. After the **revascularization** of the new liver, **metabolic alkalosis** develops in most patients, presumably because of the metabolism of lactate and citrate. The metabolic alkalosis may persist during the postoperative period.

3. Changes in glucose levels

a. Because the body's main carbohydrate store is the glycogen of the liver, it is to be expected that during the anhepatic period there is some fall in the glucose level.

b. It is necessary to give glucose IV in the later stages of the operation and in the postoperative period.

4. Changes in serum potassium

a. In the early part of the operation, a general rise in potassium concentration in plasma is seen. This is caused by:

(1) High potassium concentration in stored blood.

(2) The potassium leaks from the hepatic cells to the perfusate during the preservation of the donor liver.

b. Later, there is a fall in potassium concentration, probably due to:

(1) Reabsorption into the liver.

(2) Metabolic alkalosis, which encourages the uptake of potassium into cells.

5. Temperature changes

a. The ice-cold donor liver, at the time of insertion, is warmed by the patient's body, producing a limited fall in the patient's body temperature.

b. A warming blanket may be used to keep the patient's temperature normal.

B. The postoperative period

1. Patients who have undergone liver transplantation must receive care in an intensive care unit. Monitoring of the ECG and arterial and venous pressures is continued; measurements of blood gases, glucose, and electrolytes are made frequently; and records are kept for respiration, blood loss, and fluid balance.

2. The most notable changes during this period involve the acid-base state and serum glucose and potassium levels.

Bibliography

Duvaldestin, P., Agoston, S., Henzel, D., et al. Pancuronium pharmacokinetics in patients with liver cirrhosis. *Br. J. Anaesth.* 50:1131, 1978.

Nagel, E. Post anesthesia liver dysfunction. *Anesthesiology* 47:535, 1977.

Strunin, L. Preoperative assessment of the patient with liver dysfunction. *Br. J. Anaesth.* 50:25, 1978.

Wark, H. J., Clifton, B., and Bookallil, M. J. Halothane hepatitis revisited in women undergoing treatment of carcinoma of the cervix. *Br. J. Anaesth.* 51:763, 1979.

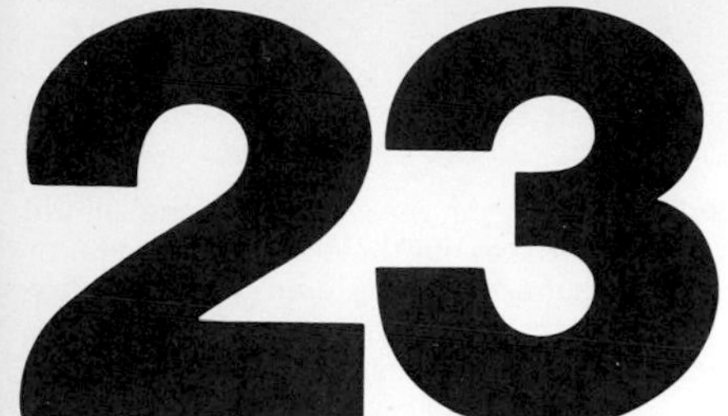

The Recovery Room and Intensive Care Unit

I. The recovery room

A. The recovery room is an essential part of hospital care that must be considered an extension of the operating room. It is ordinarily open during the day, but in a few hospitals the recovery room is prepared to keep patients overnight.

1. **The purpose of the recovery room** is to permit close, careful observation of surgical patients recovering from the immediate effects of the anesthetic drugs. This is necessary because, during the recovery period, the patient's normal protective mechanisms may be obtunded, and the sensorium is clouded.
2. **The specialized care** available in the recovery room has significantly decreased postoperative complications and mortality.
3. **Hospital personnel,** supplies, instruments, and machines are utilized more effectively in conjunction with the recovery room.
4. **It provides an excellent opportunity for study** and therapy of postanesthesia complications, because of the availability of hospital personnel and laboratory facilities.

B. The recovery room is located immediately adjacent to the operating room area and connects directly with one of the corridors leading from the operating rooms. This direct access route, avoiding the corridor and elevator lobby frequented by visitors, permits the recovery room to be kept at the same high level of cleanliness as the operating rooms. In addition, this arrangement offers a time-saving convenience to surgeons, nurse-anesthetists, and anesthesiologists.

C. In most hospitals, the ratio of 1½ recovery room litters for each operating room is adequate. **Separation of sexes** is not needed, since patients are not conscious of their surroundings until just before they are ready to be transferred to their rooms. However, movable curtains can be used to isolate patients who want privacy.

D. The medical supervision of patients in the recovery room is the responsibility of the department of anesthesiology. The recovery room is staffed by well-trained, skilled nurses; it is under the nurses' constant supervision, and an anesthesiologist is available at all times. The members of the recovery room staff must not be rotated to other parts of the hospital. Attendants, nurses' aides, and practical nurses may offer very useful services.

E. One nurse for every three patients is an adequate arrangement. However, more nurses are required when there are many high-risk patients. Well-trained practical nurses and nurses' aides may be used to supplement the staff of registered nurses.

F. Length of stay and discharge

1. **The anesthesiologist decides** the length of the patient's stay in the recovery room and the time of return to the hospital room. Each patient stays in

the recovery room until full consciousness is regained, reflexes have returned, the effects of the local anesthetic drug have been reversed, and the vital signs are stable.

2. **When the patient is ready for discharge** from the recovery room, he should be fully oriented, with stable vital signs. Excessive bleeding, drainage, or discharge should be under control. Records must be completed, with all information stated clearly, before the patient's transfer. A patient should not be discharged from the recovery room until an anesthesiologist has signed a release.

G. Supplies and equipment

1. **The installed equipment** includes central piping outlets for suction and oxygen. At every patient's location, there are outlets for oxygen and suction, a wall-mounted mercury manometer for recording BP, an electrocardioscope, adequate electrical outlets, supports for IV solutions, and a supply of disposable suction and oxygen catheters, syringes, and needles. Sufficient lighting, air conditioning, and a minimum of two telephones for the room are essential. The nurses must have a call system for summoning additional help.

2. **Other equipment and supplies** in the recovery room include:

   a. Equipment for assessment and treatment of **ventilatory inadequacy:** a self-inflating bag and masks, transparent masks, respirometers, nasopharyngeal airways, oral airways, laryngoscopes, endotracheal tubes, bronchoscopes, ventilators, oxygen tent, anesthesia machine, humidification apparatus, access to blood gas analysis facilities, thoracotomy tray, and tracheotomy set.

   b. Equipment for assessment and therapy of **heart and circulatory inadequacy:** electrocardiograph, transducers and oscillographs for direct arterial pressure measurements, venous cutdown sets, drugs for raising and lowering BP, cardiotonic drugs, appropriate fluids and needles or plastic catheters for fluid and blood replacement, and an electric defibrillator.

   c. Equipment for assessment and management of **kidney function,** such as containers for measuring urine output.

   d. **Temperature-measuring devices** and cooling and warming blankets.

   e. A complete **cardiopulmonary** resuscitation cart.

   f. **All the variety of drugs** that might be needed: narcotic analgesics, barbiturates, phenothiazines, bronchodilators, diuretics, vasopressors, antiemetics, antihistamines, antibiotics, corticosteroids, and cardiovascular agents.

   g. **Litters especially designed** for stability that permit easy access to the patient and tilting of the head up or down.

   h. **Overhead trolleys** that can be used for placement of bottles or plastic transparent bags for IV fluid and/or blood replacement.

H. General management

1. **At the completion of surgery and anesthesia,** the patient is placed on the litter or bed and taken to the recovery room, attended by the anesthesiologist or nurse-anesthetist. The side rails of the litter are elevated and the straps are fastened properly. The patient faces the nurses' station and the main door, so that he can be watched with little effort. The unconscious patient is positioned on the side to protect the airway and minimize aspiration of vomitus.

2. In the recovery room, the patient's care is turned over to the recovery room nurse. The information transmitted at this time includes:

a. The patient's name.

b. The diagnosis and the surgery performed.

c. The anesthetic technique and agents used. If relaxants and/or narcotics have been administered, this is recorded.

d. The types and quantities of fluid and blood replacement.

e. The vital signs recorded at the end of surgery.

f. Any intraoperative complications.

g. Instructions about respiration, recording vital signs, administration of analgesics, and extubation.

3. **When the patient arrives in the recovery room,** oxygen is administered through soft, flexible nasal tips inserted into the nostrils or through a transparent face mask. The patient is watched carefully, and **a complete record is kept** of vital signs and drugs administered. The patient's position is changed every hour, and he is encouraged to cough and breathe deeply at regular intervals. If the patient remains intubated, it is convenient to attach a T-piece system with humidification to the endotracheal tube. The need for oxygenation and/or ventilation must be verified by arterial blood gas analysis, since added oxygen can mask hypoventilation and allow development of increased Pco_2 and atelectasis.

4. **Analgesic drugs** are often indicated. However, these drugs should be administered with caution to avoid depression of ventilation and circulation in a patient who is still under the effects of anesthetics and surgery. Morphine, 2–3 mg (or equivalent doses of other narcotics), may be administered, preferably IV to ensure prompt relief and immediate evaluation of the effect of the narcotic.

5. **Common problems** in the immediate postoperative period may include respiratory obstruction, respiratory insufficiency, hypotension, hypovolemia, postsurgical bleeding, cardiac arrhythmias, heart failure, restlessness, emergence excitement, pain, vomiting, oliguria, convulsions, and cardiac arrest.

6. **Hypotension, inefficient ventilation,** emergence excitement, and pain are the most common problems in the recovery room and should be treated promptly.

7. Patients with **contaminated wounds** or **contagious diseases** are excluded from the recovery room.

8. **Due to radiation hazards,** patients in whom radium has been implanted for therapy of malignant tumors should be kept separate from other patients in the recovery room. The recommended distance is 35 cm for every 10 mg of radium implanted.

II. The intensive care unit

A. The recovery room in many hospitals has been expanded to include **an intensive care unit,** which in major hospitals includes a surgical intensive care unit, a medical intensive care unit, and a coronary care unit.

B. **Patients who need prolonged,** specialized surgical, medical, or cardiac care, such as for several days, are admitted to these units until they are fully recovered from their surgical and/or medical problems.

Bibliography

Bishop, V. A. A nurse's view of ethical problems in intensive care and clinical research. *Br. J. Anaesth.* 50:515, 1978.

Boutros, A. R. Arterial blood oxygenation during and after endotracheal suctioning in the apneic patient. *Anesthesiology* 32:114, 1970.

Eriksen, J., Andersen, J., and Rasmussen, J. P. Postoperative pulmonary function in obese patients after upper abdominal surgery. *Acta Anaesthesiol. Scand.* 21:336, 1977.

Marshall, B. E., and Wyche, M. O. Hypoxemia during and after anesthesia. *Anesthesiology* 37:195, 1972.

Philbin, D. M. Postoperative hypoxemia. Contribution of the cardiac output. *Anesthesiology* 32:136, 1970.

Smith, R. B., Petruscak, J., and Solosko, D. In a recovery room. *Am. J. Nurs.* 73:72, 1973.

Thompson, D. S., and Eason, C. N. Hypoxemia immediately after operation. *Am. J. Surg.* 20:649, 1970.

Wiklund, P. E. Intensive care units. *Anesthesiology* 31:122, 1969.

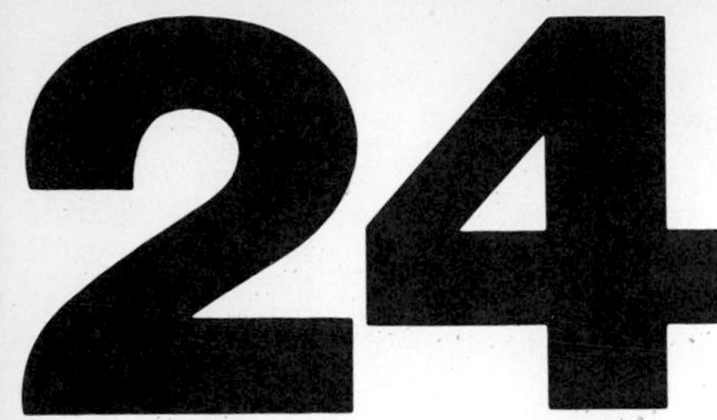

Blood Gases: Acid-Base Balance and Oxygen Transfer

When "blood gases" are measured, the blood usually analyzed is **arterial blood,** i.e., the blood available to go to the tissues. The tissues in general, and each organ in particular, may or may not actually benefit from that blood; adequate cardiac output and appropriate regional distribution are also necessary. The analysis of **mixed venous blood** provides information about the state of the blood leaving the tissues. It is, accordingly, a better guide to **tissue oxygenation, carbon dioxide level, and pH** in general, though it still does not guarantee the condition of any particular organ. This section describes methods for understanding and correcting blood gas disturbances.

I. Acid-base balance

A. Acid-base maintenance. The interior of the cell is normally maintained at a pH that is neutral for that temperature. At 37°C this is pH 6.8, or $[H^+]$ 160 nmol/liter. This contrasts with a blood pH of 7.4 or $[H^+]$ 40 nmol/liter. There is therefore a gradient favoring acid elimination from the cell.

1. Clinical **management of acid-base disturbances** consists of correcting the two components (respiratory and metabolic) to maintain the normal extracellular pH. This maintains the normal gradient across cell membranes, so that intracellular neutrality is preserved.

2. Constancy of the intracellular pH ensures that the ionized substrates are present in optimal concentrations. Major intracellular pH changes cause some substances to become significantly less ionized; in this form they can escape across the cell wall. Thus intracellular neutrality is required both for optimal metabolism and to prevent loss of metabolites.

B. PCO_2, $[H^+]$, and $[HCO_3^-]$. Carbonic acid dissociates and ionizes to produce CO_2, H^+, and HCO_3^-. These particles are in equilibrium with each other.

$$[H^+]\,[HCO_3^-] = 24.5\ PCO_2$$

1. The level of bicarbonate is therefore governed by the $[H^+]$ and PCO_2; indeed, in acid-base measurement, it is a calculated value. This equation makes it easy to anticipate some of the effects of changes in PCO_2 and $[H^+]$.

2. When the PCO_2 is constant (a pure metabolic, not respiratory, disturbance) a rise in acidity, $[H^+]$, produces a reciprocal fall in $[HCO_3^-]$; in contrast, a rise in PCO_2 (respiratory acidosis) causes some carbon dioxide and water to form carbonic acid, which ionizes to increase both $[H^+]$ and $[HCO_3^-]$.

3. This equation thus demonstrates that bicarbonate level is lowered by metabolic acidosis and raised by respiratory acidosis.

C. Respiratory acidosis. In clinical medicine, carbon dioxide is synonymous with respiratory acid. **Respiratory acidosis** is therefore easily defined as an elevated carbon dioxide level.

1. The level of respiratory acid is usually measured as a partial pressure in torr; the normal PCO_2 is 40 ± 5 mmHg. (The Système Internationale unit, the kilopascal, is used in some texts; normal PCO_2 is 5.3 ± 0.7 kPa).

2. Carbon dioxide is produced in large quantities, about 360 liters, or 16 moles, of respiratory acid per day. This massive production requires, of course, a correspondingly effective system for carbon dioxide elimination.

3. The balance between production and elimination of carbon dioxide controls the PCO_2 and allows rapid and predictable control of the pH. This powerful mechanism provides prompt compensation for metabolic disturbances.

4. Retention of carbon dioxide (respiratory acidosis) is the respiratory abnormality requiring urgent therapy.

5. The treatment is to increase ventilation by bag or ventilator. As described above respiratory acidosis (high PCO_2) directly raises the level of carbonic acid and hence also the bicarbonate concentration.

6. Any metabolic compensation (alkalosis) further raises the bicarbonate concentration. Never give bicarbonate to a patient with respiratory acidosis.

D. **Metabolic acidosis.** Metabolic acids comprise all the acids except for carbon dioxide (carbonic acid). The level of these other acids has to be assessed under the influence of carbon dioxide.

1. A useful **definition of metabolic acidosis** is "a pH that is too acid for that PCO_2." This emphasizes that changes in PCO_2 level cause predictable changes in pH and simultaneously introduces the idea that any additional, unexplained pH disturbance has a metabolic origin.

2. **The level of metabolic acids** is calculated from the PCO_2 and pH. It is expressed as the total amount of treatment (bicarbonate) that would be used to achieve correction.

3. **Metabolic acidosis.** Usually 6 mEq/liter is reported as a base excess of −6 mEq/liter. The use of the term *negative base excess* is one of the many sources of confusion and henceforth is avoided here (metabolic disturbances will, for example, be described as metabolic acidosis 10 mEq/liter, rather than BE −10 mEq/liter).

E. **Volume treated.** When bicarbonate is given, it principally neutralizes excess metabolic acids in extracellular fluid (20% of the body weight, e.g., 70 kg × 0.2 = 14 L). However, the cell wall does not totally isolate the intracellular fluid from this process.

1. As time passes, some of the bicarbonate enters the intracellular fluid. The **treatable volume** is therefore greater; 30% (or 21 liters) is commonly assumed. This corresponds to the distribution expected after 15–30 min and is therefore appropriate in emergencies.

2. After longer periods, even more intracellular neutralization occurs. The volume of distribution appears to increase (e.g., to 50%), and the effect of any bicarbonate dose therefore diminishes.

F. **Representation of acid-base balance.** Well over a hundred schemes have been devised to represent acid-base disturbances.

1. **Satisfactory schemes** allow:

   a. Acid-base disturbances to be understood.

   b. Measurement of metabolic acid level in milliequivalents per liter.

   c. Recognition of characteristic syndromes.

   d. Anticipation of the effect of therapy.

2. **Computers** conveniently print out the metabolic disturbance but provide no assistance to understanding.

3. A **suitable diagram** or nomogram assists the visual learner; however, the diagram may not be available in an emergency and is of no value to the

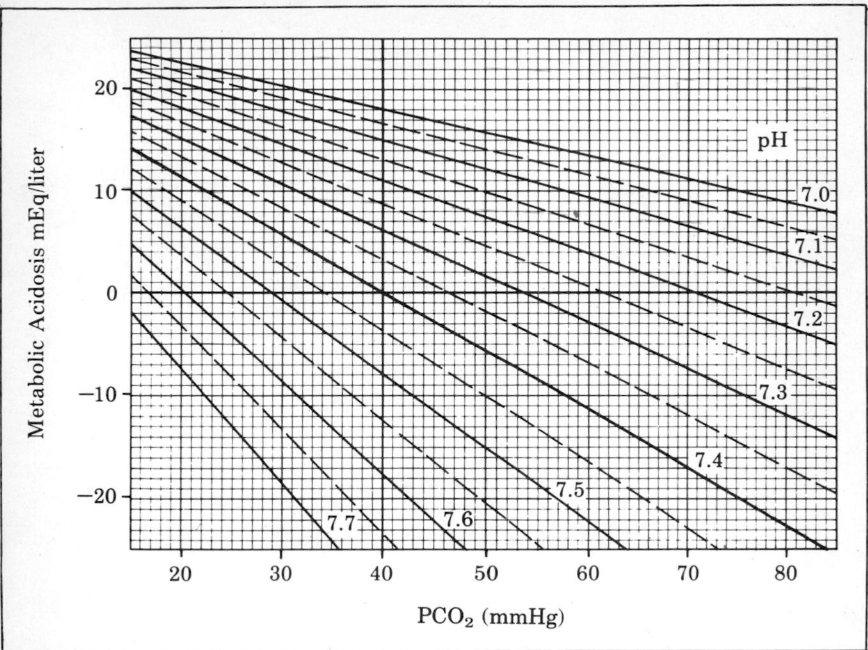

Fig. 24-1. In vivo acid-base diagram.

nonvisual learner. Therefore both an in vivo diagram and a set of simple rules are described here.

G. In-vivo acid-base diagram (Fig. 24-1)

1. The **level of metabolic acid** is read from the intersection of the PCO_2 and the pH (e.g., 10 mEq/liter in the example above). When the PCO_2 changes, the patient's position moves horizontally, staying at the same level of metabolic acid. If bicarbonate is given, the position moves vertically down, the change in metabolic acid level being proportional to the dose given.

2. **Characteristic syndromes** are easy to recognize and are shown in Figure 24-2. An acute change in PCO_2 moves the patient horizontally on the zero line (pure respiratory disturbance, zero compensation).

3. **In chronic carbon dioxide disturbances,** metabolic compensation moves the position about halfway from no compensation (zero) towards total compensation (pH 7.4). This halfway position corresponds to zone R in Figure 24-3.

4. Similar reasoning applies to metabolic disturbances that are, however, almost always associated with respiratory compensation. **Respiratory compensation** moves the patient's position sideways about halfway from no compensation (PCO_2 40 mmHg) toward total compensation (pH 7.4), i.e., to zone M in Figure 24-3.

H. Simple rules: pH 0.1 = PCO_2 12 and/or metabolic acids 6. A change in PCO_2 of 12 mmHg causes a pH change of 0.1. Thus a patient with a PCO_2 of 58 mmHg (+ 18) and a pH of 7.25 (+ 0.15) has a pure respiratory disturbance.

1. When a pH and PCO_2 do not correspond, any unexplained pH change of 0.1 corresponds to a **metabolic disturbance of 6 mEq/liter.** Thus, if at the same

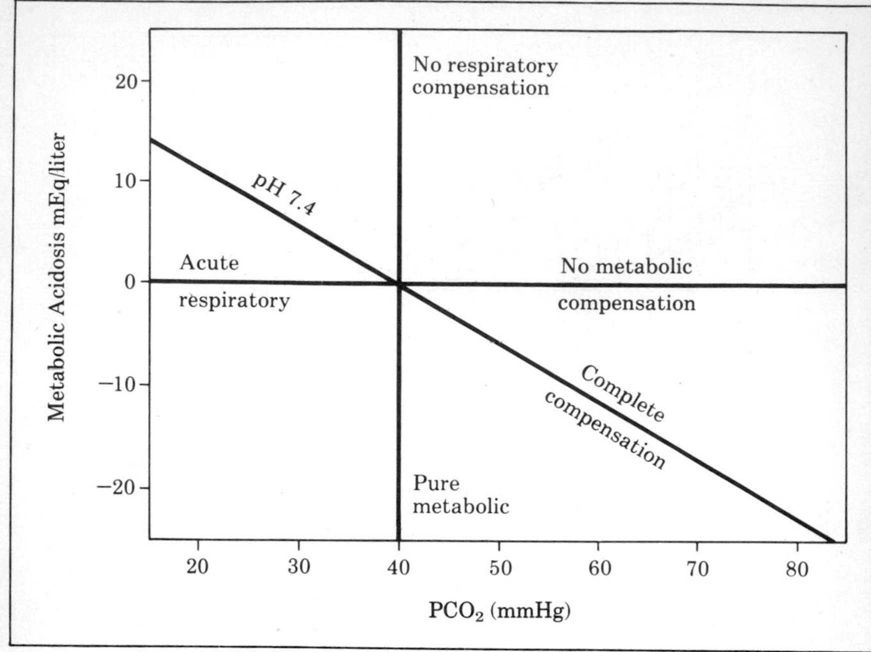

Fig. 24-2. In vivo acid-base diagram showing position of uncompensated ("pure") disturbances.

PCO_2(58) the pH were 7.1 rather than 7.25, the further 0.15 of pH indicates metabolic acidosis of 9 mEq/L.

2. **Compensated disturbances** can be recognized as they can with Figure 24-2; the patient is halfway between no compensation and total compensation. For example a patient with a PCO_2 of 64 and pH 7.3 has enough respiratory acidosis to cause pH 7.2.

3. The **compensation** (6 mEq/L of metabolic alkalosis) has moved the patient halfway toward pH 7.4. This position would therefore be typical of chronic respiratory acidosis.

4. A patient with the same acid pH (7.3), but a PCO_2 of 28 mmHg has a metabolic acidosis that dominates the respiratory alkalosis. The PCO_2 would normally cause a pH of 7.5. The **pH difference** (0.2) therefore indicates a metabolic acidosis of 12 mEq/liter. Alone, this metabolic acidosis would cause a pH of 7.2. Thus, again, the patient's pH of 7.3 is seen to be halfway toward compensation (7.4), characteristic of metabolic acidosis with compensation.

I. **Correction of respiratory acidosis.** Change the ventilation (adjust the ventilator) to correct an abnormal PCO_2. The PCO_2 multiplied by the minute volume remains approximately constant in any given situation:

$$PCO_2 \times \dot{V}_E = K$$

1. Thus, if the PCO_2 is 60 mmHg and the minute volume is 4 L/min (60 × 4 + 240), a PCO_2 of 40 mmHg will be obtained if the ventilation is increased to 6 liters/min (60 × 4 = 240).

2. **Correction of an abnormal PCO_2** is not always necessary (or possible); in a patient recovering from acute respiratory depression (e.g., drug overdose), the PCO_2 may manage to correct itself, and a patient who has chronic respi-

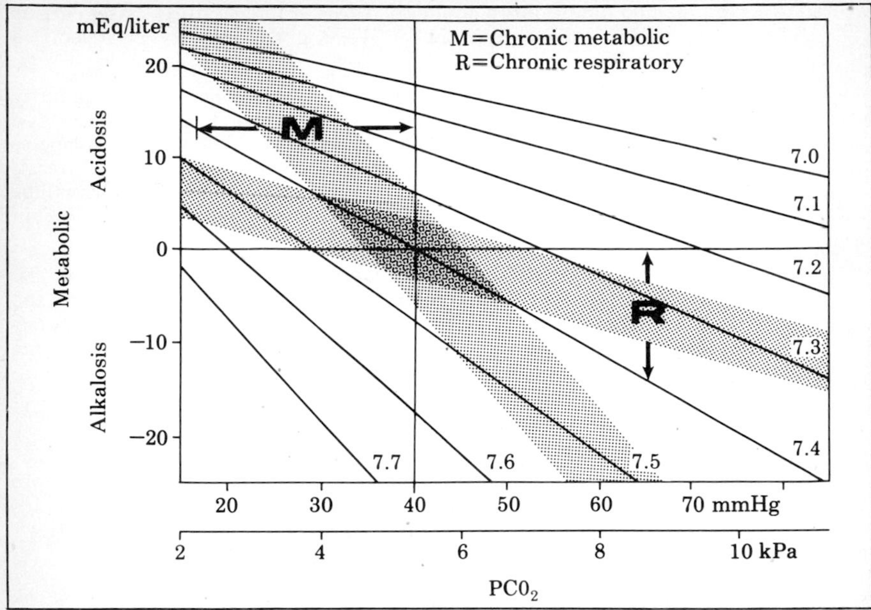

Fig. 24-3. In vivo acid-base diagram showing characteristic compensation.

ratory failure with an elevated PCO_2 should probably be allowed to stay at the PCO_2 to which he or she is accustomed.

J. **Correction of metabolic acidosis.** The treatment of metabolic acidosis should consist of correction of the underlying pathologic process (bicarbonate is poor therapy for diabetes, tissue ischemia, etc). Nevertheless, marked metabolic acidosis impairs cardiac function and may therefore require urgent neutralization.

1. **Bicarbonate added** to an acid solution initially generates carbon dioxide (i.e., it "fizzes," although, fortunately, not literally in the bloodstream). Moreover, the bicarbonate dose is initially confined to the plasma (4% of the body weight). The development of transient respiratory acidosis and the initial overtreatment of the plasma explains why it is customary to give only half a calculated dose.

2. The **calculated dose** is obtained by multiplying the level of metabolic acids by 0.3 × the weight (− BE (negative base excess) × 0.3 × weight). Thus, for a 70-kg patient with a metabolic acidosis of 10 mEq/liters (BE = − 10 mEq/L), the calculated dose is 70 × 0.3 × 10 = 210 mEq. Generally, about half this is administered.

K. **Dangers of bicarbonate therapy.** In cardiac arrest, bicarbonate may be necessary to restart the heart. However, it should be remembered the brain cells can be adversely affected.

1. The bicarbonate itself penetrates the **blood-brain barrier** very slowly. This is not the case for the carbon dioxide that has been generated in the blood. This enters the cells extremely rapidly and therefore worsens the intracellular acidosis.

2. After **recovery from metabolic acidosis** the body deals with the excess acids (lactic, pyruvic, etc.). The after effect of any bicarbonate therapy will then be an iatrogenic metabolic alkalosis.

L. Blood gases and temperature changes. At cooler temperatures, gases such as oxygen and carbon dioxide are more soluble. A given quantity is carried at a lower partial pressure.

1. **Cooling** occurs naturally as blood reaches the extremities, and the quantity of carbon dioxide that centrally produced a PCO_2 of 40 torr will now cause a lower PCO_2. This appears to be appropriate for the cells at lower temperatures and parallels the PCO_2 found in other species at lower temperatures. If this cold blood is rewarmed in a blood gas analyzer, a PCO_2 of 40 torr will be recorded. This is a convenient simplification when assessing "normality" in hypothermia.

2. When **deep hypothermia is being induced,** carbon dioxide may be administered to produce cerebrovascular dilatation and ensure uniform cooling of the brain. This high inspired PCO_2 can produce **high arterial PCO_2 levels** at low temperatures (e.g., 80 torr at 15°C). If this blood is analyzed at 37°C, the PCO_2 will be approximately 250 torr. The circulation is, of course, maintained artificially, and this marked abnormality appears to be associated with no adverse sequelae.

3. **Moderate metabolic acidosis** is commonly encountered during hypothermia and during rewarming, when perfusion recommences and tissues are rewarmed. This can commonly be left uncorrected, since the metabolic acids should be rapidly metabolized by the body when rewarming is complete.

II. Oxygen transfer

A. Factors influencing arterial oxygenation. The arterial partial pressure of oxygen (PaO_2) depends on the fractional inspired oxygen (F_IO_2), the barometric pressure (P_B), water vapor pressure (PH_2O), the respiratory quotient (RQ), the alveolar partial pressure of carbon dioxide (P_ACO_2), the degree of shunting (Qs/Qt) and/or mismatch between ventilation and perfusion (V/Q). It is hardly ever influenced by alveolar/capillary block. With so many factors determining $PaCO_2$, any single value has to be interpreted with caution.

B. Space for respiratory gases: the sum of PO_2 and PCO_2. The first essential is to estimate the inspired PO_2 (P_IO_2). The values shown are for breathing air at sea level at normal body temperature:

$$(P_B - PH_2O \times F_IO_2 = P_IO_2 \text{ (humidified)}$$
$$(760 - 47) \times 0.209 = 149 \text{ mmHg}$$

1. It is a convenient approximation to regard this as the "space available" for **the respiratory gases (O_2 and CO_2) in the alveoli.** This would be precise if carbon dioxide were produced at the same rate that oxygen is consumed. **Nitrogen,** which is neither metabolized nor excreted, would, of course, occupy the same partial pressure throughout the airways, and the remaining partial pressure would be occupied by carbon dioxide and oxygen. However, less carbon dioxide is usually produced, and, as a result, there has to be a small net inflow of air; nitrogen is slightly concentrated in the alveoli.

2. A normal person therefore has slightly less space available in the aveoli, and the sum of the P_AO_2 (100 mmHg) and P_ACO_2 (40 mmHg) is 140 mmHg.

3. A sum less than 140 torr **under normal circumstances** strongly suggests abnormal lung function. Either the alveoli are closed and venous blood is crossing the lung to the arterial blood, or there is mismatching of blood flow and ventilation, so that some alveoli receive relatively too much blood or too little air; inadequately oxygenated blood is transmitted to the systemic circulation.

4. The **two varieties of lung malfunction,** shunt and mismatch, may coexist. Commonly, one malfunction predominates, and the one that does determines the response to oxygen administration.

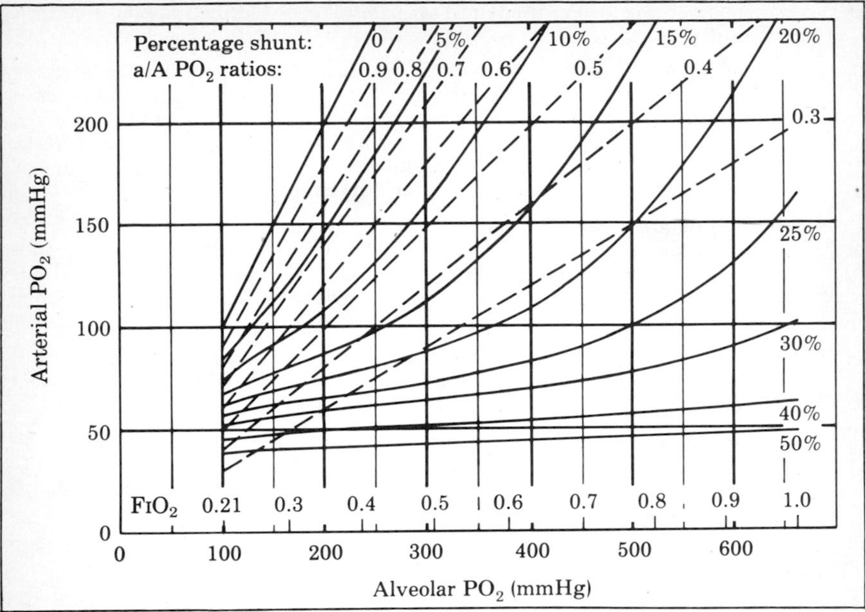

Fig. 24-4. Oxygen transfer diagram. Arterial PO_2 related to changes in inspired oxygen.

C. **Shunt.** With shunt (e.g., in atelectasis, pneumothorax, bronchial occlusion), an increased F_IO_2 has relatively little effect on the PaO_2. The blood going to normal alveoli can only take up very small amounts of extra dissolved oxygen; the blood going to abnormal alveoli continues to be shunted and, of course, receives no oxygen.

1. The heavy, curved shunt lines in Figure 24-4 show how arterial oxygenation responds to improved F_IO_2.
2. **The precise shunt value** depends on many factors, and therefore the values shown in Figure 24-4 are representative only. Fortunately, the shape of the shunt lines is much less variable, and in patients who have a shunt, the response to oxygen therapy can be satisfactorily anticipated from these lines.

D. **Mismatch.** When oxygen is administered to patients with mismatch (e.g., chronic obstructive pulmonary disease), some oxygen reaches the abnormal as well as the normal alveoli. Consequently, additional oxygen is picked up by blood that was not previously saturated, i.e., where there is a large capacity for improvement. Consequently, in patients with mismatch there is a relatively satisfactory response to oxygen therapy.

1. The interrupted lines in Figure 24-4 are lines where there is a constant ratio between alveolar and arterial PCO_2.
2. In a patient with mismatch, these lines approximately represent the change in arterial PO_2 following oxygen therapy and provide a rough guide to the response to oxygen therapy.

E. **Practical aspects.** Before a small artery is cannulated, it should be checked to ensure that distal blood flow does not wholly depend on that artery.

1. At the wrist, a **modified Allen's test** is used: With both radial and ulnar vessels compressed, the clenched (or squeezed) hand is opened. It should

remain obviously blanched until an artery is released. The maneuver is then repeated for the other artery.

2. To draw a sample, **a glass syringe** is preferred, since it does not absorb the gases. It should be rinsed with heparin solution until it fills and empties freely. The arterial pressure then passively fills the syringe, thus helping to locate the vessel. Only sufficient heparin is used to fill the tip of the syringe and the needle; excess heparin dilutes the hemoglobin estimation, and the excess acidity alters the metabolic acid measurement.
3. **Bubbles** are carefully expelled from the syringe prior to drawing blood; if any are then drawn in, they are expelled immediately afterward. This avoids errors in the measurement of PO_2 and PCO_2 caused by equilibration with the bubble. After sampling, the syringe should be capped and thoroughly rotated to mix the heparin.
4. **Analysis is done promptly** to avoid consumption of the oxygen by red cell metabolism and alteration of the PO_2 measurement. When there is a delay, the syringe should be packed in ice to reduce metabolism.
5. **Cooling** does not prevent transfer of gases to the plastic of the syringe. In practice, when experienced personnel withdraw blood and analysis is performed promptly, plastic syringes can be used satisfactorily and provide accurate values.

Bibliography

Blackburn, J. P. What is new in blood-gas analysis? *Br. J. Anaesth.* 50:51, 1978.

Grogono, A. W. Actual or standard bicarbonate. *Lancet* 2:631, 1979.

Grogono, A. W., Byles, P. H., and Hawke, W. An in-vivo representation of acid base balance. *Lancet* 2:499, 1976.

Miller, R. D., and Roderick, L. L. Acid-base balance and neostigmine antagonism of pancuronium neuromuscular blockage. *Br. J. Anesth.* 50:317, 1978.

Norman, J. An assessment of acid-base balance. *Br. J. Anaesth.* 50:45, 1978.

25 Respiratory Therapy

I. Respiratory therapy is an adjuvant therapeutic modality that contributes to improvement of pulmonary gas exchange. In anesthetic practice, respiratory therapy (a) prepares the respiratory system for the oncoming effects of anesthesia and surgery and (b) prevents and treats pulmonary complications that may occur during or after surgery.

A. **The following agents and techniques** are used to achieve the objectives of respiratory therapy:

1. Therapeutic gases.
2. Humidification.
3. Inhalation of therapeutic agents.
4. Mechanical ventilatory support in the form of either intermittent or continuous positive-pressure breathing.
5. Chest physiotherapy.

B. The improvement of the functional performance of the respiratory system resulting from respiratory therapy is the consequence of elimination of mostly reversible obstructive factors along the airways: (1) edema, (2) secretions, (3) infection, and (4) spasm.

C. **The function of the respiratory system** is adversely affected by:

1. Obstructive factors (e.g., chronic bronchitis, emphysema, and bronchospasm).
2. Restrictive factors (e.g., thoracic cage deformities, obesity, tight abdominal binders, and muscle paralysis).
3. Circulatory factors (e.g., circulatory failure and low output syndromes).
4. All or any combination of these factors may coexist in a given situation; the proper therapeutic approach would depend on the main causative factor.

II. **Airway obstruction**

A. Airway obstruction is always associated with **increased resistance,** which eventually increases the work of breathing. Such an increase demands higher oxygen consumption, which the respiratory system may not be able to provide. **Evaluation** of increased resistance is important for correctly determining the therapeutic approach.

1. **Slight resistance.** The patient can sustain indefinitely an increased respiratory effort sufficient for maintenance of alveolar ventilation. Blood gases remain normal.
2. **Moderate resistance.** The patient must make a considerable effort to maintain close-to-normal blood gases. Patients with chronic bronchitis and ob-

structive lung disease belong in this group. These patients need very close observation and care, since they may decompensate rapidly.

3. **Severe resistance.** This patient is not able to cope with the increased resistance; in these circumstances, ventilation deteriorates, PCO_2 rapidly increases, PO_2 usually deteriorates more than the PCO_2 rises, and the life of the patient is threatened.

4. **Complete respiratory obstruction.** In this situation neither the patient nor artificial ventilation can achieve sufficient ventilation to sustain life.

B. **Certain concepts concerning the airways** need to be emphasized:

1. **In healthy persons,** resistance during inspiration and expiration is about equal; however, resistance becomes greater during expiration when breathing is forced or deep. If such resistance during expiration is excessively high, this signifies airway collapse and weak airway walls. In these cases, air trapping is taking place in the lungs.

2. **Rapid reversal of obstruction** signifies bronchospasm or mucous plug, which can be corrected with appropriate therapy. This situation is not likely to occur in chronic obstructive lung disease.

3. **Weak or paralyzed muscles** of the larynx, pharynx, and neck may appear to cause obstruction of the airway.

C. **The ultimate success** of respiratory therapy depends on:

1. Understanding the nature of the respiratory disturbance.

2. Selecting appropriate treatment for a particular disturbance.

3. Monitoring for possible adverse systemic effects of the treatment selected.

III. Therapeutic gases

A. Oxygen

1. Excluding anesthetic gases and gases used for investigational purposes, respiratory therapy utilizes oxygen almost exclusively, with occasional rare use of carbon dioxide or helium. Oxygen combines with the blood in two ways:

   a. **As a physical solution.** In this instance, oxygen dissolves in the aqueous part of the blood. The amount dissolved depends on the partial pressure of the oxygen (Henry's law); at PO_2 of 100 torr, the amount dissolved is 0.3 ml. For every increase in PO_2, there is an increase of dissolved oxygen in a linear proportion. This is the principle of **hyperbaric oxygenation.**

   b. **As a chemical solution.** Oxygen combines chemically with hemoglobin: 1 g of hemoglobin combines with 1.34 ml of oxygen. Again, the chemical combination of oxygen with hemoglobin depends on PO_2. However, this combination, unlike the physical solution, is not linear but, rather, follows an S-shaped curve. At a PO_2 of 100 torr, saturation is almost maximal, and further increase in PO_2 does not affect the percentage saturation. Most oxygen in blood is carried in combination with hemoglobin.

2. **Causes of arterial hypoxemia**

   a. Low inspired oxygen.

   b. Hypoventilation.

   c. Diffusion and ventilation perfusion abnormalities.

   d. Circulation problems (stagnant hypoxia).

   e. Histotoxicity.

3. **Indications for oxygen therapy.** The most common indications for oxygen therapy are prevention and correction of arterial hypoxemia.

a. **Arterial hypoxemia** may be present in a patient with intact respiratory and circulatory mechanisms. High-altitude hypoxemia is the most common example.

b. **Arterial hypoxemia secondary to alveolar hypoventilation or venous admixture.** It is extremely important to treat the hypoventilation or venous admixture in conjunction with the administration of oxygen.

c. **Oxygen therapy may be used** to alleviate ischemic or anemic effects (stagnant and anemic hypoxia).

d. **Carbon monoxide poisoning** is also treated with oxygen.

e. **Denitrogenation** and clearance of gas loculi (after air embolus, pneumoperitoneum, pneumothorax, pneumoencephalography, or intestinal obstruction) also require treatment with oxygen.

4. **Dangers associated with administration of oxygen**

a. **Ventilatory depression** is extremely important to consider when dealing with patients who have been ventilating in response to hypoxic drive. An elevated $PaCO_2$ will identify such patients. **Elimination of the hypoxic drive** may lead to severe hypoventilation and apnea. All patients with chronic hypoxia should be treated with great caution. Absence of cyanosis does not prove satisfactory ventilation. Arterial blood gases are the most valuable diagnostic tool.

b. **Pulmonary damage** may occur if lung tissue is exposed to high oxygen concentrations over a long period of time. The most desirable inhaled oxygen concentration (FIO_2) is the one that provides an arterial PO_2 between 70–100 torr; therefore, to avoid damage to lung tissue, the administered oxygen must be titrated against the arterial PO_2.

c. **Pulmonary collapse** may result if a section of the lung is filled with oxygen and then subjected to airway obstruction.

d. **Retrolental fibroplasia** (vascular obliteration and fibroblastic infiltration in the retina) is another form of oxygen toxicity that occurs in neonates, especially the premature, who are exposed to high oxygen concentration.

e. There is always **risk of fire** and explosion.

5. **Sources of oxygen for therapy**

a. **Central distribution.** Oxygen is piped throughout the hospital, from a central location at a pressure of 50 psi.

b. Oxygen is also available **compressed in cylinders** at pressures of 1000–2000 psi.

6. **Quantitation of oxygen** takes place in the flowmeter, following which the gas is conducted to the humidifying system before it finally reaches the patient. The humidifying system is either a nebulizer, which produces particulate mist, or a plain humidifier, in which oxygen is either bubbled through or drawn over water.

7. **Oxygen is administered by:**

a. **Nasal cannulas or nasal catheters.** The flow of oxygen should not be greater than 6–8 L/min.

(1) High flows will dry the mucosa of the upper airways, causing uncomfortable dryness as well as encrustation secretions. In addition, there is the possibility of stomach inflation, which may cause nausea and vomiting.

(2) Oxygen so given has a concentration of 30–40%.

b. **Masks** should fit fairly tightly and cover the nose and mouth. With a flow of 6–8 L/min, oxygen concentration is slightly higher than when oxygen is administered with nasal cannulae. Several types of masks or mask-bag combinations are available.

(1) The most commonly used mask is the **partial rebreathing mask-bag combination,** in which partial rebreathing of exhaled gases occurs from the reservoir bag.

(2) Most of the exhaled gases and carbon dioxide are eliminated from the mask through side holes by utilizing a high flow of oxygen. This is an important point to remember when this therapy is given to a patient with high PCO_2, since a low flow of oxygen in such a patient may cause carbon dioxide rebreathing and retention.

(3) Further, a low oxygen flow will allow air to enter through the holes, resulting in dilution of oxygen and lower-than-desired oxygen administration.

(4) **The nonrebreathing mask** eliminates virtually all the exhaled gases through the exhalation valve. Oxygen flow should be at least equal to the minute volume of ventilation to prevent air dilution through the safety air-inlet valve.

(5) There are other types of masks that, utilizing the **Venturi principle,** provide various degrees of air mixture.

(6) Masks also have been modified to provide oxygen and humidity for patients with **tracheostomies.**

c. **Face tents** are more comfortable than the tight-fitting masks and are suitable for routine use in the recovery room.

d. **Oxygen hoods and tents** are used much less today than formerly. One variation of these is the **Croupette,** which is extensively used in pediatrics. The Croupette is essentially a small oxygen tent that provides humidity and heat in addition to oxygen. The **Isolette** is a very small, confined space that provides a controlled atmosphere and temperature regulation by the use of a thermostat.

e. **Endotracheal tubes** (through the nose, mouth, or tracheal stoma).

B. Carbon dioxide

1. Inhalation of CO_2 increases both the rate and the depth of respiration. **The therapeutic value of CO_2 depends** on its potent stimulating effects on the respiratory center. Respiratory stimulation begins in seconds following the inhalation of even low concentration of CO_2, and maximal stimulation usually is attained within 5 min.

2. **CO_2 stimulates respiration** by acting on:

   a. The medullary brainstem respiratory integration centers.

   b. Peripheral arterial chemoreceptors.

3. **Indications for CO_2 administration**

   a. CO_2 is used in research and diagnosis.

   b. A practical method of increasing PCO_2 is the addition of dead space and reinhalation of expired CO_2.

4. **Contraindications**

   a. Coma.

   b. Stupor.

   c. Severe hypertension.

   d. Cardiac disease and arrhythmias.

e. Chronic pulmonary insufficiency.

f. Increased intracranial pressure.

5. **CO_2 is commercially available** in cylinders, either pure or mixed with oxygen in 5–10% concentrations.

C. **Helium**

1. **The therapeutic value of helium** is based on its physical characteristics. It has the ability to lower the specific gravity of any mixture of gases of which it forms a part. Although a helium-oxygen mixture has a lower density than air, it has a higher viscosity.

2. **Gases with high viscosity,** in passing through narrow orifices, lose their streamlined flow pattern and become turbulent; a turbulent flow always requires higher pressure to move a given gas mixture through the orifices. In small airway obstruction (such as in asthma, where helium formerly was indicated), because of the high viscosity, helium is unlikely to be of any benefit.

IV. Humidification

A. **Normally the inspired air** is warmed to body temperature and, by means of a highly efficient system provided by the mucous membranes of the nose and pharynx, becomes completely saturated with water vapor as it reaches proximal bronchi.

1. **The cilia,** which are part of the columnar cells of the lining of the respiratory tract, beat in a coordinated fashion, propelling the mucus toward the glottis.

2. **The proper functioning** of this ciliary epithelium depends on the percentage of the inspired air's saturation with water vapor. If the air that comes in contact with this epithelium is less than 70% saturated, ciliary activity becomes impaired, and propulsion of the mucus, debris, or foreign bodies toward the glottis becomes inefficient.

B. **Humidity is expressed** as either absolute or relative.

1. **Absolute humidity** is the amount of molecular water in a given volume unit of gas (grams per cubic meter).

2. **Relative humidity** is the amount of molecular water actually present in the unit volume of gas as compared to the maximal amount that the unit volume of gas could contain (expressed as a percentage).

C. Inspired air is always fully saturated below the carina. This humidity is supplied by the mucosa of the upper airways and nasopharynx. **Artificial humidification** is indicated in the presence of moisture deficits in the upper airways. **Deficits in humidity** can be caused by:

1. Dehydration.

2. Interference with the normal activity of the mucous membrane by an allergenic or injective process.

3. Temporary or permanent bypass of the humidifying mucous membranes by either endotracheal or tracheostomy tubes.

D. **Devices** providing humidification:

1. **Humidifiers** expose the gas, prior to inhalation, to a large surface area of water.

2. **Aerosol generators** produce water droplets of sufficiently small size to remain in suspension long enough to reach the periphery of the respiratory tract. There are two ways of producing aerosol:

a. High-pressure gas nebulizers, which disperse the water into particles.

b. Ultrasonic nebulizers. The principle of this nebulizer is subjection of the liquid to intense ultrasonic vibration in a stream of carrier gas. Aerosol generators, particularly the ultrasonic nebulizers, produce very fine particles that may penetrate the terminal bronchioles.

3. **Condenser humidifiers.** These devices replace the function of the nose. The principle of these humidifiers is that the expired gas loses heat to the element; with the fall in the temperature of the gas, water condenses on the metal surface of the device. Inspired gas at low humidity, when it comes in contact with the condenser humidifier, is warmed and absorbs the condenser water. This method is used primarily in tracheotomized patients in whom thick secretions are a problem.

4. **All these various devices** used in inhalation therapy must be processed, cleaned, and sterilized properly. The incidence of cross-infection where such care is not taken is very high, endangering the lives of patients as well as the personnel caring for them. Each institution or hospital must adopt a policy to ensure that clean, aseptic techniques are followed to the letter.

V. Inhalation of therapeutic agents

A. **Therapeutic agents** are deposited at various parts of the tracheobronchial tree by means of inhalation. After nebulization, these agents are conducted through the nebulizer output to the tracheobronchial system, where they exert their effect. **Deposition** of these agents depends on:

1. The **particle size.** In the absence of turbulence, particles of less than 0.5–2 microns may enter even the smallest airway.

2. The presence of **turbulence.** Increased turbulence will deposit the particles at more proximal airways.

B. **The choice of therapeutic agent** depends on the pathophysiologic factors compromising the patency of the airway.

1. **In general, airways are compromised** by bronchospasm, edema in the airway, and retention of secretions.

2. **Bronchospasm** is an exaggerated increase in the bronchial smooth muscle tone. Bronchial smooth muscle tone is determined by:

a. Local tissue gas tensions.

b. Local hormones, such as histamine, serotonin, and prostaglandins.

c. Autonomic tone (vagal stimulation causes bronchoconstriction).

3. **Bronchodilators** are medications that relieve the bronchospasm. They can be given either systemically or by inhalation. They are particularly useful in patients with paroxysmal attacks of bronchospasm.

a. **Bronchodilators** are either epinephrine-like (catecholamines) or aminophylline-like (xanthine derivatives).

b. Recently, **beta-adrenergic receptors** at the bronchial level have been further subdivided into $beta_1$ and $beta_2$ receptors.

(1) **Stimulation of $beta_1$ receptors,** in addition to bronchodilation, causes tachycardia, palpitation, hypertension, insomnia, and tremor. Typical representatives of this group of stimulants are isoproterenol, epinephrine, and ephedrine.

(2) **Stimulation of $beta_2$ receptors** causes mainly bronchodilation, with minimal or no effect on the heart. Drugs that belong in this group are isoetharine (Bronkosol), metaproterenol (Alupent, Metaprel), and terbutaline (Bricanyl).

4. **Bronchodilators available** for inhalation use are:

   a. **Racemic epinephrine** (Vaponefrin) stimulates both alpha and $beta_1$ receptors. The alpha-stimulating properties decrease the edema of the bronchial mucosa. The usual dose is 0.125–0.25 ml/3 ml of water every 4–6 hr. This agent is **contraindicated** in the presence of hyperthyroidism, hypertension, various types of heart disease, and sensitivity to this medication.

   b. **Isoproterenol** (Isuprel) is purely a $beta_1$ stimulator and has bronchodilating potency 10 times that of epinephrine. The fact that it has no alpha-stimulating properties causes bronchial mucosa edema, which eventually may lead to the so-called locked lung syndrome. It has a strong influence on the cardiovascular system. The recommended dose is 0.25–0.5 ml/3 ml of water.

   c. **Metaproterenol** (Alupent, Metaprel) is predominantly a $beta_2$ stimulant. The recommended dose is one to two whiffs every 4–6 hr.

   d. **Isoetharine** (Bronkosol) is a combination of a purely $beta_2$ stimulant, isoetharine, and phenylephrine. The recommended dose is 0.25–0.5 ml/3 ml of water every 3–4 hr.

   e. **Aminophylline-like drugs** (xanthine derivatives) are best used systemically. There is some indication for their use by aerosol in severe cases of bronchospasm.

   f. **Terbutaline.** Can be given parenterally or orally.

   g. **Steroids.** Depending on the severity of muscle spasm they can be given as a bolus or in an IV solution.

C. **Clearing of secretions**

1. **Retention of secretions** compromises the patency of the airway. In the presence of dehydration, secretions become encrusted and adhere to the mucosa, forming a mechanical obstruction that, if not removed, will eventually cause complete obstruction and atelectasis. In view of these factors, effective removal of these secretions is extremely important.

   a. In the same way, in patients with **chronic bronchitis,** the increased number of goblet cells (mucin-producing cells) secrete very thick, tenacious secretions that, because of the destruction of the ciliary epithelium, adhere to the bronchial wall.

   b. **Most patients with chronic bronchitis** have emphysema, and the coughing mechanism may be impaired to a certain extent, leaving the patient in a state of chronic retention of these secretions.

   c. **A superimposed infection** may precipitate an exacerbation of the chronic respiratory failure, posing a threat to life.

2. **Respiratory therapy,** in addition to general measures such as hydration, antibiotics, and elimination of offending factors, contributes considerably to the elimination of the secretions. Essentially, respiratory therapy offers three modes of treatment: liquefaction of secretions, mucolytic agents, and surface tension–reducing agents.

   a. Of these three methods, by far **the simplest and most effective** is liquefaction with simple saline.

   b. Among the **mucolytic agents,** the most popular are acetylcysteine (Mucomyst) and pancreatic dornase (Dornavac).

      (1) **Acetylcysteine** is very effective in dissolving and liquefying mucus. At times, such liquefaction is so great, the patient is practically

drowned in his own secretions. **The disadvantages** and side effects of acetylcysteine are:

(a) It is ineffective in the presence of a high oxygen concentration.

(b) It is ineffective on fibrin, blood, or purulent material.

(c) It has an antagonistic effect on certain antibiotics.

(d) It may cause bronchospasm and allergic reactions.

(2) Pancreatic dornase, an enzyme extracted from beef pancreas, is effective in clearing purulent secretions. Like acetylcysteine, it also may cause allergic reactions.

c. Certain agents have the property of thinning the mucus by **reducing the surface tension.** Such agents are Alevaire (a combination of 0.125% tylopaxol, 2% sodium bicarbonate, and 5% glycerin) and Tergemist (a combination of a detergent, ethasulfate, and potassium iodide). The use of these agents is controversial, and they have no distinct advantage over normal saline inhalations.

VI. Ventilatory support. This important area of respiratory therapy is discussed in detail in Chapter 27.

VII. Chest physiotherapy. See also Chapter 26.

A. Chest physiotherapy aims **to clear the tracheobronchial secretions** and expand the lungs without using mechanical means, stimulation, or aspiration.

B. Three methods are used:

1. Postural drainage is the use of an inverted position to drain otherwise dependent and trapped segments of the lungs. Postural drainage is helpful in certain parts of the lung, where disease is somewhat localized. However, only watery, purulent supernatant of lung abscesses or bronchiectasis can be brought up in this way. This position is ineffective for thick, purulent, and/or tenacious secretions of advanced chronic suppurative diseases of the tracheobronchial tree.

2. Pounding (vibration-percussion) is clapping of the open cupped hand over the chest in vigorous repetitive blows. This type of percussion is used only over that topographic area of the chest where clinical and radiologic findings suggest there is underlying collapse or retained secretions. The pounding is directed toward, and localized to, only that area of disease.

3. Assisted cough and deep breathing. The patient is trained preoperatively in deep breathing and coughing. For the purpose of this training, **cough** can be divided artificially into three phases. These should be demonstrated to the patient, and he should practice coughing faithfully at least 10 times per hour before surgery:

a. Deep inspiration.

b. A powerful Valsalva maneuver.

c. Termination in a belch-like explosion.

C. Assisted respiration after thoracotomy or laparotomy consists of application of support or actual compression on the involved side. With the therapist's fingers spread widely, the anterior and posterior portions of the chest wall are compressed. The fingers spread and relax somewhat with each inspiration and actively compress during exhalation. The therapist then follows progressive respiratory movements, compressing more with exhalations and encouraging deeper inspirations.

Bibliography

Ali, J., Weisel, R. D., Layug, A. B., et al. Consequences of postoperative alterations in respiratory mechanics. *Am. J. Surg.* 128:376, 1974.

Dohi, S., and Gold, M. I. Comparison of two methods of postoperative respiratory care. *Chest* 73:592, 1978.

Meyers, J. R., Lembeck, L., O'Kane, H., et al. Changes in functional residual capacity of the lung after operation. *Arch. Surg.* 110:576, 1975.

Mueller, R. A. Recent developments in the physiology of bronchomotor tone and the pharmacology of bronchodilators. *Int. Anesthesiol. Clin.* 15(2):137, 1977.

Wahba, W. M., Don, H. F., and Craig, D. B. Post-operative epidural analgesia: Effects on lung volumes. *Can. Anaesth. Soc. J.* 22:519, 1975.

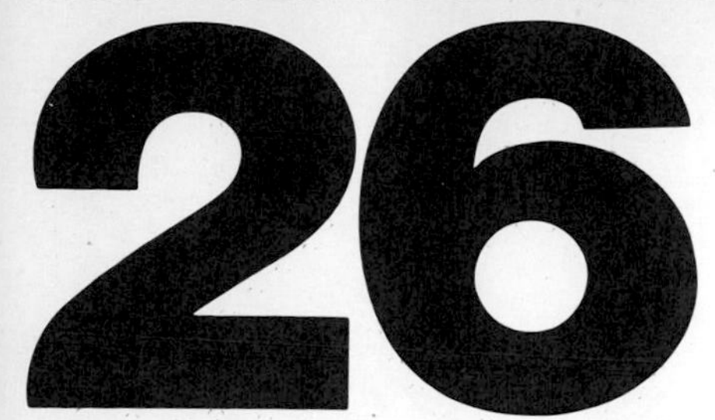

Chest Physiotherapy

I. The subject of this chapter is the use of physical means to effect improved **pulmonary ventilation.** A brief description of the basic modalities and technical aspects of chest physiotherapy will be presented. It is important to keep in mind that this is only one aspect of patient care. For optimal results, the **chest physiotherapists** should coordinate the activities that will be discussed with those of the **respiratory therapist** (see Chap. 25), all under the guidance of competent **medical supervision.**

II. **Physical techniques**

A. **Deep-breathing** exercises.

B. **Cough** stimulation.

C. **Positioning** (postural drainage).

D. **Vibration** (gross and ultrasonic).

E. **Percussion.**

III. **Indications.** Physiotherapy should be considered as an adjunct in the following situations:

A. As preoperative **prophylaxis** when ventilatory difficulties might be anticipated in the postoperative period.

B. **In the treatment** of acute respiratory disease of the lungs and air passages.

C. **In the management** of chronic obstructive respiratory disease of pulmonary origin.

D. To **train patients** to participate in their own respiratory therapy.

IV. **Gross anatomy of the bronchopulmonary tree and passages. The physical techniques** in chest physiotherapy may be more intelligently utilized through full understanding of the divisions and angulation of the bronchopulmonary segments (Fig. 26-1).

A. At the approximate level of the **sixth thoracic vertebra,** the **trachea** divides into a **right** and a **left bronchus.**

1. **The carina,** marking the division, is situated slightly to the left of the midline.

2. **The right bronchus** is shorter and broader and extends in a relatively straight line (approximately 25 degrees from the midline).

3. **The left bronchus** is longer and narrower and extends to the left in an acute angle (approximately 45 degrees from the midline).

B. **The right upper lobe bronchus** branches just below the origin of the right main stem bronchus.

1. **The right main stem bronchus** continues down to divide into the **middle** and **lower lobe bronchi.**

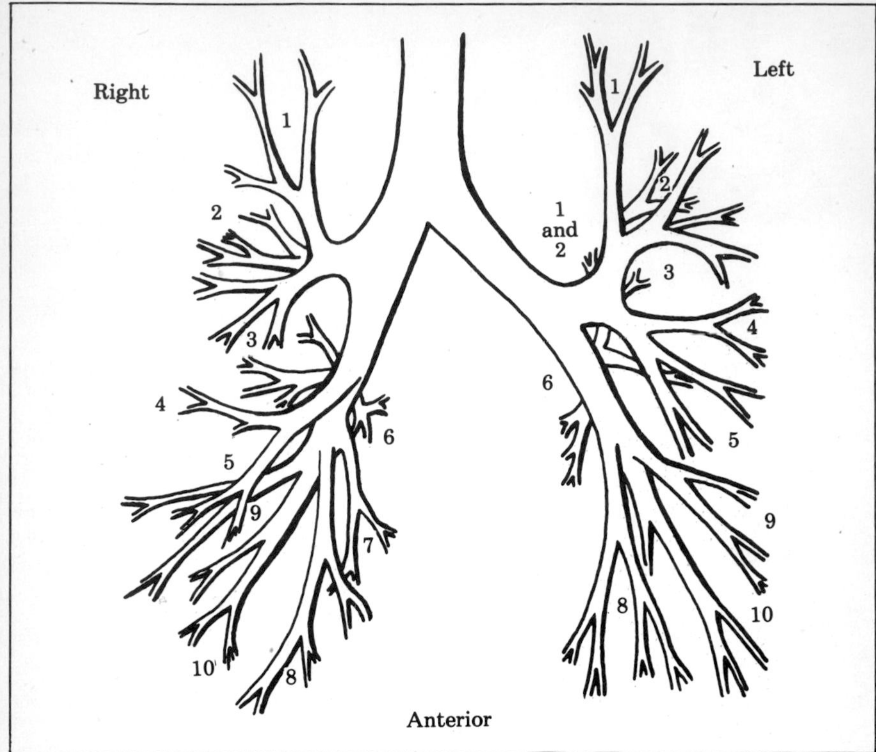

Fig. 26-1. Diagram illustrating the bronchopulmonary nomenclature (as approved by the Thoracic Society). Upper lobes: 1, apical bronchus; 2, posterior bronchus; 3, anterior bronchus. Right middle lobe: 4, lateral bronchus; 5, medial bronchus. Right lower lobe: 6, apical bronchus; 7, medial basal (cardiac) bronchus; 8, anterior basal bronchus; 9, lateral basal bronchus; 10, posterior basal bronchus. Left lingula: 4, superior bronchus; 5, inferior bronchus. Left lower lobe: 6, apical bronchus; 8, anterior basal bronchus; 9, lateral basal bronchus; 10, posterior basal bronchus.

2. **The right upper lobe** divides into apical-anterior, apical-posterior, anterior, and posterior segments.

3. **The right middle lobe** divides into medial and lateral segments.

4. **The right lower lobe** divides into apical, medial basal, anterior, lateral, and posterior segments.

C. **The left main stem bronchus** terminates in the upper and lower bronchi, leading to the upper lobe and lower lobe division of the left lung.

1. **The left upper lobe** divides into apical-anterior, apical-posterior, anterior, posterior, and lingula segments.

2. **The left lower lobe** divides into apical, anterior, lateral, and posterior segments.

V. **Positioning of the patient.** Since each of these divisions enters the next larger (cephalad) segment at varying angles, it is absolutely mandatory to **position the patient properly,** as follows, to achieve optimum drainage during therapy.

A. Right lung

1. **Right upper lobe, posterior segment.** The patient is placed a quarter turn from the prone position, left arm outstretched behind.

2. **Right upper lobe, anterior segment.** The patient is placed in the supine position, with arms extended above the head and the foot of the bed elevated 30 cm.

3. **Right upper lobe, apical-anterior and apical-posterior segments.** The patient is placed in a semisitting position, a quarter turn from the prone position, with the left arm outstretched behind. Alternate positioning can be achieved by sitting the patient upright and tilting him forward, then sideward.

4. **Right middle lobe, medial and lateral segments.** The patient is placed a quarter turn from the supine position, with the right side elevated and the foot of the bed elevated 30 cm.

5. **Right lower lobe, anterior, apical, and medial basal segments.** The patient is placed in the supine position, with the foot of the bed raised 45 cm. The patient should be rotated a quarter turn anteriorly and posteriorly.

6. **Right lower lobe, posterior and lateral segments.** The patient is placed in the prone position, with a pillow under the abdomen and the foot of the bed raised 45 cm. The alternate position, as discussed in **B.8,** also can be used for patients who can tolerate the added stress.

B. Left lung

1. **Left upper lobe, posterior segments.** The same position as in **A.3** but with the right arm outstretched. The alternate positioning described also may be used.

2. **Left upper lobe, anterior segment.** Positioning is as in **A.3** but with a quarter turn being taken from the supine position. Alternate positioning is the same as in **A.3.**

3. **Left upper lobe, anterior segment.** The patient is placed in the supine position.

4. **Left upper lobe, lingula.** The patient is placed a quarter turn from the supine position, with left side elevation, and the foot of the bed raised approximately 30 cm.

5. **Left lower lobe, apical segment.** The patient is placed in the prone position, and the patient's back is flattened by placing a pillow under the abdomen.

6. **Left lower lobe, lateral basal segment.** The patient is placed on the side, with the foot of the bed raised 45 cm. A pillow is put under the patient's waist to keep the spinal column straight.

7. **Left lower lobe, anterior segment.** The patient is placed in the supine position, with the foot of the bed raised 45 cm.

8. **Left lower lobe, posterior segment.** The patient is placed in the prone position, with a pillow under the abdomen and the foot of the bed raised 45 cm. An alternative position (involves much more rigorous stress, not tolerated by very ill patients) is to jackknife the patient over the side of the bed, with the forearms resting on a pillow on a low stool or on the floor. An angle of at least 45 degrees at the hips is required for maximum drainage.

VI. Specific modalities of chest physiotherapy

A. Deep-breathing exercises

1. The emphasis is on **diaphragmatic respiration.** The objective is to teach proper use of the diaphragm to accomplish:

   a. Adequate **distribution of gases** in the basal segments of the lungs.
   b. Utilization of ancillary as well as primary **muscles of respiration,** with a view to decreasing the energy requirements of respiratory effort.

2. An additional benefit is the **support** diaphragmatic respiration gives the **cough effort** by improving the mechanics of the force of the cough.
3. Of particular importance is the effort the patient must put forth. While it is extremely important to obtain deep respiration, **hyperventilation** to the point of producing **hypocapnia** must not be permitted.
4. Also, **aerophagia** must be avoided to prevent either gastric distention and regurgitation or distention of the intestines.

B. **Coughing.** The obvious purpose of cough training is efficient **removal of foreign bodies,** including excessive **secretions,** from the respiratory tract. The objective of a productive cough, i.e., bringing up mucus and other debris of the tracheobronchial tree, must be pursued. However, it is important to **avoid exhausting** the patient by too-prolonged and too-forceful efforts.

C. **Postural drainage** involves placement of patients into previously described positions, making it possible to facilitate **gravitational drainage of secretions** that adversely affect ventilation. It further assists in distribution of gases and thus prevents and/or aids in reversing atelectasis. Caution is advised in employment of extreme positions, and particular attention must be given to the effects of positional changes on the cardiovascular system.

D. **Vibration.** The theory of this modality is that the use of vibratory motions over the chest wall during the expiratory phase of respiration helps to loosen and mobilize the moderately thick secretions within the lung. However, the potentialities of ultrasound and other physical technologic applications are more promising. There is no evidence that manual vibration accomplishes any purpose.

E. **Percussion.** Clapping with cupped palms, or pounding with the fist or the blade of the hand, over the chest wall overlying the area of pathology is the best description of this technique. Thick **secretions are loosened** from bronchial tube walls. Air turbulence within the air passages adds to the dislodging of the secretions. This is done throughout both inspiratory and expiratory phases of respiration.

F. All the modalities described **require planning.** It is manifestly impossible to utilize all the techniques in sequence.

   1. The patient should receive two or three treatments, using differing therapeutic approaches, each day. The duration of each treatment should be 15–20 min initially, with subsequent timing based on the patient's energy output.
   2. Additionally, the final approach should be based on the patient's response to each therapeutic modality used.

G. In situations involving markedly **viscid secretions,** consultation and a combination of these techniques with therapeutic bronchoscopy can be of major value.

H. At no time should chest physiotherapy be initiated or continued without **medical direction.** Evaluation of the results of treatment on a daily basis will lead to the most efficient therapy, based on cost-benefit considerations. This evaluation can be accomplished by **arterial blood gas** studies combined with **radiologic** and **auscultatory studies.**

Bibliography

Ali, J., and Khan, T. A. The comparative effects of muscle transection and median upper abdominal incisions on postoperative pulmonary function. *Surg. Gynecol. Obstet.* 148:863, 1979.

Bartlett, R. H., Gazzaniga, A. B., and Geraghty, T. R. Respiratory maneuvers to prevent postoperative pulmonary complications. *J.A.M.A.* 224:1017, 1973.

Black, J., Kalloor, G. J., and Collis, J. L. The effect of the surgical approach on respiratory function after esophageal resection. *Br. J. Surg.* 64:624, 1977.

Hedstrand, U., Liw, M., Rooth, G., et al. Effect of respiratory physical therapy on arterial oxygen tension. *Acta Anaesthesiol. Scand.* 22:349, 1978.

Wallace, P. G. M., and Norris, W. The management of postoperative pain. *Br. J. Anaesth.* 47:113, 1975.

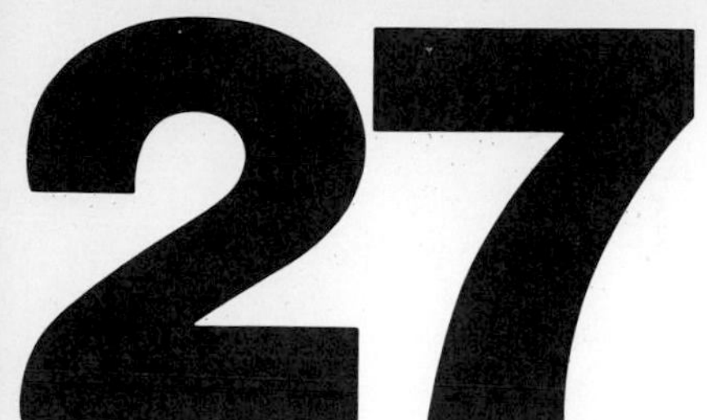

Respiration and Respiratory Care

I. Physiology

A. The primary function of the lungs is the loading of mixed venous blood with oxygen and the elimination of excess carbon dioxide. Thus the lungs convert venous blood to arterial blood.

B. Pulmonary gas exchange involves a number of processes:

1. **Ventilation,** including both volume and distribution of air reaching the alveoli.
2. **Diffusion,** by which carbon dioxide and oxygen pass across the alveolocapillary membrane.
3. **Pulmonary capillary blood flow,** which must be adequate in volume and distributed to all ventilated alveoli.

C. Gas exchange should be accomplished with minimal expenditure of energy by both the respiratory and circulatory systems. For **adequate inspiration,** sufficient force must be applied to the lungs (by expansion of the thorax) to stretch elastic components and overcome frictional resistance in the pulmonary tissues and airways.

D. During **normal respiration,** the work of breathing accounts for 2–4% of the total metabolic rate but may require up to 30% during exercise.

II. Anatomy

A. The respiratory tract is composed of the conducting airway (nose, mouth, pharynx, larynx, trachea, bronchi, and bronchioles) and alveoli (Fig. 27-1). Rapid exchange of oxygen and carbon dioxide between gas and blood occurs only in the alveoli and not in the conducting airway.

B. Bronchi

1. **The main bronchi** maintain their patency by rings of cartilage, which are incomplete posteriorly.
2. **The right main bronchus** is wider and more nearly vertical than the left.
3. **The average angle** between the right bronchus and the long axis of the trachea is 25 degrees, and that of the left and the long tracheal axis is 45 degrees.
4. A little over 2 cm from its origin, the **right main bronchus** gives off the right upper lobe bronchus.
5. **The left main bronchus** bifurcates about 5 cm from its origin into upper lobe and lower lobe bronchi.

C. The terminal bronchiole contains smooth muscles, spirally arranged, and spasm of these muscles may impair the gas exchange. In fact, loss of elasticity in the muscles may lead to **emphysema,** with resulting collapse of the terminal bronchiole.

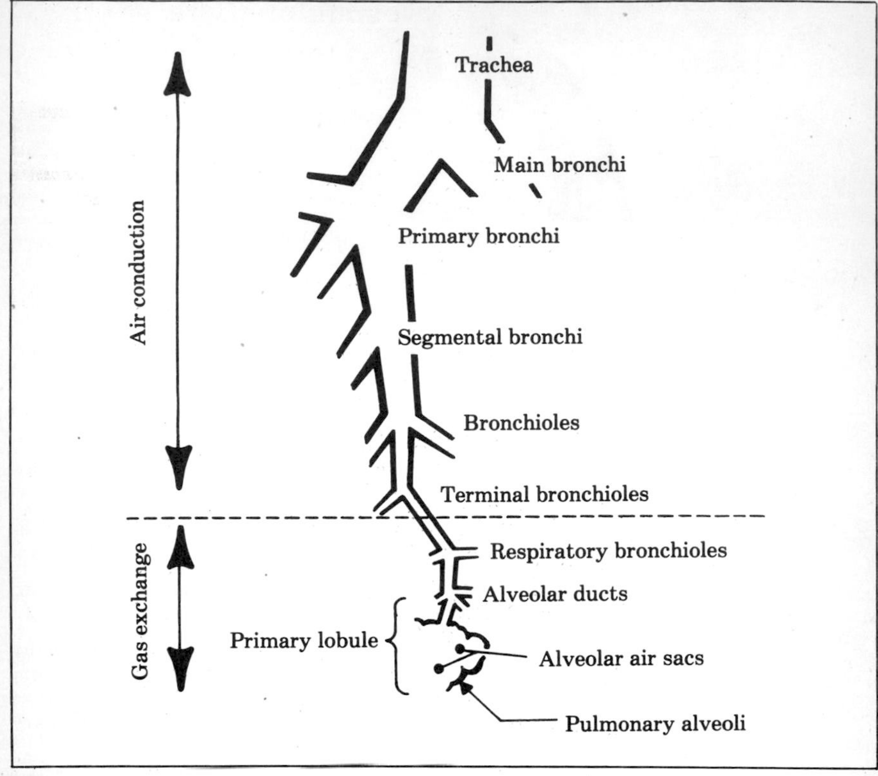

Fig. 27-1. Schema of respiratory tract anatomy.

D. **The alveoli** are lined with flattened epithelium. Large alveolar cells in the lining epithelium secrete a substance, **pulmonary surfactant,** which causes variation of surface tension with changing alveolar volume. **Surface tension** occurs when there is a surface separating liquid from gas.

1. The conception that there is a surface tension of the film of fluid between the layers of pleura, which was thought in the past to be an important force in helping to keep the lungs inflated, must be abandoned. Until the pleura is opened, there is no "surface," since there is no cavity.

2. If in the alveoli (diameter about 40 microns) there were a normal surface tension of biologic fluids of, say, 40 dynes/cm, there would be a pressure difference across the surface of 40 cm H_2O in a direction that would tend to collapse the alveoli. In fact, the constituents of the surface film in the alveoli, probably mainly mucoprotein, reduce the effective surface tension to about 1 dyne/cm, and thus the pressure difference across the surface is reduced to about 1 cm H_2O, which is a negligible amount.

III. Pulmonary circulation

A. **Pulmonary blood volume** is the volume of blood between the beginning of the pulmonary artery and the end of the pulmonary veins. It is about 900 ml for an adult.

B. Pulmonary capillary blood volume is the volume of blood in the capillary bed at any given moment, which is 75–100 ml in a resting adult. However, it increases during exercise, hypervolemia, and pulmonary congestion and decreases in patients with destructive lesions of the pulmonary parenchyma.

C. Causes of uneven pulmonary capillary blood flow

1. **Physiologic.** Uneven blood flow occurs in large part because of the effect of gravity and therefore is minimal when a person is supine or prone, greater in a lateral position, and maximal when erect. Thus when a person stands, more blood is present at the bases of the lungs than at the apices; and when the person is in the lateral position, more blood is present at the lower-lying lung.

2. The **pathologic** causes of uneven capillary blood flow affecting the lungs and circulation are many. Some of these are:

   a. Embolism or thrombosis of parts of the pulmonary circulation.

   b. Partial or complete occlusion of some of the arterioles by arteriosclerotic lesions.

   c. Endarteritis.

   d. Reduction of part of the pulmonary vascular bed by destruction of lung tissue by fibrotic obliteration of pulmonary vessels.

   e. Regional congestion of vessels such as occurs in some types of heart failure.

IV. The lung volumes

A. Measurement of resting ventilation is seldom of value, although it is accepted that it might help to establish the diagnosis of ventilatory failure in the absence of methods of measurement of $PaCO_2$.

B. The vital capacity (VC) is the volume of gas expired by a maximal effort following maximal inspiration. It can be measured directly by the use of simple volume recorders, such as Wright's spirometer.

1. The VC of healthy persons varies with sex, height, weight, and age.

2. **A number of formulas** have been worked out to predict vital capacity. A simple, rapid means of calculating the predicted **VC (in milliliters)** is:

   a. Males: height (in cm) × 25
   Females: height (in cm) × 20

   or

   b. 70 per kilogram of body weight

3. **The VC of healthy persons may vary** as much as 20% from the average values. It varies with a patient's position (it may be 300 ml less when lying down than when standing), and it may vary from time to time even in the same person. For these reasons, a "low" VC obtained during the first examination cannot be regarded with certainty as abnormal unless it is 20% less than the average or predicted value. Only the volumes of serial measurements may have prognostic value.

4. **VC may be reduced** in a number of lung diseases (atelectasis, pneumonia, bronchiolar obstruction, or pulmonary edema), in some nonpulmonary causes (depression of respiratory center or limitation of expansion of the lungs due to pleural effusion), and in limitation of descent of the diaphragm, as in ascites and abdominal tumors.

5. **VC may be normal or decreased** in emphysema; when decreased, it is the result of a large residual volume (RV), but the total lung capacity (TLC) may be increased.

C. **The functional residual capacity (FRC)** is the volume of gas in the lungs at the end of a complete expiration. It is the only one of the four volumes (total lung capacity, VC, IC, and FRC) that cannot be measured by direct spirometry and must be determined by indirect methods.

1. **Increased FRC** is commonly assumed to represent structural emphysematous changes in the lungs. Actually, it represents hyperinflation, not emphysema. **Hyperinflation** may result from:

   a. Structural changes, such as occur in emphysema.

   b. Partial obstruction to the airway, as in asthma.

   c. Deformity of the thorax.

   d. Compensatory overinflation of the lung following surgical removal of lung tissue.

2. **When FRC is increased,** the rate of uptake of anesthetic gases is reduced, and elimination of inhalation anesthetics is prolonged (more marked with anesthetics of high solubility in blood).

D. **Typical lung volume values.** See Table 27-1.

V. Measurement of ventilatory capacity

A. The assessment of **ventilatory capacity** is generally of greater value than the measurement of resting ventilation.

B. The maximum volume of air that the patient can breathe within 1 min is known as the **maximum breathing capacity.**

1. The patient is asked to breathe as quickly and deeply as possible for a period of 15 sec (through a spirometer), and the volume of air moved is then multiplied by 4. This test is exhausting for the patient and requires considerable practice.

2. A simpler test, the **forced expiratory volume (FEV),** is preferred, because the ventilatory capacity is usually closely related to the expiratory ability of the patient (an exception is the rare cases of inspiratory obstruction exclusively). A close correlation has been demonstrated between FEV at 1 sec and MBC. One can estimate MBC by multiplying FEV_1 by 35.

C. The most popular method of expressing the **expiratory ability** is to measure the volume exhaled in the **first second,** designated $\mathbf{FEV_{1.0}}$. The $FEV_{1.0}$ is normally greater than 75% of the vital capacity (this ratio is reduced in obstructive but not in restrictive disease).

VI. Mechanics of breathing

A. **During aspiration,** active muscular contraction provides the force necessary to overcome:

1. **Elastic recoil of the lungs** and thorax.

2. **Frictional resistance** during movements of the tissues of the lungs and thorax.

3. **Frictional resistance to air flow** through the fine tubes and ducts of the tracheobronchial tree.

4. **At the end of inspiration,** potential energy created by contraction of the inspiratory muscles is stored in the elastic tissues, and, when the inspiratory muscles relax, the elastic tissues recoil. If nonelastic tissue resistance and airway resistance are minimal, the **elastic recoil** causes the lungs and thorax to return rapidly to the resting level, although expiration is completely passive. In contrast, if expiratory resistance is great, active contraction of the expiratory muscles will be needed unless the time for the expiration is prolonged.

Table 27-1. Lung Volumes in Healthy Recumbent Subjects (in ml)

Lung Volume	Males 20–30 yr 1.7 m^2	Males 50–60 yr 1.7 m^2	Females 20–30 yr 1.6 m^2
Inspiratory capacity (IC)	3.600	2.600	2.400
Expiratory reserve capacity (ERC)	1.200	1.000	800
Vital capacity (VC)	4.800	3.600	3.200
Residual volume (RV)	1.200	2.400	1.000
Functional residual capacity (FRC)	2.400	3.400	1.800
Total lung capacity (TLC)	6.000	6.000	4.200

B. Compliance of lungs and thorax

1. The greater the muscular force applied, the more the lungs are stretched and the greater the volume change on inspiration.
2. The slope of the line that results from plotting the external force (pressure) against the increase in volume serves as a measure of the distensibility of the lungs and thorax. If the slope is more vertical, the tissues are more distensible; if it is more horizontal, the tissues are less distensible. This phenomenon is called **mechanical compliance** or, more simply, **compliance of the tissue,** and it is defined as the **volume change per unit of pressure change.** Its units are L/cm H_2O.
3. Since the lungs and thoracic cage are acting together as a unit, they require more force for expansion to a given volume than does either component alone:

$$\frac{1}{\text{Total compliance}} = \frac{1}{\text{Lung compliance}} + \frac{1}{\text{Thoracic cage compliance}}$$

C. Compliance is reduced in some pathologic conditions—pulmonary edema, pleural effusion, pulmonary fibrosis, atelectasis, pneumonia—and in diseases of the thoracic cage (kyphoscoliosis, pectus excavatum).

D. Airway resistance

1. **A driving pressure** is necessary **during inspiration** to pull air through the upper airway, bronchial and bronchiolar resistances in the alveoli, and during expiration to push alveolar gas out through these tubes. Here the following equation applies:

$$\text{Resistance} = \frac{\text{driving pressure}}{\text{flow}}$$

2. **The driving pressure across the airway** is the atmospheric pressure minus alveolar pressure during inspiration, and alveolar pressure minus atmospheric pressure during expiration. The units are cm H_2O/L/sec.
3. The airway resistance **is created** by friction between molecules of the gas and the walls of the airway.
   a. **When the flow is laminar,** airway resistance varies directly with the length of the tube and the viscosity of the gas and inversely with the fourth power of the radius of the lumen of the tubes.
   b. **When the flow is turbulent,** the airway resistance is independent of the viscosity of the gas and varies directly with its density.
4. In patients, airway resistance is always **increased** during an **asthmatic attack** and even in the symptom-free interval between attacks. It also is

increased in emphysema (due to collapse of fine airways during expiration) and in other disorders in which fibrous tissue, tumors, or effusions constrict or obstruct airways.

VII. Dead space

A. Anatomic dead space is the internal volume of the conducting airway, from the nose and mouth down to the alveoli. This volume of air is called **wasted ventilation,** because it does not enter the perfused alveoli to be effective in blood gas exchange.

B. During a quiet inspiration, **the tidal volume** (V_T) is 450 ml. Of this, approximately 150 ml never reaches perfused alveoli, and this portion of the tidal volume is called **anatomic dead space** (V_D). To determine the alveolar ventilation with each breath (V_A), subtract the anatomic dead space (V_D) from the tidal volume (V_T). The alveolar ventilation per minute ($\dot{V}_A$) can then be calculated: it is equal to the alveolar ventilation per breath multiplied by the respiratory frequency/min (f): $\dot{V}_A = V_A \times f$. Deep breathing causes a greater fraction of the V_T to enter the alveoli and shallow breathing, a smaller fraction.

1. **The V_D is decreased** by a third when an endotracheal tube is placed and is **increased** in masks and conducting tubing used for inhalation anesthesia.
2. **Alveolar dead space** (V_{DA}) is the ventilation of nonperfused or underperfused alveoli. It is increased in pulmonary embolism and in low-flow states of hemorrhage or marked hypotension.
3. **Physiologic dead space** is the sum of V_D and V_{DA}. Because in normal subjects V_{DA} is minimal, V_D is essentially equal to the physiologic dead space. The term **physiologic dead space** is misleading; it is not physiologic but, rather, pathologic.

VIII. Respiratory failure. Respiratory insufficiency may arise from the following causes, several of which may be present at the same time:

A. Central factors affecting the areas of respiratory control in the medulla and pons: depression due to drugs; depression due to retained metabolic products, as in carbon dioxide retention, diabetes mellitus, and uremia; damage by injury or cerebrovascular accident; invasion by neurologic disease; the raising of intracranial pressure by the presence of a tumor; or the immediate aftereffects of neurosurgery.

B. Neuromuscular disorders, including brainstem and cervical spinal cord lesions, poliomyelitis, myasthenia gravis, the myopathies, and partial or complete paralysis following the use of relaxant drugs, as in the treatment of tetanus or in the immediate postoperative phase.

C. Metabolic abnormalities also may cause neuromuscular derangement, as, for example, in porphyrinuria or metabolic acidosis.

D. Diseases of the lungs or air passages, including conditions such as emphysema and bronchitis, especially when acute infection is superimposed; acute bronchospastic states; and acute inflammatory conditions (pneumonia).

E. Injury or disorders of the muscles of respiration or their attachments. These include stove-in chest, fractures of the ribs, kyphoscoliosis, ankylosing spondylitis, and myopathies.

F. Acute obstruction of air passages

1. The causes of the obstruction may be **intrinsic,** as from aspirated foreign material; excessive secretions; new growth of the pharynx, larynx, or lower airways; inflammatory conditions of the floor of the mouth and glottis; or paralysis of the vocal cords due to injury or disease.
2. The causes of obstruction may be **extrinsic,** as in the case of a neoplasm compressing the airway or hematoma formation.

G. Abnormalities of pulmonary circulation, including pulmonary embolism or low-flow states.

H. Other conditions, such as spontaneous pneumothorax or pleural effusion.

IX. The anesthesiologist and respiratory failure

A. Although the **anesthesiologist** is the most competent person to care for patients with respiratory failure, a **team of physicians** with special knowledge (including an internist and a neurologist) will provide the best care, since in each case not only is respiratory support needed but also the cause of the respiratory failure must be treated.

B. The approach to patients with **lesser degrees of respiratory impairment** or with temporary impairment—as in the postoperative period—generally will not be a problem. Special problems will arise in patients with respiratory insufficiency for whom respiratory support may be needed for days or weeks.

X. Mechanical ventilation

A. A mechanical ventilator is a device for changing the pressure within the patient's airway in cyclic fashion, so that gas enters and leaves the lungs.

1. Application of external negative pressure to the chest

a. Cabinet ventilators are designed to provide artificial respiration by exerting negative and positive pressure alternatively on the whole body area. The whole body is enclosed in an airtight tank or cabinet. The airtight seal is effected at the patient's neck.

b. The pressure in the cabinet can be varied, as can the respiratory rate and cycle.

c. The pressure in the cabinet is usually held at 12–18 cm H_2O below atmospheric pressure, so that air flows into the chest and expands the lungs and thorax.

d. The apparatus is cumbersome, nursing care is difficult, and an airtight seal around the neck is not easily obtained. In addition, the pressure difference is applied to the whole body surface and affects the peripheral circulation. Some of these drawbacks are minimized by the use of a **cuirass ventilator** (surrounding the chest and abdomen). This device is more portable and more mobile than other ventilators but is less efficient, because it is not easily adjusted or applied.

2. Intermittent pressure ventilators. It is convenient to classify intermittent pressure ventilators according to their primary cycling mechanism:

a. Pressure-cycled ventilators.

b. Volume-cycled ventilators (pressure limited).

c. Time-cycled ventilators (pressure limited).

d. The first group may be classified as preset pressure ventilators, and the second and third, as preset volume respirators.

B. Pressure-cycled machines

1. In these ventilators, the **inspiratory phase** ends when the pressure in the circuit reaches some critical value. The cycling mechanism is activated by changes in the patient's lungs at a pressure set by the anesthesiologist.

2. The length of the inspiratory period is adjusted by varying the flow rate. The higher the flow rate, the quicker the cycling pressure is reached.

3. Any obstruction in the lungs, decreasing lung volume or compliance or increasing muscle tone or coughing, will allow cycling pressure to be reached more rapidly, and inspiration will become shorter. Thus the inspiratory volume will be reduced.

4. **Removal of obstruction,** decreasing muscle tone, or increasing compliance, will increase the length of inspiration and the inspiratory volume.

5. **For accurate timing** of inspiratory and expiratory phases, the pressure-cycling device demands a circuit with no leaks, although well-designed machines with large flow rates can compensate for leaks.

C. **Volume-cycled machines** are pumps that utilize bellows or pistons and deliver preset volumes to the lungs irrespective of the pressure produced. These machines can compensate for pulmonary changes but not for leaks. A pressure-limiting valve must be used to avoid building up dangerous pressures ("safe" inflation pressures are generally given as 20–30 cm H_2O).

D. **Time-cycled machines** are preset volume machines in which inspiration ends after a preset time, the time being determined entirely by the ventilator.

E. **Triggers**

1. Any intermittent positive-pressure breathing machine may be fitted with a triggering device. If a patient initiates an ineffectual spontaneous inspiration during the expiratory phase of automatic ventilation, arrangements can be made (by the use of permanent magnets or microswitches) so that a small pressure difference produced by the patient will trigger an inspiration by the machine.

2. A small inspiration of 5 ml of air may be sufficient to trigger the machine.

F. **Humidification**

1. During **short-term** use of mechanical ventilation, humidification of inspired gas is important because the nose and pharynx, the natural humidifiers of inspired air, are bypassed by the endotracheal or tracheostomy tube. With inadequate humidification, the tracheal mucosa dries, and the function of cilia is impaired.

2. Humidification is essential in **long-term** treatment. The water loss from the lungs is proportional to the minute volume of ventilation and is usually expressed as loss of water in the units ml/L of minute volume of the ventilator. The average loss per hour in a nonrebreathing system is 11–13 g.

XI. Management of patients during mechanical ventilation

A. **Indications for tracheal intubation** and ventilation.

1. **Mechanics**

   a. Respiratory rate > 35 breaths/min.

   b. VC < 15 ml/kg of body weight.

   c. FEV_1 < 10 ml/kg of body weight.

   d. Inspiratory force < 25 cm H_2O.

2. **Oxygenation**

   a. PaO_2 < 70 torr (FIO_2 50–60%, mask or T-piece).

   b. A − aDO_2 (torr) > 450 after 10 min of 100%.

3. **Ventilation**

   a. $PaCO_2$ > 55 torr (except in patients with chronic hypercapnia).

   b. V_D/V_T < 0.60.

B. **A tidal volume of 10 to 15 ml/kg,** which is higher than normal, is chosen for an adult to prevent atelectasis. A larger tidal volume also permits a slower rate (10–14 respirations per minute in adults) to achieve a proper ventilatory pattern.

1. In the presence of normal lungs, the **Radford nomogram** can act as a guide, and PaO_2 and $PaCO_2$ will permit adjustments of the tidal volume.
2. Commonly, in the early stage of mechanical ventilation, **arterial hypotension** occurs as the result of several factors:
   a. The effects of positive pressure on the circulation (diminished venous return), which are more severe in hypovolemic patients.
   b. The sudden reduction in $PaCO_2$.
   c. The use of different drugs.
   d. A significant fall in **cardiac output** does not occur provided (1) positive pressure is limited to a small portion of the respiratory cycle, (2) the expiratory period is made as long as possible, and (3) there is no other cause of hypovolemia.
   e. The addition of **subatmospheric pressure** in the expiratory period reduces the mean pressure in the system and thus may improve cardiac output.

C. **Subatmospheric (or negative) pressure** during the expiratory phase may be of use in improving ventilation in some patients with respiratory disease, but there is danger that "**air trapping**" may occur. The bronchial walls may collapse before the alveoli empty, or collapsed alveoli may tend to stick and thus require a higher inflation pressure to reexpand them.

D. Sometimes it is desirable either to **retard the outflow of gas** during expiration or **to maintain a positive pressure** through the entire respiratory cycle **(continuous positive-pressure ventilation).** Continuous positive-pressure ventilation helps to maintain the patency of collapsed alveoli and reduces the alveolar-arterial (A–a) gradient for oxygen (in shock lung syndrome, for instance). It is also of value in the presence of pulmonary edema, probably by diminishing the venous return to the heart.

E. Another mode of augmented ventilation is **intermittent mandatory ventilation,** in which patients are allowed to breathe on their own, and at certain intervals a mandatory inspiration is provided by the ventilator. The use of intermittent mandatory ventilation in the weaning process seems to be of great advantage.

F. **Accumulation of secretions** in the respiratory tract must be avoided. General body hydration by intravenous infusion and humidification of the inspired air loosens thick secretions. Antibiotics, bronchodilators, and physiotherapy as prophylaxis are also of use.
   1. **Aspiration of secretions** through the endotracheal or tracheostomy tube must be done under strict **aseptic conditions.** It is wise to preoxygenate the patient before suctioning, and to avoid hypoxemic episodes and alveolar collapse, suction must not last more than 5–10 sec.
   2. **After suction,** vigorous inflation of the lungs will reexpand collapsed alveoli.

G. **An orotracheal, nasotracheal, or tracheostomy tube** may be used.
   1. The choice between the first or the second is rarely a problem. Each has its advantages and disadvantages.
   2. A decision to perform **tracheostomy** early may be considered. If it is obvious that a patient will need artificial ventilation for a long time, tracheostomy is done at the beginning. Otherwise, an endotracheal tube is introduced; this can be replaced by a tracheostomy tube later.
   3. **When tracheostomy is to be avoided,** the endotracheal tube may be left in place, even for weeks. However, it must be changed at regular intervals.
   4. **Cuffs** must be deflated, if possible, once an hour for 3 min. A cuff with a large surface area, requiring low pressure, is preferred.

H. Prolonged oral or nasotracheal intubation may cause laryngeal stenosis. **Stenosis of the trachea** may develop after both tracheostomy and intubation. Probably the first lesion is the ulceration of the mucosa, which later involves the deeper structures, with formation of tissue granulation and then scarring.

I. Patients on mechanical ventilation must be **monitored** continuously: measurements of blood gases (a $PaCO_2$ of 40 torr in the arterial blood or perhaps a little less); measurement of pH (the aim being to maintain the pH of the blood at 7.4 or a little higher, since alkalosis is much less harmful than acidosis); and measurements of respiratory volumes.

J. Water and electrolyte replacement must be done very carefully and **dietary requirements** must be met in patients undergoing long-term mechanical ventilation. These patients require at least 2000 calories daily, which can be administered through a feeding tube as carbohydrates (in the form of lactose in milk) and proteins (mainly obtained from milk, supplemented if necessary by raw egg). Vitamin supplements may be added. IV feeding is indicated only when gastric stasis develops, as shown by the large volume of fluid aspirated through the feeding tube before injection of the food, and when diarrhea occurs.

K. Care of the eyes is important because they may exfoliate, even in the absence of trauma, simply because they are dry. Also, the **care of bladder and bowels** is important in many patients.

L. Nursing care and physiotherapy are of paramount importance; a friendly, human approach to these patients will minimize the problems posed by their respiratory care.

M. Weaning from a respirator should be done as soon as possible. However, a decision to wean should be based on measurements of the shunt, dead space, VC, and compliance.

1. Criteria of weaning ability

a. Tests of mechanical capability

(1) VC $>$ 10–15 ml/kg body weight.

(2) FEV_1 in 1 sec $>$ 10 ml/kg body weight.

(3) Peak inspiratory pressure > -20 to -30 cm H_2O.

(4) Resting minute ventilation $<$ 10 L/min (can be doubled with maximal voluntary ventilation).

b. Tests of oxygenation capability

(1) $A\text{-}aDo_2$ on 100% O_2 $>$ 300–350 torr.

(2) Shunt fraction ($\dot{Q}S/\dot{Q}T$) $<$ 10–20%.

(3) Dead space/tidal volume (VD/VT) $<$ 0.55–0.6.

2. After a period when the patient is without mechanical ventilation, during which oxygen is breathed, he or she is **watched closely** for cyanosis, tachypnea, tachycardia, and assessment of general condition. During this period, heavy sedation is to be avoided.

3. In some instances it will be possible to stop the respirator entirely once and for all. In others, it will be necessary to wean the patient slowly, giving perhaps a half hour of rest every 4 hr to start with and then increasing the periods of normal breathing until the patient is no longer dependent on the machine.

N. The next part of the recovery process—**when the patient is able to swallow**—is to remove the feeding tube and attempt to feed the patient in the normal manner. It is vital that the cuffed tracheostomy tube remain in situ during feeding, for the cuff of the tube is still the patient's main protection against aspiration of fluid or food.

O. The last stage in the patient's return to normal is **the closure of the tracheostomy.** This should be done only when the patient is able to cough vigorously without assistance. It should not precede the recovery of normal swallowing.

Bibliography

Leventhal, S. R., Orkin, F. K., and Hirsh, R. A. Prediction of the need for postoperative mechanical ventilation in myasthenia gravis. *Anesthesiology* 53:26, 1980.

Loh, L., Sykes, M. K., and Chakrabarti, M. K. The assessment of ventilator performance. *Br. J. Anaesth.* 50:63, 1978.

Moore, D. C. Intercostal nerve block for postoperative somatic pain following surgery of thorax and upper abdomen. *Br. J. Anaesth.* 47:284, 1975.

Rehder, K. Anesthesia and the respiratory system. *Can. Anaesth. Soc. J.* 26:451, 1979.

Rigg, J. R. A., and Jones, N. L. Clinical assessment of respiratory function. *Br. J. Anaesth.* 50:3, 1978.

Stenquist, O., Sonander, H., and Nilsson, K. Small endotracheal tubes. Ventilator and intratracheal pressure during controlled ventilation. *Br. J. Anaesth.* 51:375, 1979.

Stoddart, J. C. Postoperative respiratory failure. An anesthetic hazard? *Br. J. Anaesth.* 50:695, 1978.

Vejlsted, H., Hansen, M., and Jacobsen, E. Postoperative ventilatory response to carbon dioxide following neurolept anesthesia. *Acta Anaesthesiol. Scand.* 21:529, 1977.

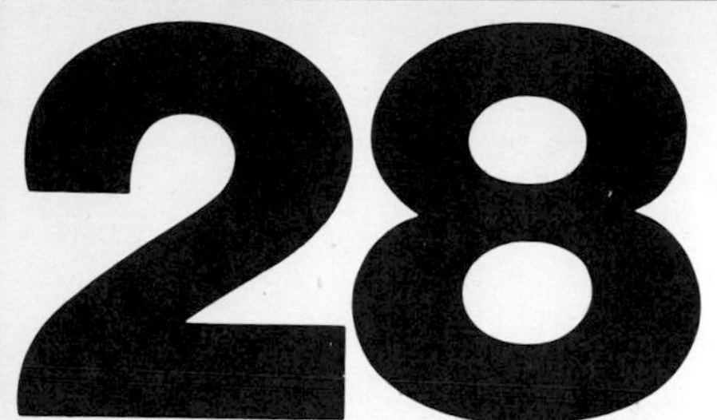

Diabetes and Anesthesia

I. **Diabetic patients** (over 4 million in the United States) are exposed to elective and emergency surgery with increasing frequency. Improved long-term diabetes management has reduced the risks involved to the point where these patients essentially differ very little from those who are not diabetic. Nevertheless, the diabetic patient is a candidate for certain **potential complications** related to the severity and chronicity of the diabetes.

A. **The first step of management of anesthesia** in diabetic patients is assessment of the control of the disease, followed by evaluation of the diabetic complications and their degree of severity.

B. **Primary care.** Very useful information can be obtained by establishing good communication with the patient and the physician caring for that patient. **In the case of a hospitalized patient,** a careful study of the available records is extremely important. The effort spent in this task is both generally worthwhile and clinically rewarding.

C. **Diabetes is a multisystem disease** that is classified in the following manner:

1. **The genetic type** is the classic form of diabetes and by far the most common. It is subdivided into **ketosis-prone** and **ketosis-resistant** varieties. Approximately 80% of diabetic patients who belong in the genetic type category are ketosis-resistant (adult- or maturity-onset diabetics). The rest are ketosis-prone (juvenile diabetes), the so-called brittle diabetes, which is extremely resistant to treatment.

2. **The pancreatic type** is attributed to direct destruction of pancreatic islet cells by a variety of factors:

   a. Inflammation.

   b. Cancer.

   c. Hemochromatosis.

   d. Surgery.

3. **Endocrine diabetes** is associated with a variety of endocrinopathies:

   a. Hyperpituitarism.

   b. Hyperthyroidism.

   c. Hyperadrenalism (Cushing's syndrome, primary aldosteronism).

   d. Pheochromocytoma.

   e. Pancreatic alpha cell tumor.

   f. Diabetes of stress.

   g. Diabetes of pregnancy.

4. **Iatrogenic diabetes** may occur as a result of the administration of certain drugs, such as corticosteroids, benzthiazide diuretics, and estrogen-progesterone combinations.

II. Pathophysiology

A. The major differentiating factor between the two subdivisions of **genetic diabetes** is the **presence or absence of pancreatic insulin.**

1. **The ketosis-prone diabetic** patients produce essentially no insulin, whereas the **ketosis-resistant diabetic** patients do, but in varying quantities.

2. **The quantity of insulin in ketosis-resistant diabetic patients** will determine not only the severity of their disease but also the mode of their lifetime diabetic management and treatment. These patients control their diabetes with diet alone, oral hypoglycemic agents, or exogenous insulin. Combining these modalities and switching from one type of treatment to another may be done as the situation requires.

3. **Approximately 10% of diabetic patients belong to the ketosis-prone group.** Their management depends on exogenously administered insulin.

B. Diabetic patients suffer from certain **complications** that are attributed to the secondary metabolic effects of diabetes. Because the longevity of diabetic patients has been prolonged, there is sufficient time for development of these associated pathologic states, which modify and increase the anesthetic risk status of the patient.

1. **Accelerated arteriosclerosis.** Of deaths due to cardiovascular-renal diseases, 60% are associated with diabetes.

   a. **During the preoperative assessment,** diagnostic findings pertinent to the cardiovascular state of the patient must be analyzed carefully. Although these findings may not be entirely objective, they do have clinical and prognostic value. Without critical consideration of these factors, **anesthetic management** can become casual and technically hazardous.

   b. A patient who has had diabetes for a long time and who also has **angina and heart failure** tolerates any **hypotension** extremely poorly during either induction or maintenance of anesthesia. Therefore the primary concern of the anesthesiologist in planning the anesthetic management of such a patient is to avoid techniques that may cause hypotension. If it does occur, the anesthesiologist must know how to treat it effectively. Hypertension and tachycardia are equally detrimental. These conditions disturb the oxygen supply/consumption balance, leading to ischemia.

2. A large number of diabetic patients suffer from **cataracts,** which are the leading cause of blindness in diabetes. **Retinopathies, neuropathies,** and **nephropathies** also tend to develop. Preoperative awareness of the existence of these complications will help in the proper selection of anesthetic agents and techniques.

3. **Diabetic neuropathy** may present itself in many forms. The distal, symmetrical, and primarily sensory form is the most common.

   a. **Etiology.** There is strong evidence suggesting that the accumulation of certain sugar alcohols (such as sorbitol) in the peripheral nerves may be responsible for the nerve damage. Tissues like nerve, lens, retina, kidney, blood vessels, and islet cells, which are exposed to high blood glucose levels, permit the penetration of glucose within their cells. This excess sugar is shunted into the normally quiescent sorbitol pathway, causing an increase in sorbitol, leading to osmotic phenomena that affect the Schwann cell and demyelinize the peripheral nerves in a segmental fashion.

   b. **Symptoms.** Numbness and tingling, with relatively little pain, are the main symptoms, usually confined to the feet and lower legs. Muscle weakness is usually mild, but in some cases weakness in the legs with only minor sensory disturbances may predominate.

c. **Autonomic neuropathy** in diabetes is recognized with increasing frequency. This type of neuropathy is particularly serious, since several **cardiovascular reflexes** are sympathetically mediated. Preoperative recognition is extremely important. The usual manifestations are postural hypotension, resting tachycardia, painless or silent myocardial infarction, gastrointestinal and bladder (urinary) dysfunction, and impotence.

d. **Cardiovascular reflexes** are extremely important, and their preoperative assessment is warranted. The usual clinical tests are a Valsalva maneuver, beat-to-beat (R–R interval) heart rate variation, the cardiac response to standing, and the blood pressure response to sustained muscular exercise.

4. **Obesity,** which is strongly associated with diabetes (especially in the ketosis-resistant, or maturity-onset type), may complicate the situation further by adding a **respiratory** component to the whole picture. Of course, obesity itself, in the presence of complicated major surgery, may call for postoperative ventilatory support; postoperative hypoventilation in the obese diabetic patient may be an intolerable insult. In the presence of **chronic obstructive lung disease,** additional objective pulmonary evaluation is mandatory.

C. **Negative findings** in a young diabetic patient during the preoperative assessment **do not exclude the existence of pathologic changes.**

1. From the physiologic point of view, the **chronological age of a diabetic patient** has very little significance.

2. The **young diabetic patient** may not be physiologically young; on the contrary, such a patient may have advanced physiologic changes characteristic of a much older person, with the full spectrum of possible pathologic changes. Patients in their early twenties may be seen suffering from severe arteriosclerotic heart disease similar to that present in 70- or 80-year-old nondiabetic patients.

3. A good clinical rule of thumb in **estimating the physiologic age of the diabetic patient** is to add to the chronological age the length of the clinically known disease. **For example,** a 50-year-old patient with diabetes dating back 20 years has a physiologic age of 70.

III. Treatment

A. **The treatment** of a diabetic patient is as varied and multifaceted as the disease itself. Essentially, there are three modalities of diabetic management:

1. Diet only.
2. Oral hypoglycemic agents.
3. Insulin.

B. **A patient on a special diet only** needs close followup with no additional antidiabetic medications. These patients have very mild diabetes that is easily controlled by diet alone. **A preoperative blood sugar (fasting)** value should be taken, and it must be considered as a baseline.

1. **On the morning of surgery,** these patients may have **acetone in urine with no sugar.** Most probably this represents **starvation ketosis,** which can be treated easily with IV glucose.

2. **If stress (surgical or obstetrical)** disturbs the diabetic state of the patient, insulin may be needed temporarily. **The amount of insulin** required can be estimated by the **sliding-scale technique:** For every 1+ sugar in the urine, 5 units of regular insulin are given. However, this may not be an ideal way to estimate insulin requirements for the following reasons:

a. **The glucose threshold** is not standard for every patient and may change, and considerable variations are possible.

b. **A patient may have very high blood sugar** but little spilled in the urine.

c. In general, **a single daily injection** of 10–20 units of NPH or Lente insulin will suffice to reduce the blood sugar below 200 mg/100 ml. Patients with **iatrogenic diabetes** fall in this category.

d. Another group of patients are adversely affected by certain physiologic processes, such as **pregnancy.** In these patients, who are completely asymptomatic initially, signs of diabetes develop later in pregnancy.

(1) These are patients with prediabetes, most of whom remain diabetic after delivery. However, in a few, the glucose tolerance test during the puerperium shows normal values. They will continue as **latent diabetic patients** for years, or until another pregnancy again provokes clinical diabetes.

(2) In these patients, **from the fourth month of gestation onward,** the renal threshold for glucose falls. As a result, glycosuria becomes an unreliable guide for diabetes management, and, because of the excessive loss of sugar, the patient may be in a state of carbohydrate starvation. This situation, if uncorrected, eventually may lead to glyconeogenesis from proteins and fat, with the production of ketone bodies.

e. Recently, **the administration of insulin** has been changing. There is evidence to suggest that small, continuous doses of insulin are preferable to one preoperative injection. Some suggest that insulin be constantly administered at a rate of 1 unit/hr in patients receiving less than 20 units of insulin daily and at a rate of 2 units/hr in patients receiving more than 20 units of insulin daily. Insulin administered in this fashion is being given, on a limited scale, by **continuous infusion pumps.** Furthermore, when the technology becomes available, infusion from these pumps is to be regulated by an analyzer that senses the blood sugar level and responds by pumping the appropriate amount of insulin.

C. **Patients on oral hypoglycemic agents** have physiologically active beta cells, whose activity will determine the efficacy of the treatment and the type of medication used.

1. There are two types of oral hypoglycemic agents, **sulfonylureas** and **biguanides.**

a. **Sulfonylureas** exert their action by stimulating the beta cells and thereby increasing the output of endogenous insulin. Furthermore, they inhibit glucose formation and release from the liver. The commercially available sulfonylurea derivatives are:

(1) Tolbutamide (Orinase).

(2) Chlorpropamide (Diabinese).

(3) Acetohexamide (Dymelor).

(4) Tolazamide (Tolinase).

b. **Biguanides** act mainly by inceasing the anaerobic metabolism of sugar. Phenformin (DBI) is the commercial preparation from this group.

2. These two groups of oral hypoglycemic agents have different sites of action, and their combined use frequently produces a potentiated effect on the blood sugar.

3. There are **three ways** to plan for anesthesia in a diabetic patient on oral hypoglycemic agents:

a. **For minor surgery** on a mildly diabetic patient, an oral hypoglycemic agent may be omitted.

b. **If surgery is to take place in the morning** and some type of regional anesthesia is planned, medication may be withheld until supper.

c. **If surgery is major** and the patient is going to be on IV fluids for a few days, he or she should be switched temporarily to insulin.

4. **In evaluating a diabetic patient on oral hypoglycemic agents for anesthesia,** keep in mind that the effects of barbiturates and other sedatives and hypnotics may be prolonged. Certain analgesics (phenylbutazone, oxyphenylbutazone, probenecid, and salicylates), bacteriostatic sulfonamides, and monoamine oxidase inhibitors may potentiate their action, resulting in prolonged hypoglycemia. This is especially true with **chlorpropamide,** which may have a hypoglycemic effect for as long as 60 hr. For this reason, patients whose diabetes is controlled preoperatively with chlorpropamide may not require insulin the day of surgery. In addition, since these patients are going to receive nothing by mouth, IV glucose will offer some protection against possible hypoglycemia.

D. **Diabetic patients on insulin** require specific adjustments in insulin dosage. This adjustment depends largely on the type and hour of surgery. **For minor procedures** scheduled in the early hours of the day, such adjustments can be minimal. However, in the great majority of cases, this is not possible, because **surgical schedules** are not always maintained on time. Thus a diabetic patient scheduled for operation in the early morning may not arrive in the operating room until late in the afternoon. Of course, the opposite also is possible. Therefore it is not good practice to adjust insulin and oral intake with the assumption that surgery is to be performed at a predetermined time. **A better rule** is to keep a diabetic patient on NPO status and adjust the insulin accordingly. **Blood sugars** are to be monitored constantly during the procedure. Stress hormones increase the blood sugar much more in diabetic than in nondiabetic persons.

1. **Several methods of insulin adjustment** have been recommended. The most popular are:

a. **Total daily insulin is divided into two doses.** Half is given preoperatively, and at the same time 5% D/W is started IV to provide coverage for the insulin already administered. The rest of the insulin is given in the postoperative period, after the blood and urine sugar have been checked.

b. **Insulin is reduced by one-third of the total daily dosage.** On the day of surgery, the patient receives one-third of the original daily dosage of insulin, which is also covered by 5% D/W given IV. The second one-third is given after surgery. Further supplementation with regular insulin, if necessary, is carried out by the sliding-scale technique.

c. **No preoperative insulin is given.** Since the patient is on an NPO regimen, there is a possibility of occurrence of hypoglycemia on the day of surgery. To avoid this situation, all insulin is withheld until the postoperative period, when it is given by the sliding-scale technique. However, this precaution is not justified, because glucose can be given IV. Furthermore, the stress of surgery and anesthesia will raise blood sugar by means of sympathetic activation.

d. **Another method** that has been tried is the following: **On the morning of surgery,** all long-acting and intermediate-acting insulin is withheld and, instead, 10–15 units of regular (crystalline) insulin is added to 1000 ml of 5% D/W, which is given IV. **Proponents** of this method claim that interruption of IV glucose obviates the need for further administration of insulin and protects the patient against hypoglycemia. However, **this opinion is challenged** by the fact that insulin, which is heavier than water, settles to the bottom of the flask and is infused ahead of the glucose. Thus the patient again faces the possibility of hypoglycemia. **Another argument against** this technique is that insulin may stick to the glass, or part of it may be diluted, so to speak, in the IV tubing, and the patient may get an inadequate amount of insulin.

2. **Pregnant diabetic patients require large amounts of insulin** because of the increased resistance secondary to hormonal changes (estrogen, progesterone, corticosteroids, and placental lactogen). This is true until delivery. Once delivery has occurred, the patient's insulin requirement diminishes considerably, and therefore the amount of insulin should be reduced. As a result, **hypoglycemia on the day of the delivery is common.** If the patient has received a large dose of insulin during the day of delivery, she needs to be protected by administration of IV glucose. Occasionally a patient may need 50% glucose to prevent or treat **postpartum hypoglycemia.**

E. **Emergency surgery in poorly controlled diabetes.** The patient in this situation has **metabolic acidosis,** is dehydrated, has deranged fluid and electrolyte balance, and may be in a coma. Except for life-threatening emergencies, when no time can be spared, all diabetic patients in this category will profit considerably from intensive preoperative treatment. Frequently **diabetic acidosis may mimic acute abdomen,** and preoperative correction of the diabetic acidosis may change the clinical picture completely.

IV. Anesthesia management

A. **Most inhalation anesthetics** increase blood sugar. This has been attributed to increased sympathetic activity evoked by these agents. In addition, most of these anesthetics have an inhibitory effect on the release and utilization of insulin.

1. **Cyclopropane and ether** increase blood sugar more than do any other inhalation agents. **Halothane** and **methoxyflurane** do so to a lesser extent. No change in blood sugar has been noted with thiopental combined with nitrous oxide and narcotics or with the newer inhalation agents, such as enflurane (Ethrane) and isoflurane (Forane).

2. **The rule** that hyperglycemia is normally followed by increased insulin release does not apply in anesthesia.

B. **The choice of anesthetic agent and technique for the diabetic patient** is dictated by the patient's general condition. **Factors** determining the general condition of a diabetic patient are:

1. The type of diabetes.
2. The duration of diabetes and the adequacy of control.
3. The patient's general nutritional state.
4. The presence of certain very common diabetic complications, which may be cardiovascular, renal, or neurologic in origin.
5. Obesity and pulmonary problems.
6. The patient's drug history.

C. Both **general** and **regional anesthesia** can be given safely, provided the administrator of the anesthetic is very familiar with the potential complications of each technique and agent for a given patient. Diabetes should not be considered as a simple endocrinopathy but rather as a multisystem disease with its own peculiarities.

1. **Premedication.** Diabetic patients must not be premedicated heavily with narcotics; one-half to two-thirds of the usual dose is advisable. Atropine can be avoided and should be given only when there is clear indication for its use.

2. **For simple procedures in the lower extremities,** light **general anesthesia** induced with thiopental and maintained with nitrous oxide is adequate. Nitrous oxide can be potentiated with small amounts of a short-acting

analgesic such as fentanyl (Sublimaze). The majority of diabetic patients suffer from peripheral neuropathies, which reduces the amount of anesthetic needed considerably.

3. **For prolonged vascular procedures in the lower extremities,** hyperbaric **spinal anesthesia** with tetracaine (Pontocaine) mixed with phenylephrine provides an exceptionally complete anesthesia for 5–7 hr.

   a. The **disadvantages** of this technique are:

      (1) Long immobilization of the awake patient on the operating table.

      (2) The extent of sympathetic blockade, with associated hypotension.

      (3) Blockade (motor) of the abdominal muscles, which produces a sensation of breathlessness that even in the presence of adequate ventilation may agitate the patient, especially one with a barrel chest.

   b. These **side effects** of spinal anesthesia **can be alleviated by:**

      (1) Sedating the patient after the establishment of anesthesia; diazepam in small doses seems suitable.

      (2) Treating the hypotension with vasopressor drugs, plasma volume expanders, or a combination of the two.

      (3) Administering oxygen by nasal prongs.

4. **In the presence of hypovolemia,** the indication for spinal anesthesia should be very carefully evaluated, and, if no alternative technique is available, volume expansion before spinal anesthesia, under central venous pressure control, is indicated. In this context, one may consider the prophylactic use of vasopressor agents to buy time while such volume expansion is under way.

5. In the average diabetic patient, **judicious use of inhalation anesthetics** poses no great problem. **Nitrous oxide combined with muscle relaxants and analgesics** affects the diabetic patient least.

   a. **Potent inhalation agents,** such as halothane or enflurane, are best reserved for specific indications.

   b. **The use of muscle relaxants** (depolarizing and nondepolarizing) follows the same general rules as for nondiabetic patients.

6. **Narcotics or analgesics,** during surgery or after, should be given in doses that would not compromise either respiration or circulation. The overall physical condition of the patient and the anticipated length of the procedure must be the determining factors for a given analgesic.

7. **Lumbar peridural (epidural, extradural) anesthesia** may be chosen as an alternative to spinal (subarachnoid) anesthesia. The physiologic changes of peridural anesthesia are essentially similar to those of spinal anesthesia (see Chap. 15 and 16).

8. **Anticoagulants and regional anesthesia.** The administration of spinal or peridural anesthesia in the presence of anticoagulants is **contraindicated.** The peridural space, with its rich venous plexuses, can be traumatized easily, and bleeding is inevitable when coagulation is prolonged because of anticoagulant drugs.

   a. **Bleeding** is most likely to occur during continuous peridural anesthesia, since the insertion of a peridural catheter increases such a risk. In these circumstances **in younger patients,** nonclotting blood in the peridural space may escape to the paravertebral space through the patent intervertebral foramina. **In elderly patients,** however, where the intervertebral foramina are blocked because of arthritic changes associated with deposition of calcium, blood in the peridural space will stay, will eventually clot, and will become an organized hematoma.

b. **An organized hematoma** in the peridural space will behave like a space-occupying lesion, with similar symptoms. **Surgical treatment** is mandatory after myelographic documentation of the presence of the hematoma.

c. **Certain medications** (aspirin, Persantine, Indocid, etc.) decrease platelet adhesiveness in these patients; bleeding time is unusually prolonged. If regional anesthesia is contemplated, discontinuation of these medications is mandatory. In the same context, preoperative check of bleeding time will objectively determine the need to change from regional to general anesthesia.

Bibliography

Alberti, K. G. M. M., and Thomas, D. J. B. The management of diabetic during surgery. *Br. J. Anaesth.* 51:693, 1979.

Duchen, L. W., Anjorin, A., Watkins, P. J., et al. Pathology of autonomic neuropathy in diabetes mellitus. *Ann. Intern. Med.* 92:301, 1980.

Ewing, D. J., Campell, I. W., and Clarke, B. F. Assessment of cardiovascular effects in diabetic neuropathy and prognostic implications. *Ann. Intern. Med.* 92:308, 1980.

Levin, M. E., Boniuk, I., Anderson, C. B., et al. Prevention of diabetic complications. *Arch. Intern. Med.* 140:691, 1980.

Patel, A. U., Stark, D. C. C., and Miller, R. Anesthetic management of a diabetic patient susceptible to malignant hyperpyrexia. *Mt. Sinai J. Med.* (N.Y.) 45:495, 1978.

Taitelman, U., Reece, E. A., and Bessman, A. N. Insulin in the management of the diabetic surgical patient. Continuous IV infusion vs. subcutaneous administration. *J.A.M.A.* 237:658, 1977.

Thomas, D. J. B., and Alberti, K. G. M. M. Hyperglycemic effects of Hartmann's solution during surgery in patients with maturity onset diabetes. *Br. J. Anaesth.* 50:185, 1978.

Watkins, P. J., and Mackay, J. D. Cardiac denervation in diabetic neuropathy. *Ann. Intern. Med.* 92:304, 1980.

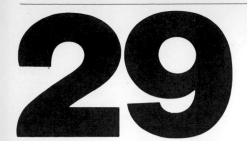

Pollution, Fires, Explosions, and Electrical Hazards

I. Atmospheric pollution in the operating room

A. Operating room personnel appear to be exposed to an increased health hazard due to waste anesthetic gases. The known hazards to exposed persons include:

1. An increased incidence of spontaneous abortion.
2. An increase in the number of congenital abnormalities in the children born to exposed females and males.
3. An increased incidence of liver and kidney diseases.
4. An increase in cancer.

B. Spontaneous abortion

1. Women who are regularly exposed to the operating room environment are subject to an increased risk of spontaneous miscarriage during the first trimester of pregnancy. The incidence is 1.5 to 2 times that in unexposed personnel.
2. The highest incidence of miscarriage is observed among female anesthesiologists, nurse-anesthetists, and operating room nurses and technicians.

C. Congenital abnormalities. Infants of women who work in the operating room have an increased incidence of congenital abnormalities. The risk is 2 times greater in female anesthesiologists than in unexposed female pediatricians.

D. Liver and kidney diseases have been demonstrated to occur more frequently in personnel working in the operating room than in unexposed control groups. The risk in exposed personnel is 2 times higher than in the unexposed, again with the highest increase among anesthesiologists.

E. Cancer. There is an increased incidence of cancer in persons working in the operating room. The rate is about double the expected incidence, with, as usual, the highest increase found in anesthesiologists.

F. Control of risk of exposure to waste anesthetics

1. **The main sources** of atmospheric pollution from waste anesthetic gases distributed within the operating room are the pop-off valve and the ventilator. Other sources are poorly fitted components of the breathing system, spilled liquid anesthetic drugs, and worn-out seals in high-pressure hose connectors.
2. Because **all operating room personnel are exposed** to increased health hazards associated with operating room atmospheric pollution, efforts should be made to reduce the levels of waste anesthetic vapors and gases as much as possible.
3. **Use of a proper scavenging system** plus meticulous attention to its use will greatly decrease the amounts of waste anesthetic gases in the operating

room. Installation, maintenance, and monitoring of a scavenging system to handle anesthetic gases and vapors in all anesthesia areas are therefore strongly recommended.

4. **No scavenging system is 100% effective.** Waste anesthetic gases are always present in the area of anesthesia administration. These can be removed to some degree by an effective air conditioning system, depending on both the rate at which fresh air enters the anesthesia area and the patterns of air currents within the operating room.

II. Fires and explosions

A. **The risk of fire and explosion** in the operating room is always present, and every precaution should be taken to prevent both. These accidents are extremely rare, but they are dramatic and receive wide publicity when they do occur.

B. **More and more new electrical equipment** is filling the operating room, adding new sources of potential fire or explosion. There are electrocardioscopes, electrocautery machines, diathermy machines, electric tables, electric saws and drills, hypothermic units, extracorporeal circulation machines, portable x-ray machines, and numerous monitoring devices incorporating electrical circuits.

C. Because of their chemical composition, the following **combustible anesthetic agents** present a possible hazard of fire and explosion in anesthesia locations: cyclopropane, diethyl ether, divinyl ether, ethyl chloride, ethylene, and fluroxene (the latter is nonflammable in concentrations up to 4% in oxygen or nitrous oxide–oxygen).

D. Sources of ignition

1. **Production of a fire or explosion** depends on three factors: a flammable substance, a supply of oxygen, and a source of ignition. The sources of ignition in the operating room are:
   a. **Sparks** from both fixed and portable electric appliances.
   b. Sparks from the accumulation of **static electricity.** Through friction, electrical charges are built up on surfaces, resulting in differences in electrical potential. The potentials are discharged with a spark that crosses the gap between differently charged surfaces.
   c. **Percussion sparks** from the striking together of hard, metallic surfaces.
   d. **Open flames** and objects heated above the ignition temperature of the combustible gases in use. An electrocautery machine, a diathermy machine, or a sterilizer may become hot enough to ignite a flammable mixture.
2. **Oxygen** is not combustible or explosive, but it supports combustion. The risk in using an oxygen tent is not explosion but the accelerated rate of burning of any fire that may originate from another source of flame. Thus a blanket set afire by a cigarette or match will burn vigorously in an oxygenated environment. In addition, grease or oil should never be placed on equipment supplying oxygen, and the valves on oxygen systems should be opened slowly.

E. Anesthesia locations

1. **The anesthesia area** is considered hazardous.
2. **The National Fire Protection Association** specifies conductive floors, efficient ventilation, and explosion-proof wiring and fixtures for anesthesia locations. In addition, it requires that all materials used in the operating rooms be conductive. **The recovery room,** in which the use of flammable anesthetics is prohibited, is not considered a hazardous area and is not required to have conductive flooring and explosion-proof equipment.
3. **Conductive materials** are those that provide a path by which electrostatic charges can be carried to the ground—in the operating room, the conductive

floor. These conductive materials have low electrical resistance, and they are composed of metal or materials with added conductive agents, such as carbon black, graphite, or acetylene black. Safe limits in terms of resistance of the conductive floor are 25,000 ohms minimum and 1,000,000 ohms maximum, as measured between two electrodes placed 3 ft apart at any points on the floor.

4. **Nonconductive materials** are those that block the path of electrostatic flow to the ground. Examples are wood, wool, oil, synthetics, silk, glass, plastics, nonconductive rubber, and air.

F. Preventive measures

1. **The operating room floor** must be conductive, and all furniture and equipment should be constructed of metal or some other electrically conductive material. Anesthesia-machine parts, such as breathing tubes, bags, and masks, must be made of good-quality conductive rubber.
2. **No woolen blankets** should be permitted in the operating room. Mattresses, pillows, and pads used on operating tables and litters must be covered with conductive sheeting.
3. **All personnel** in anesthesia locations should be attired in cotton uniforms and grounded by conductive shoes.
4. **Overgarments** worn by operating room personnel must not be made of synthetic materials, wool, or silk unless worn in contact with the skin.
5. **The patient** should have an electrical connection with the conductive floor by means of a conductive strap in contact with the skin, with one end fastened to the metal frame of the operating table.
6. **Electrocautery machines,** electrocoagulators, and other electrical equipment employing an open spark must not be used during surgery carried out under anesthesia with flammable agents.
7. **The National Fire Protection Association states** that equipment operating on < 0.5 amp and < 8 V, such as endoscopic instruments, is considered safe for use in anesthesia areas.
8. **Smoking and open flames** are absolutely forbidden in the operating room, and flammable germicides should never be used for preoperative skin preparation in the surgical area.
9. **Maintenance of over 50% relative humidity** will reduce the hazard of fire and/or explosion due to anesthetic agents. Static charges accumulate easily in a dry atmosphere.
10. **The storage room** for combustible agents should be a special area that is ventilated sufficiently to dissipate any gases that may be released by accident. Oxygen and nitrous oxide should not be stored with flammable anesthetics, because both support combustion.
11. The risk of fire and explosion due to flammable anesthetic gases and vapors can be eliminated by forbidding the use of flammable anesthetics in the operating room.

III. Electrical hazards

A. Fundamental concepts in electrical safety

1. **Electrocution** occurs when a person becomes the component that closes a circuit in which a lethal current can flow.
2. **The contacts** that connect the person into the circuit are of two kinds: (1) sustained and (2) casual.
   a. **For sustained or deliberate contacts,** such as electrodes placed on the skin or heart, the path of the current from the person to the ground on the

one hand, and the path from the person to the electrical power source on the other hand, should offer infinitely high impedance to electrical current. Sustained connections to the person should be isolated from the ground and the electrical power system.

b. **Casual contacts** are inevitable and occur unpredictably from multiple sources. All exposed conducting surfaces should be maintained at the same potential to reduce the hazard of casual contacts.

3. **Grounding.** The National Electrical Code defines **grounding** as a conducting connection, whether accidental or intentional, between an electrical circuit or equipment and the earth, or some conducting body that serves in place of the earth, serving to drain off excess electrons.

B. Safe practice

1. **Avoid placing the patient** in a position too close to a circuit in which lethal electrical current can flow.
2. **Sustained, deliberate connections.** Avoid making these connections between the patient and the power line or ground.
3. **Casual connections.** Maintain these connections equipotential by proper individual grounding.

Bibliography

Beymen, F. M., Knopp, T. J., and Rehder, K. Nitrous oxide exposure in the operating room. *Anesth. Analg.* (Cleve.) 57:216, 1978.

Cohen, E. N. Occupational disease among operating room personnel: A national study. Report of an ad hoc committee on the effects of trace anesthetics on the health of operating room personnel. American Society of Anesthesiologists. *Anesthesiology* 41:321, 1974.

Cohen, E. N. Toxicity of inhalation anesthetic agents. *Br. J. Anaesth.* 50:665, 1978.

Ericson, A., and Kallen, B. Survey of infants born in 1973 or 1975 to Swedish women working in operating rooms during their pregnancies. *Anesth. Analg.* (Cleve.) 58:302, 1979.

Ferstanding, L. L. Trace concentrations of anesthetic gases: A critical review of their disease potential. *Anesth. Analg.* (Cleve.) 57:328, 1978.

Geraci, C. L. Operating room pollution. Governmental perspectives and guidelines. *Anesth. Analg.* (Cleve.) 56:775, 1977.

Hull, C. J. Electrocution hazards in the operating theatre. *Br. J. Anaesth.* 50:647, 1978.

Lecky, J. H. The mechanical aspects of anesthetic pollution control. *Anesth. Analg.* (Cleve.) 56:769, 1977.

Sass-Kortsak, A. M., Wheeler, I. P., and Purdham, J. T. Exposure of operating room personnel to anaesthetic agents. An examination of the effectiveness of scavenging systems and the importance of maintenance programs. *Can. Anaesth. Soc. J.* 28:22, 1981.

Snow, J. C., Norton, M. L., Saluja, T. S., et al. Fire hazard during CO_2 laser microsurgery of the larynx and trachea. *Anesth. Analg.* (Cleve.) 55:146, 1976.

Spence, A. A., and Knill-Jones, R. P. Is there a health hazard in anesthetic practice? *Br. J. Anaesth.* 50:713, 1978.

Vickers, M. D. Fire and explosion hazards in operating theatres. *Br. J. Anaesth.* 50:569, 1978.

Virtue, R. W., Escobar, A., and Modell, J. Nitrous oxide levels in operating room air with various gas flows. *Can. Anaesth. Soc. J.* 26:313, 1979.

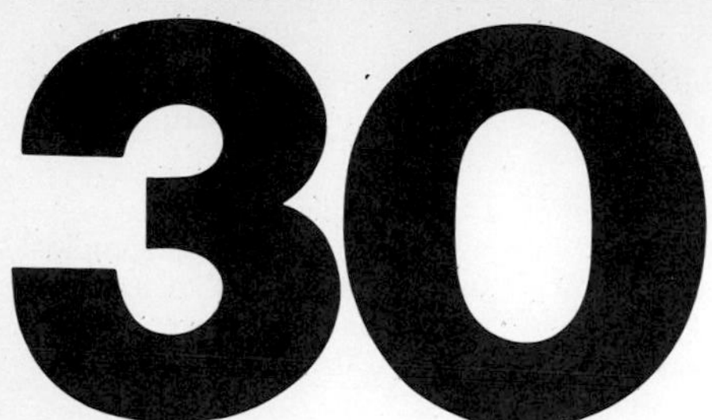

30 Complications During Anesthesia and the Recovery Period

The complications discussed in this chapter will be limited to respiratory, cardiovascular (except cardiac arrest), ophthalmic, and ulnar nerve complications, postanesthesia shivering, and hypothermia. Cardiac arrest is covered in Chapter 8. Complications during laryngoscopy and endotracheal intubation are discussed in Chapter 13. Complications due to intravenous barbiturates are reviewed in Chapter 11, and those due to muscle relaxants, in Chapter 12. Complications resulting from blood transfusion are discussed in Chapter 21. Complications due to local and regional anesthesia, spinal anesthesia, and epidural and caudal anesthesia are reviewed in Chapters 14, 15, and 16 respectively. Finally, complications resulting from pollution, fire, explosion, and electrical hazards are covered in Chapter 29.

I. Respiratory complications

A. Hypoventilation may occur intraoperatively and during the immediate postoperative period.

1. **Etiology.** Hypoventilation may be caused by preanesthetic and anesthetic drugs, narcotics, muscle relaxants, or reduction in body temperature (particularly in infants). Pain from thoracic or abdominal incisions markedly decreases maximal breathing capacity; some degree of hypoxia and hypercapnia results or follows.

2. **Therapy** of hypoventilation—regardless of cause—requires establishment of a free airway and maintenance of adequate artificial respiration.

   a. Ventilation can be assisted by a mask or endotracheal tube with a self-inflating bag, the breathing bag of the anesthesia machine, or a mechanical ventilator.

   b. If respiratory depression is due to **narcotics,** administration of a narcotic antagonist, such as naloxone, is indicated. If hypoventilation is due to **tubocurarine** or **pancuronium,** injection of neostigmine with atropine is indicated.

3. **Administration of oxygen,** by a disposable face mask or by soft nasal tips inserted into the patient's nostrils, is recommended for every patient during the early postoperative period.

B. Respiratory obstruction

1. **Etiology.** Respiratory obstruction may be due to soft tissue obstruction, excessive secretions, blood, gastric contents, laryngeal spasm, tumors, inflammation, foreign bodies, hypertrophic tonsils and adenoids, and kinking or blockage of the endotracheal tube. The most common site for airway obstruction to occur in the postoperative period is the upper airway.

2. **The signs** of respiratory obstruction include (a) inadequate tidal exchange, (b) retraction of the chest wall and supraclavicular and suprasternal spaces, (c) excessive abdominal movements, (d) use of accessory muscles of respiration, (e) noisy respiration, and (f) cyanosis. The presence of tracheal tug during anesthesia or the recovery period may indicate either deep anes-

thesia, residual neuromuscular blockade, and/or hypoxia with carbon dioxide retention, the latter caused by inadequate respiration or by ventilatory obstruction.

3. **Therapy** includes insertion of a nasal or pharyngeal airway (if tolerated), elevation of the mandible forward and upward by pressure behind the angles of the mandible, and artificial ventilation. It may be necessary to free the airway of secretions by frequent suctioning. If the patient's airway cannot be maintained, then tracheal intubation is indicated. Rarely, a tracheotomy may be necessary.

C. **Apnea** may develop due to airway obstruction, peripheral respiratory depression, or central respiratory depression. **Therapy should be instituted immediately** by artificial ventilation—mouth-to-mouth, mouth-to-nose, mouth-to-mask, mouth-to-airway, or mouth-to-endotracheal tube. A self-inflating bag, a reservoir bag of the anesthesia machine, and/or a mechanical ventilator are very useful. A tracheotomy may be necessary.

D. **Vomiting and aspiration** of gastric contents may occur during induction and maintenance of anesthesia or during the recovery period, especially in patients undergoing abdominal procedures. This condition can be disastrous and must be treated immediately.

1. **Signs and symptoms**

   a. **Aspiration of large volumes** can result in death from drowning; **smaller volumes** induce coughing, laryngospasm, bronchospasm, and pulmonary edema with resulting hypoxia.

   b. **Aspiration of acidic fluid** gastric contents results in **chemical pneumonitis,** whereas aspirated particulate material may cause atelectasis, pneumonia, or lung abscess. The lesions are due to a pH of less than 2.5. Chemical pneumonitis should be suspected when there is persistent cyanosis, tachycardia, and tachypnea, along with development of expiratory wheezing following vomiting or regurgitation. A chest x-ray is indicated to support the clinical diagnosis.

2. If aspiration has occurred, **therapy** includes endotracheal intubation, suctioning of the trachea, oxygenation, hydrocortisone, 500–1000 mg, aminophylline, and antibiotics. Respiration should be assisted or controlled. For blockage of bronchopulmonary segments, therapeutic bronchoscopy is indicated.

E. **Pulmonary complications** occur in 30% of patients who have abdominal or thoracic surgery and is the most frequent cause of morbidity and mortality in the postoperative period. The high rate of complications following upper abdominal surgery is related to low vital capacity and reduced ability to cough and clear secretions. These functional abnormalities are secondary to abnormal pulmonary patterns, pain, position of recumbency, surgical muscle injury associated with upper abdominal incisions, and the effects of anesthetic agents and techniques.

1. **Arterial hypoxemia** is a frequent finding after major surgery. Most often it is subclinical and can be detected only by measuring blood gases.

2. Every effort should be made to prevent the familiar **progression of atelectasis,** tachypnea, hypoxia, fever, and pneumonitis.

F. **Atelectasis** is the result of obstruction of a conducting airway, with subsequent absorption of air from the distal part of the lung. This may occur during or following local, regional, or general anesthesia.

1. **Signs and symptoms.** Asymmetrical movements and retraction of the chest, absence of breath sounds over a segment of the lung area, increasing difficulty in breathing, tachycardia, tachypnea, fever, and cyanosis.

2. The **diagnosis** is made by chest x-ray and by strong presumptive evidence.

3. **Treatment.** Chest physiotherapy, bronchial suction through a catheter or bronchoscope, coughing, deep breathing, positive-pressure inflation of the lungs, expectorants, surfactants and mucolytic agents, and bronchodilators.

G. **Pneumothorax** may be caused by rupture of lung tissue (such as an emphysematous bleb following excessive coughing), vigorous positive-pressure respiration, or direct trauma to the apex of the lung during tracheotomy, thyroidectomy, neck dissection, insertion of a subclavian central venous pressure catheter, or supraclavicular brachial plexus block. In addition, pneumothorax may appear during partial airway obstruction with deep respiration: During this period, air may be sucked into the superior mediastinum, which causes rupture into one or both pleural spaces. In the case of **vigorous positive pressure,** gas spreads from the ruptured alveolus to the perivascular or peribronchial space, to the hilus, to the mediastinum and root of the neck, to the subcutaneous tissue, and then to the pleural space (or retroperitoneally or intraperitoneally through the aorta or esophagus).

1. The **diagnosis** is made by physical examination, chest x-ray, and arterial blood gas analyses.

2. **Treatment.** Aspiration of the air through a puncture made with a large-bore needle in the pleura at the midclavicular line in the second or third anterior space, together with placement of a chest tube connected to water-seal drainage bottles.

H. **Gastric distention** can cause airway embarrassment. This can happen in a paralyzed patient with airway pressure above 25 cm H_2O in spite of the existence of a clear airway, and it may lead to postoperative vomiting, respiratory and surgical difficulties, or hiccups.

I. **Hiccups**

1. **Hiccups** are intermittent spasms of the diaphragm, accompanied by a sudden closure of the glottis.

2. **Hiccups may occur** during induction and/or maintenance of anesthesia, with inhalation or with IV anesthetics, and can be most distressing to both surgeon and anesthesiologist, especially when the hiccups persist in spite of application of a variety of therapeutic methods.

3. **Therapy** is aimed mainly at removing the contributory causes: gastric distention, diaphragmatic irritation, or upper abdominal visceral stimulation.

   a. Assisted respiration is necessary, and, if the hiccups persist, a relaxant drug can be used with tracheal intubation and controlled ventilation.

   b. **Therapeutic methods.** Nasopharyngeal stimulation, deepening of established general anesthesia, muscle relaxant drugs, carbon dioxide inhalation, gastric decompression, and unilateral phrenic nerve block.

J. **Fever** occurring within the first postoperative 24 hr suggests pulmonary **atelectasis;** within 48 hr, a **urinary tract infection;** and after 72 hr, a **wound infection.** Postoperative fever resulting from thrombophlebitis may appear at any time. Any postoperative increase in body temperature, as little as 1°F above normal or lasting more than 2 days, must be considered important, and studies should be done to determine the cause.

II. **Cardiovascular complications**

A. **Hypotension** can be caused by narcotics, anesthetics, hypoxia, reflexes, surgical handling, hemorrhage, adrenocortical insufficiency, position changes, heart disease, transfusion of incompatible blood, allergic hypersensitivity, or air embolism.

1. **Narcotics** injected preoperatively, intraoperatively, and/or postoperatively may decrease BP by depressing the vasomotor center, reducing muscle tone, depressing ventilation, and dilating peripheral vessels.

2. **Overdosage of inhalation and/or IV anesthetics** is one of the main causes of hypotension during anesthesia.

   a. **BP may be decreased** when the anesthetic is administered in excess of the amounts usually tolerated, especially during induction of anesthesia. BP can be decreased even though the amount given is within the acceptable range. Such relative overdosage can be avoided if a minimal dose of anesthetics is used during induction of anesthesia, particularly in patients with heart disease, obesity, hypertension, decreased blood volume, loss of weight, cachexia, or chronic debilitating disease.

   b. **Treatment of overdosage** includes immediate cessation of the inhalation anesthetic, and, if barbiturates have been given, general supportive measures include an adequate airway, efficient respiration, infusion of lactated Ringer's solution, and vasopressors.

3. **Adrenocortical insufficiency** (see Chap. 1, sec. **III.B**). Hypotension and shock due to adrenocortical insufficiency are much easier to prevent than to treat. Many patients will be treated unnecessarily (but harmlessly) to protect the few who may be at risk. Hypotension due to other causes should be ruled out. The **therapy** of adrenocortical crisis includes IV administration of hydrocortisone with either isotonic saline or saline in dextrose. Norepinephrine is also used with great caution.

4. Severe hypotension due to **myocardial ischemia or infarction** may develop during anesthesia and surgery. Diagnosis is made by strong presumptive evidence and therapy should not be delayed until the diagnosis is definitively established within a few days.

5. **Signs of incompatible blood transfusion** under anesthesia (see Chap. 21, sec. **V.B.3**) are hypotension, generalized oozing from wounds, hemoglobinuria, and cyanosis. Later signs are jaundice, oliguria, and anuria.

6. **Prevention and treatment of hypotension**

   a. Excessive amounts of preanesthetic and anesthetic drugs should be avoided.

   b. Surgical manipulations should be done as gently as possible.

   c. Administration of fluids and blood replacement should be accomplished early.

   d. The central venous pressure should be monitored.

   e. Prompt drug treatment with vasopressors (see Chap. 18).

   f. If hypotension is due to hypoxia, oxygen should be given first and vasopressors last.

B. **Hypertension** may occur during anesthesia and the recovery period as a result of pain, hypoxia, hypercapnia, hypervolemia from overtransfusion, reflex stimulation, increased intracranial pressure, pheochromocytoma, and drugs (e.g., ketamine, vasopressor amines, or succinylcholine). The use of an IV drip of trimethaphan or nitroprusside, followed by administration of a long-acting antihypertensive drug, if needed, should be reserved for last-resort emergency therapy.

C. **Cardiac arrhythmias.** See Chapter 7, section **VII.**

III. **Ophthalmic complications**

A. During anesthesia, **in many patients the eyelids do not cover the eyes** completely, particularly if muscle relaxants are used. Because of this, if no preventive measures are taken, an injury to the eye—by direct trauma, drying of the cornea, or irritation by the liquid or vapors of the anesthetic drugs—may follow administration of general anesthetic agents.

1. **A corneal abrasion** is the most common eye complication that occurs during general anesthesia and recovery. It is painful, may progress to inflammation of the uveal tract, and, in the presence of contamination, may lead to a serious infection.
   a. **A corneal abrasion may be caused** either by a face mask placed inadvertently on the open eyes or by the hands and fingernails of the anesthesiologist during laryngoscopy and intubation. Most often this complication occurs during **head or neck surgery,** particularly during craniotomy, and in neurosurgical or orthopedic procedures that require the patient to remain in the prone position.
   b. In addition, corneal abrasion may occur during surgery involving the **facial nerve,** as in mastoidectomy, tympanoplasty, or parotidectomy.
   c. **During the surgical procedure,** the arm of an assistant, instruments, or the surgical drapes or head towels may rest on the patient's open or partly open eyes, producing conjunctivitis, corneal abrasion, or ulceration.
2. **If the eye is merely left open** during anesthesia, the protective action of tears is absent, the cornea becomes dry, and the epithelium may be damaged.
3. **The anatomic position of the eye** is another factor: The risk of drying is greater in a person with prominent eyes (proptosis or exophthalmos). In addition, injury to the eye may be caused by allowing secretions to pass into the eye or by spillage of sterilizing solutions during preparation of the skin for surgery on the head or neck.

B. **Pressure on the eyeball** can result in **blindness** by occluding the arterial supply to the eye, especially during induced hypotensive techniques. **During the recovery period,** the eye may be injured by bedclothes, the face mask, or the patient's fingers.

C. **Diagnosis.** A corneal abrasion causes pain, lacrimation, and blepharospasm. The pain is severe and is aggravated by blinking and by motion of the eyeball. The patient may complain of a sensation of a foreign body in the eye. Following examination of the cornea with an eye loupe under good light, sterile strips impregnated with fluorescein dye are used to delineate the epithelial injury; the abraded cornea takes a deeper green stain than does the undamaged cornea.

D. **Treatment.** Local application of an antibiotic ointment and an eye pressure patch. In addition, a cycloplegic and mydriatic solution is instilled to prevent synechiae and to relieve the pain associated with spasm of the iris and ciliary muscle.

E. **Prophylaxis.** Ophthalmic complications may be best prevented by ensuring that the patient's eyes are completely covered during anesthesia. This can be accomplished by holding the eyelids closed with adhesive or cellophane tape. However, when this is not practical, as during the recovery period, application of a bland ophthalmic preparation will reduce any drying effect.

IV. Postanesthesia shivering

A. Following cessation of **thiopental, halothane, or enflurane anesthesia,** a few patients may show spasticity of some somatic muscles and shivering over the entire body with tremors of the head, shoulders, body muscles, and upper and lower extremities. This may be explained as a thermal reaction due to the low room temperature during anesthesia and surgery in the operating room. It results in a greater oxygen demand. **Another factor** to be considered, although a minor one, is the large loss of ventilatory heat during general anesthesia with high flows in a semiclosed or partial rebreathing system. Young adults are particularly susceptible to this type of heat loss.

B. Therapy includes covering the patient with hot blankets and maintaining the room temperature at 24° C. Administration of 5–10 mg of chlorpromazine IV will aid in correcting symptoms only.

V. Ulnar nerve paralysis

A. Motor weakness and paresthesia may occur in the distribution of the ulnar nerve from pressure on the nerve at the elbow region. It may happen in an emaciated patient whose elbow is fastened on a firm object. This also may occur if the nerve is compressed between the bone and the edge of the operating table, or if the patient's arm is abducted and the elbow is compressed against the edge of the operating table.

B. Prevention includes securing the arm close to the side of the body in the horizontal position and supporting it properly.

C. When weakness, numbness, or paralysis occurs in the distribution of the ulnar nerve, a detailed neurologic examination should be made and **treatment** instituted immediately, including physiotherapy and proper support of the arm.

VI. Malignant hyperthermia

A. Malignant hyperthermia is a fulminant hypermetabolic crisis triggered by anesthetic drugs.

1. Malignant hyperthermia is **rare** but potentially life-threatening and occurs during general anesthesia, with a 60% **mortality.** The higher the maximum temperature and the longer the duration of anesthesia, the higher the mortality. Therefore early detection and rapid treatment are the keys to successful reversal.

2. **The incidence** has been reported to be 1 in 15,000 administrations of anesthetics in children, and 1 in 50,000 in adults. The majority of cases occur in children, adolescents, and young adults. Males are victims more often than females.

3. The **cause** remains uncertain and controversial. The predisposing factor is inherited by 50% of victims' offspring. Although the reaction is known to be hereditary, the site and nature of the defect remain to be elucidated fully. Fifty percent of the patients have relatives in whom malignant hyperthermia developed under general anesthesia, which suggests an autosomal dominant trait. Muscular rigidity occurs in three-fourths of the patients; a great number of patients who manifest rigidity have preexisting muscle or musculoskeletal disease.

   a. Malignant hyperthermia most often develops following the administration of **halothane and succinylcholine.** It may occur, however, with almost all forms of general anesthesia. It has not been reported during local or regional anesthesia.

   b. A previous uncomplicated anesthetic experience does not exclude the appearance of malignant hyperthermia during subsequent general anesthesia.

B. Clinical signs and laboratory findings

1. **The clinical signs** include tachycardia, tachypnea, fever over 40° C, arrhythmias, cyanosis, dark venous blood in the surgical field, red urine, hot skin, and prolonged generalized skeletal muscle rigidity.

2. **Tachycardia and tachypnea** are the earliest signs and are due to the intense metabolic and respiratory acidosis. Respiratory acidosis is present because of a marked increase in carbon dioxide production. **Arrhythmias** stem from the hyperkalemia associated with this syndrome.

3. The **laboratory findings** include metabolic and respiratory acidosis, hypoxemia, hyperkalemia, hypermagnesemia, myoglobinemia, and elevated lac-

tate and pyruvate levels. **Additional findings** include myoglobinuria, hypocalcemia, impaired blood coagulation, muscle biopsy abnormalities, oliguria, dehydration, peripheral vascular failure, and elevated serum enzymes SGOT, LDH, SGPT, and CPK. In normal situations, these intracellular enzymes are present in small quantities in the serum. The increase in levels of these enzymes in the serum during malignant hyperthermia indicates that an injury to muscles has occurred, thus permitting the enzymes from the intracellular space to escape into the extracellular fluid.

4. **Acute renal failure,** hemolysis, and brain damage may occur later in the course of this syndrome.

C. **Diagnosis.** The importance of early diagnosis and early termination of anesthesia lies in the fact that the chances of cardiopulmonary collapse and eventual death increase statistically in proportion to the duration of anesthesia.

1. **One must suspect this complication** in the presence of tachycardia (unexplained), tachypnea, arrhythmias, abnormal response to succinylcholine, generalized or localized muscular rigidity, and/or rapid rise in body temperature.

2. **Routine monitoring** of the electrical activity of the heart and the body temperature is recommended for all anesthetized patients, especially children and young adults. The probe of the electronic thermometer for continuous body temperature monitoring may be rectal, esophageal, or tympanic.

3. **Once the diagnosis is made,** indexes to be monitored include ECG, temperature, arterial blood gases, electrolytes, hematocrit, urine output, and central venous pressure.

D. **Therapy.** Emphasis is placed on the vital importance of early detection, early cessation of anesthesia (and of surgery, if possible), and early application of therapeutic measures, which include:

1. **Hyperventilation** with 100% oxygen through an endotracheal tube.

2. **Dantrolene** (Dantrium), 1–2 mg/kg IV. This may be repeated every 5 to 10 min for a total dose of 10 mg/kg. Each vial of dantrolene for IV administration should be reconstituted by adding 60 ml of sterile water for injection, and the vial shaken until the solution is clear.

3. IV administration of sodium bicarbonate (2 to 4 mEq/kg) to correct metabolic acidosis.

4. Prompt measures to **control temperature** by rapid external and internal cooling.

   a. **External cooling methods** include immersion of the patient in an ice-water bath. If this method is not immediately feasible, then effective body cooling can be achieved by packing the patient with ice and using hypothermia blankets.

   b. **Internal cooling methods** include rapid IV infusion of cold fluids, together with gastric, wound, and rectal lavage. Extracorporeal cooling with the heart-lung bypass machine also has been used for rapid cooling of the patient with malignant hyperthermia.

5. IV injections of **diuretics** (furosemide and mannitol).

6. IV drip of procainamide (1 g diluted in 500 ml of NaCl) for the treatment of arrhythmias.

7. **Hyperpotassemia** is treated by infusion of buffers and dextrose with insulin.

E. **If a patient survives** an episode of malignant hyperpyrexia under general anesthesia and needs subsequent anesthesia and surgery, the **choice,** if at all possible, should be local or regional anesthesia (lidocaine should be avoided). If nerve block anesthesia cannot be used and general anesthesia is absolutely indicated, the use of nitrous oxide, oxygen, barbiturates, narcotics, pancuronium, and preoperative oral doses of dantrolene with meticulous body-temperature monitoring seems to be a rational technique.

F. The following should be avoided in susceptible persons: local anesthetics of the amide type (lidocaine, mepivacaine), halogenated drugs, ketamine, and depolarizing muscle relaxants (succinylcholine).

G. Standard treatment regimen

1. Stop anesthesia and surgery immediately.
2. Hyperventilate the patient with 100% oxygen.
3. Administer dantrolene IV and procainamide IV (if required for arrhythmias) as soon as possible.
4. Initiate cooling.
5. Correct acidosis.
6. Treat hyperkalemia.
7. Secure monitoring lines. Monitor the ECG, temperature, Foley catheter, arterial pressure, central venous pressure, and electrolytes.
8. Maintain urine output.
9. Monitor the patient until the danger of subsequent episodes is past.
10. Administer oral dantrolene if indicated.

Bibliography

Batra, Y. K., and Bali, I. M. Corneal abrasions during general anesthesia. *Anesth. Analg.* (Cleve.) 56:363, 1977.

Bond, V. K., Stoelting, R. K., and Gupta, C. D. Pulmonary aspiration syndrome after inhalation of gastric fluid containing antacids. *Anesthesiology* 51:452, 1979.

Cameron, M. G. P., and Stewart, O. J. Ulnar nerve injury associated with anaesthesia. *Can. Anaesth. Soc. J.* 22:253, 1975.

Cross, D. A., and Collins, J. R. Hypertension and anesthesia. Cause for concern. *South. Med. J.* 71:161, 1978.

Frazer, J. G., Crumrine, R. S., and Izant, R. J. A preplanned treatment of malignant hyperpyrexia. *Anesth. Analg.* (Cleve.) 55:713, 1976.

Gal, T. J., and Cooperman, L. H. Hypertension in the immediate postoperative period. *Br. J. Anaesth.* 47:70, 1975.

Gold, M. I. Treatment of bronchospasm during anesthesia. *Anesth. Analg.* (Cleve.) 54:783, 1975.

Gronert, G. A. Malignant hyperthermia. *Anesthesiology* 53:395, 1980.

Gronert, G. A., Thompson, R. L., and Onofrio, B. M. Human malignant hyperthermia. Awake episodes and correction by dantrolene. *Anesth. Analg.* (Cleve.) 59:377, 1980.

Harrison, G. G. Control of malignant hyperthermia syndrome by dantrolene. *Br. J. Anaesth.* 47:66, 1975.

Liebenschutz, F., Mai, C., and Pickerodt, V. W. A. Increased carbon dioxide production in two patients with malignant hyperpyrexia and its control by dantrolene. *Br. J. Anaesth.* 51:899, 1979.

Malatinsky, J., and Kadlic, T. Inferior vena caval occlusion in the left lateral position. *Br. J. Anaesth.* 47:1118, 1975.

Masson, A. H. B., and Millar, R. A. Symposium on the postoperative period. *Br. J. Anaesth.* 47:89, 1975.

Patton, C. M., Moon, M. R., and Dannemiller, F. J. The prophylactic antiemetic effect of droperidol. *Anesth. Analg.* (Cleve.) 53:361, 1974.

Paul, D. R., Hoyt, J. L., and Boutros, A. R. Cardiovascular and respiratory changes in response to change of posture in the very obese. *Anesthesiology* 45:73, 1976.

Proger, S., and Snow, J. C. Hyperpyrexia, hepatic necrosis, and myocardial infarction after cardiac surgery. *J.A.M.A.* 228:504, 1974.

Snow, J. C., Healy, G. B., Vaughan, C. W., et al. Malignant hyperthermia during anesthesia for adenoidectomy. *Arch. Otolaryngol.* 95:442, 1972.

Snow, J. C., Kripke, B. J., Norton, M. L., et al. Corneal injuries during general anesthesia. *Anesth. Analg.* (Cleve.) 54:465, 1975.

Stirt, J. A., and Sullivan, S. I. Aminophylline. *Anesth. Analg.* (Cleve.) 60:587, 1981.

Sy, W. P. Ulnar nerve palsy possibly related to use of automatically cycled blood pressure cuff. *Anesth. Analg.* (Cleve.) 60:687, 1981.

Weber, I., and Hirshman, C. A. Cimetidine for prophylaxis of aspiration pneumonitis: comparison of intramuscular and oral dosage schedules. *Anesth. Analg.* (Cleve.) 58:426, 1979.

Special Anesthesia Problems in Surgical Specialties

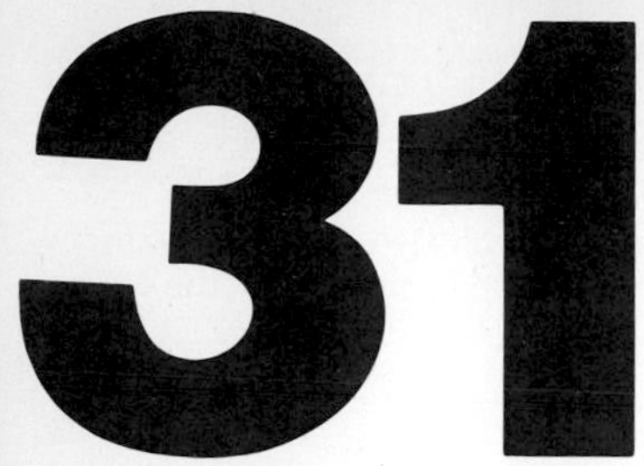

Anesthesia in Thoracic Surgery

I. Problems

A. Open pneumothorax

1. **Normally,** the lungs are kept inflated by the pressure difference between the atmosphere and the pleural space and by the adhesion of two layers of the pleura. When one side of the chest is opened, the pressure difference is lost, and the lung on the affected side collapses due to recoil of its elastic tissues.

2. **Ventilation** is affected by:

   a. **Collapse** of the lung.

   b. **Paradoxical breathing.** The movement of the lung on the open side is called **paradoxical** because air passes out of the lung on the affected side with each **inspiration** and is drawn from it into the sound lung. During **expiration** the reverse occurs: The lung on the open side expands, and the V_D/V_T ratio increases. The air passing from one lung to another is called **pendulum air.**

   c. **Shifting of the mediastinum or mediastinal flap.** If the opening in the chest is 6 to 8 times larger than the tracheal diameter and the mediastinum is mobile, the difference in pressure between each pleural cavity (greater negative pressure with inspiration on the sound side) tends to move the mediastinum toward the sound lung, pressing on the sound lung and interfering with its efficiency. **When the patient lies on the side,** this pressure is increased by the weight of the heart. The result is a to-and-fro motion of the mediastinum, which also causes an intermittent obstruction of the superior and inferior venae cavae, diminished venous return, and hypotension. **Hyperpnea** makes the mediastinal movement worse.

   d. The problems of open pneumothorax **can be avoided** with controlled intermittent positive-pressure ventilation.

B. Tension pneumothorax

1. This may occur when a **bulla** on the lung surface ruptures and the pleura covering the perforation forms a one-way valve that allows gas to pass into the pleural space only during inspiration or as a result of traumatic rupture of the lung, trachea, or bronchi. The result is increasing pleural pressure with a shift of the mediastinum.

2. **Therapy.** Immediate insertion of a 16-gauge needle in the second interspace anteriorly in the midclavicular line, followed by placement of a larger drain connected to a water-seal drainage bottle. The use of nitrous oxide is not advisable because of differential gas solubility (nitrous oxide–nitrogen).

C. Control of secretions

1. Profuse tracheobronchial secretions complicate management.
2. The following serious conditions challenge the anesthesiologist in controlling secretions:

a. Chronic pulmonary abscess.

b. Empyema associated with bronchopleural fistula and excessive bleeding during resection of a pulmonary segment.

c. Secretions or blood from the diseased lung, which is uppermost in the lateral position, may trickle over the carina and infect or flood the normal lung.

3. **Measures to control secretions**

a. Preoperative therapy.

b. Physiotherapy.

c. Antibiotics.

d. During the operation, removal of secretions with intermittent suction.

e. Positioning the patient on the operating table in the prone position, so that secretions are either retained in the diseased lung or drain readily toward the mouth.

f. The use of endobronchial tubes to prevent the spread of secretions to the healthy lung.

D. **Blood loss**

1. Two major IV lines should be inserted for all but the simplest lung resection. One IV line should serve for **uninterrupted blood transfusion.** The other is for administration of **drugs.**

2. **In high-risk patients,** one of the two lines could be a central venous pressure line. This should be planned in advance, because it is difficult to install a central venous pressure line via an external jugular vein or internal jugular vein in a patient in the lateral position. If the external jugular vein is chosen, the right side is the better choice. A **J-wire** is a useful tool to pass the catheter through the external jugular vein–subclavian vein junction.

3. **Watch** for sources of **unseen hemorrhage** from the intercostal vessels in the posterior end of the incision, as well as for collection of blood in the paravertebral space and on the surgical packs.

4. In case of a **disastrous hemorrhage** from the central veins, when the chest is already open, direct intraaortic or intraventricular transfusion is readily accessible.

E. **Cardiac embarrassment.** A too-vigorous retraction may interfere with cardiac contraction or venous return and cardiac output.

F. **Hilar reflexes.** Dissection around the hilus may produce cardiac irregularities because of stimulation of nerves; to obviate these, occasionally it may be necessary to infiltrate the hilus with local anesthetics.

G. **Atelectasis**

1. Lung areas can become atelectatic from uniform ventilation or compression of retractors.

2. At a convenient time, it is desirable to inflate the collapsed lung.

3. As in any other procedure, the basic rule in anesthesia for thoracic surgery must be kept in mind: Anesthesia administered without continual observation of what is going on in the operative field is poor anesthesia.

H. **Opposite pneumothorax.** During pneumonectomy and dissection of hilar glands, contralateral pneumothorax occasionally occurs.

II. Anesthetic management

A. Choice of anesthesia and agents

1. **General anesthesia** with controlled ventilation is the most practical approach to the anesthetic management of thoracotomy.
2. **For induction of anesthesia,** an IV agent is used (thiopental or thiamylal).
3. **For maintenance of anesthesia,** there are many combinations of anesthetic drugs. The anesthesiologist's knowledge of the anesthetic agent is more important than the choice of the agent. **Inhalation anesthetic drugs,** such as nitrous oxide with halothane or enflurane, are preferable to IV anesthetics. Their use results in an increase in inspired oxygen concentration. In endobronchial anesthesia, the nitrous oxide may be eliminated without danger of allowing the patient's consciousness to return.
4. **Tubocurarine or pancuronium** is used to control respiration. This control should be maintained until all muscle layers are closed and the water-seal drainage has been established.

B. Positioning of the patient on the operating table

1. **The lateral position** is most commonly used.
2. **The head** should be properly supported, so that the cervical and thoracic spinous processes are in the same horizontal plane.
3. **A pad** should be placed on the chest wall below the scapula to distribute weight between the shoulder and the chest wall.
4. **The upper arm** is positioned on an arm support.
5. **Sandbags** are placed in front of and behind the upper chest to form a rigid support that leaves the lower chest and abdomen free to move.
6. **The knees are flexed,** the lower knee more than the upper, and a **pillow** is placed between them lengthwise to prevent both knees and ankles from touching.
7. **A strap or a large adhesive tape** reaching over the patient's hip from one side of the table to the other should be sufficiently secure to stabilize the patient on the table satisfactorily.

C. The operative field

1. **During thoracotomy,** the anesthesiologist must cooperate with the surgical requirements.
   a. To avoid puncture of the lung, **positive-pressure ventilation** should cease while the surgeon is opening the pleura.
   b. When adequate collapse of the lung has been achieved to allow surgical manipulation, a shallow ventilation with a slightly increased rate will maintain gas exchange. During this period, the anesthesiologist carefully observes the surgical field and adjusts the degree of inflation and the frequency of the patient's respiration to the surgeon's movements.
2. **Compromise** between the surgeon's desire for the best exposure and the anesthesiologist's interest in a generous ventilation is achieved by the use of packs and retractors. The surgeon should halt periodically to allow expansion of the collapsed segments of the lung. Repeated arterial blood gas determinations will indicate the need for expansion.
3. A few surgeons prefer not to use the clamp when the **bronchus is transected** (in the lateral position, the bronchus is the last structure cut).

a. The patient should be ventilated with **100% oxygen** prior to the preparatory period of hypoventilation during suturing of the bronchial stump.

b. When this is accomplished, **the pleural cavity** is filled with saline solution, and a positive pressure is exerted on the bag to test the integrity of the suture line.

4. **Prior to the closure of the pleura,** the remaining lung is inflated and inspected for atelectasis. Sustained moderate positive pressure with the breathing bag and the gentle manipulations by the surgeon will reinflate residual atelectatic areas.

5. **When the pleura is being closed,** synchrony between inflation and surgical manipulation is required to prevent the lung from being punctured by the surgical needle.

6. **After chest drains are connected** to water-seal drainage bottles, and the chest wall is airtight, all air should be removed from the pleural cavity by more vigorous inflation of the lung.

D. Monitoring

1. Precordial or esophageal stethoscope.
2. Electrocardiogram.
3. Esophageal or tympanic membrane temperature.
4. Central venous pressure when major blood loss is expected in high-risk patients.
5. An intraarterial pressure line is useful in long operations; in laterally positioned patients, in whom hypotension may cause peripheral vasoconstriction; and in situations where the positioning of the upper arm may interfere with determination of the blood pressure by cuff.
6. An arterial line is mandatory for repeated determinations of blood gases in cases of one-lung anesthesia.

III. Anesthetic management of specific pathologic lung conditions and surgical procedures

A. Pneumonectomy

1. **Preoperative evaluation.** About 60% of patients with an operable carcinoma of the lung will require a pneumonectomy. If a lesion is considered resectable, an evaluation of the patient's **cardiopulmonary function** is necessary. Other considerations important in the preoperative evaluation are:

a. Severe anemia, diabetes, arteriosclerosis, blood coagulopathies, and hypoadrenalism.

b. In a patient who has had a **myocardial infarction** within the previous year, pneumonectomy carries a 50% mortality risk.

c. It is important to determine in advance the pulmonary function that the patient will have after the lung is removed. **Split-function** criteria suggesting inoperability are:

(1) **On balloon occlusion of the pulmonary artery** during supine exercises using a bicycle ergometer, the main pulmonary artery pressure is 35 torr or greater. Balloon occlusion of the pulmonary artery is performed by placing a double-lumen cardiac balloon catheter in the pulmonary artery of the lung to be resected. The balloon is inflated until it blocks blood flow to the involved lung. Proximal to the balloon there is a lumen that allows one to monitor the proximal main pulmonary artery pressure after blood flow is blocked.

(2) Under the same conditions, if the arterial oxygen tension falls to 45 torr or less.

(3) If the calculated postoperative forced expired volume of 1 sec (FEV_1) is less than 0.8 L.

2. Double-lumen **endobronchial intubation** is not necessary for most pneumonectomies.

3. **Arrhythmias** are more frequent after pneumonectomy than following most other operations.

B. Upper lobectomy with resection of a segment of the main bronchus is usually performed in carcinoma of the lung; thus the main bronchus will be open for some time during surgery. **Endobronchial anesthesia** of the healthy lung is indicated.

C. Endobronchial or one-lung anesthesia

1. In this technique, anesthetic gases may be excluded from one lung.

2. **Indications**

a. To prevent spread of infected secretions from the pathologic to the normal lung during thoracic surgery.

b. Copious bleeding from a traumatized, inflamed lung.

c. A ruptured bronchus.

d. Expanding lung cysts.

e. To improve operative conditions by producing a quiet, unventilated lung on the side being operated on, as well as facilitating access to the aorta and the esophagus.

3. **Physiology of one-lung anesthesia**

a. **Carbon dioxide clearance.** The arterial carbon dioxide pressure is not expected to rise, provided the ventilation volume of the one lung is maintained at the same level as that originally distributed to the two lungs. This means that more pressure will have to be applied during inspiration.

b. **Arterial oxygenation** is affected by the following factors:

(1) **Shunting of blood** through the unventilated lung. Factors that influence blood flow through the collapsed lung are:

(a) **The distribution of pulmonary flow** prior to operation. In diseases involving fibrosis or destruction of lung tissue, circulation to the pathologic lung is considerably reduced.

(b) **The position of the patient.** In the lateral position, especially in the paralyzed patient or in the event of a thoracotomy, most of the blood passes through the lower-lying lung under the influence of gravity. This **gravitational effect** is minimized once the lung has collapsed during one-lung anesthesia and lies at the level of the heart.

(c) **The pressure in the airway.** The mediastinum tends to sink under its own weight into the lower thorax during expiration, thus reducing the volume of the lower-lying lung and producing atelectasis.

i. This can be corrected by maintaining a **positive pressure in the airway** during expiration (positive end-expiratory pressure—PEEP).

ii. **The effect of PEEP** is twofold: (a) If the functional residual capacity of the ventilated lung was previously low and was restored to normal with PEEP, the pulmonary vascular resistance should fall, producing increased blood flow through the ventilated lung. (b) If functional residual capacity is increased with PEEP over an initially normal value, pulmonary vascular resistance should be increased, and a higher proportion of the blood flow will be shunted through the unventilated lung.

(2) **Oxygenating efficiency** of the ventilated lung can be compromised by aspiration, severe bilateral pulmonary disease, or pulmonary damage secondary to heart disease. The use of relatively large tidal volumes will prevent atelectasis in the dependent, ventilated lung.

(3) **Cardiac output.** A fall in cardiac output causes a decrease in PaO_2 with the same level of shunt fraction (QS/QT).

(4) **It is recommended** that no less than 95% inspired oxygen be administered during one-lung anesthesia. The PaO_2 must be checked following 10–15 min of one-lung anesthesia; if the PaO_2 is more than 200 torr, the functional inspired oxygen concentration (FIO_2) can be reduced, keeping the PaO_2 at 100–120 torr. If the PaO_2 is less than 100 torr, oxygenation may be improved by inflating the unventilated lung with oxygen at intervals of 5–10 min.

D. Techniques of endobronchial anesthesia

1. **The Carlens double-lumen tube** consists of a double-lumen tube with two cuffs. One cuff is on the distal end, which is positioned into the left bronchus. The second cuff is on the portion that remains in the trachea proximal to the opening for the right bronchus. A rubber hook is provided to be engaged on the carina. The tube is manufactured in four sizes: 35, 37, 39, and 41 French.

   a. **During intubation** the tube is introduced with the hook directed posteriorly and is rotated counterclockwise through 90 degrees. Then it is advanced until the hook is engaged on the carina, and the endobronchial portion is placed into the left main bronchus.

   b. **Modification of this technique** consists of using a straight laryngoscope blade. The tube is passed through the larynx with the tip pointing anteriorly. As soon as the tip passes the vocal cords, the tube is rotated 180 degrees. This brings the carinal hook anteriorly, where it slides along the laryngoscope blade (Fig. 31-1).

   c. It is advisable to **tie the rubber hook to the tube** with a No. 3 black silk suture. The knot is tied in such a manner that it can be released by gently pulling its proximal end as soon as the hook passes the vocal cords. In this way, a larger-size tube can be used.

   d. **The left cuff is inflated first,** using the minimal amount of air necessary to prevent a leak. A connection is made to the left side only. The left chest only should be inflated with the squeezing of the breathing bag. Following this, the tracheal cuff is inflated, and the right chest is checked.

2. **The White double-lumen tube** is very useful when it is necessary to amputate the left main bronchus. This tube is almost a mirror image of the Carlens tube. The endobronchial part is introduced into the right main bronchus. The bronchial cuff has a slit that communicates with the right lumen of the tube. This slit is in opposition to the orifice of the right upper lobe bronchus, thus permitting ventilation of the right upper lobe.

3. **The Robert Shaw tube** is a right and a left double-lumen tube. Three sizes are available: large, medium, and small. It has a larger lumen than the

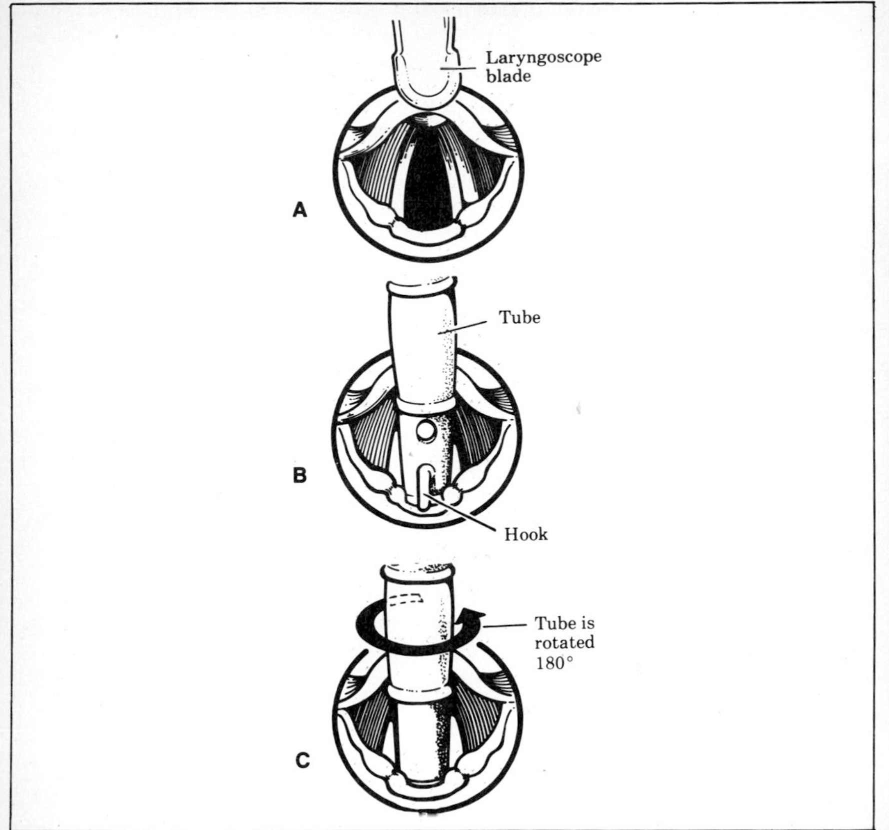

Fig. 31-1. Modification for insertion of the Carlens double-lumen tube. **A.** A straight laryngoscope blade is inserted to expose the vocal cords. **B.** The tube is passed through the larynx with the tip pointing anteriorly. **C.** As soon as the tip passes the vocal cords, the tube is rotated 180 degrees. This brings the carinal hook anteriorly, where it slides along the laryngoscope blade.

Carlens tube, and the shape of the tube is molded more accurately to the anatomy of the upper airway, trachea, and main bronchi. There is **no carinal hook,** and intubation can be performed more easily without it.

4. **The Gordon-Green tube** is used for right endobronchial intubation. It was designed for right endobronchial anesthesia for left lung surgery. It is a single-lumen tube and has two cuffs, one to occlude the bronchus and one to occlude the trachea, and a small carinal hook. The bronchial cuff is fenestrated to ensure right upper lobe inflation.

E. Esophagectomy

1. For cancer of the thoracic esophagus, **esophagectomy** and **esophagogastrectomy** are performed with the patient in the lateral position, with the left side uppermost, and a posterolateral thoracic incision.
2. The anesthesiologist should monitor the cardiovascular system and the operative field, because the possibility of **exerting pressure on the heart** is great.

3. The use of **one-lung anesthesia** improves operating conditions but is not absolutely indicated.

F. Tracheal resection for benign stricture or for tumors

1. **Premedication.** Where the accessory muscles of respiration are required for the maintenance of adequate ventilation, only atropine is given. In all other patients, pentobarbital and atropine are given. With the sedated patient, breathing becomes quieter and easier.

2. **Monitoring.** A radial artery line is used for sampling blood gases and monitoring arterial pressure. A chest stethoscope is attached on each side of the chest.

3. **Management of anesthesia**

   a. **Alternatives.** One of the following two techniques may be applied:

      (1) Bronchoscopic examination with a **ventilating bronchoscope** is carried out with the patient under **topical anesthesia.** The bronchoscope is passed through the stricture, securing the airway. **General anesthesia** is induced with thiopental and halothane or thiopental and enflurane. Maintenance of anesthesia is accomplished through the sidearm of the bronchoscope with assisted respiration.

      (2) Slow, cautious induction of anesthesia is carried out with **thiopental and halothane.** After topical anesthesia of the oropharynx, larynx, and trachea, bronchoscopy is performed, and the exact site, size, and nature of the stricture are determined. Following this, the bronchoscope is removed and the patient is intubated with a normal-size orotracheal tube placed in the trachea above the lesion.

   b. **Positioning of the patient**

      (1) The **supine position** is convenient for an anterior cervical incision with a median sternotomy, if necessary.

      (2) The **right thoracotomy position** is suitable for approach to the lower part of the trachea or resection of carinal lesions.

   c. **Following surgical exposure** of the exterior of the involved portion of the trachea, **alternative 1** (with the bronchoscope in the trachea) allows better evaluation of the extent of the disease and determination of the proper level for caudal transection.

   d. **Tracheal transection**

      (1) **The distal tracheal segment** is intubated through the surgical field with a sterile cuffed endotracheal tube, and at the same time the bronchoscope (as in **alternative 1)** is withdrawn.

      (2) **The endotracheal tube** is connected to the anesthesia machine by sterile, corrugated-rubber breathing tubes.

      (3) **If the distal tracheal stump** is too short to hold an endotracheal tube, the tube is advanced into the left main bronchus, through which only the left lung is ventilated (the approach is usually through a right thoracotomy in these cases).

   e. **Excision of the diseased segment of the trachea**

      (1) Following excision, the trachea is anastomosed.

      (2) Before anastomosis is completed, the distal endotracheal tube is removed, and the original orotracheal tube (as in **alternative 2**) is advanced beyond the suture line.

      (3) If the bronchoscope was used, as in **alternative 1,** the patient is reintubated with an orotracheal tube, which can be difficult. A catheter

can be passed into the trachea from the surgical field and retrieved in the mouth. This can serve as a guide over which the endotracheal tube can be slid into position, or the endotracheal tube can be attached to the catheter and drawn into position.

f. **The patient's neck** is flexed during anastomosis of the trachea and is maintained in this position for 1 week.

g. **The final extubation** is performed in the operating room with the patient awake and able to maintain his or her own upper airway.

G. Thymectomy

1. In a patient with myasthenia gravis, **thymectomy** is performed when the disease has reached a stable state in regard to anticholinesterase drugs and control of pulmonary infection.

2. **Surgical approach**

   a. **Transcervical incision** is simple and expeditious. Disruption of the chest cage is avoided, and postoperative care is facilitated.

   b. **Median sternotomy** in the case of a large thymoma.

3. **On the day of the operation,** the morning dose of anticholinesterase medication is given IM or is omitted. The IM dose should correspond to half the dose administered by mouth.

4. **Premedication.** Respiratory depressant drugs are omitted. Atropine is used to counteract the effects of the anticholinesterase drugs.

5. **Induction of anesthesia**

   a. A minimal sleep dose of IV barbiturate with nitrous oxide, oxygen, and halothane or enflurane is given.

   b. If the patient is very weak, induction of anesthesia is accomplished only with inhalation anesthetics.

   c. When anesthesia has been established and the jaw is relaxed (which is much easier to achieve in these patients), endotracheal intubation is performed.

   d. In the presence of an existing **tracheotomy,** general anesthesia is induced through the tracheotomy tube, which is replaced later by an orotracheal tube.

6. **Maintenance of anesthesia** is carried out only with inhalation anesthetic agents.

7. **Postoperative care**

   a. **All patients** are provided with ventilatory support in the postoperative period via a low-pressure, cuffed orotracheal, nasotracheal, or tracheotomy tube (in the case of a preexisting one).

   b. If possible, **tracheotomy** should not be performed for 48 hr following surgery. By that time, the sternotomy wound is relatively well sealed.

   c. **No anticholinesterase drugs** are given until the patient can breathe with a minimum of incision pain.

   d. Patients are **weaned from the ventilator** when tidal volume is normal, vital capacity is approximately 3 times the tidal volume, and inspiratory force exceeds 20 cm H_2O negative pressure.

H. Bronchopleural fistula

1. Bronchopleural fistula may follow a postoperative infection of a lobectomy or pneumonectomy. It also may occur because of malignant or tuberculous invasion of the bronchial stump.

2. **Surgical treatment**
   a. Rib resection and drainage of the pleural space.
   b. Thoracoplasty.
   c. Thoracotomy and closure of the fistula (in early postoperative cases).
3. **Problems**
   a. **Pleural fluid** can flood the bronchial tree and spill over into the unaffected lung, especially when the patient coughs or is placed in the supine or lateral position.
   b. There may be an **inability to inflate** the lungs or a paralyzed patient because air is leaking.
   c. **Tension pneumothorax** may occur if the fistula is relatively small and positive-pressure ventilation is employed.
4. **Preoperative preparation.** As much pleural fluid as possible should be aspirated before surgery, or a chest drain tube should be inserted.
5. **Management of anesthesia**
   a. The patient is placed in **Fowler's position** (the head of the bed is raised 45 cm above horizontal).
   b. A Carlens tube is inserted under topical anesthesia, with the patient breathing spontaneously. **For a left-sided fistula,** a Gordon-Green tube can be used.
   c. When the sound lung has been isolated, induction and maintenance of anesthesia are accomplished with thiopental, oxygen, halothane or enflurane, and muscle relaxant drugs.
   d. Occasionally (when the chest drain tube is in place and connected to suction), endotracheal intubation may be performed under general anesthesia with succinylcholine.

I. **Emergency lung conditions**

1. **Removal of a lung cyst**
   a. **A lung cyst** that requires emergency treatment develops a one-way valvular orifice, allowing the air to be trapped in the cyst when the intrathoracic pressure rises during coughing or straining.
   b. **Consequences**
      (1) The surrounding lung tissue is compressed, and the ventilatory capacity of the contralateral lung is decreased by the mediastinal shift.
      (2) The mediastinal displacement causes circulatory impairment.
   c. **Special points** to remember until the pleural cavity has been opened:
      (1) No coughing and/or straining must be allowed. These may result in a further rise of tension in the cyst.
      (2) Assisted or controlled ventilation is contraindicated.
      (3) Nitrous oxide is to be avoided (the differential solubility of nitrous oxide–nitrogen causes further expansion of the lung cyst).
   d. **Management of anesthesia**
      (1) The patient is preoxygenated before topical anesthesia of the oropharynx, larynx, and trachea.
      (2) Induction of anesthesia is carried out with a sleep dose of thiopental, halothane or enflurane, and oxygen or with only an inhalation anesthetic.

(3) Intubation and maintenance of anesthesia must be carried out with the patient breathing spontaneously until the pleura is open.

(4) In a dire emergency, a large-bore needle may be inserted through the chest wall into the cyst to release the air and the pressure.

2. **Hemoptysis**

a. **Hemoptysis may result** from:

(1) Bronchial adenoma, carcinoma, bronchiectasis, or a tuberculous cavity.

(2) An inadvertent biopsy of a vascular malformation or bronchial adenoma.

b. **Problems**

(1) **The seriously ill patient,** in shock from apprehension and blood loss.

(2) **Hypoxia** from a combination of atelectasis, lung destruction, and spread of blood in the bronchial tree.

c. **Surgical treatment** is lobectomy or segmental resection.

d. **Anesthetic management**

(1) General anesthesia is accomplished with an inhalation anesthetic drug (halothane or enflurane), oxygen, and a muscle relaxant.

(2) There are several alternatives to confine the **bleeding** in the affected area and to prevent **drowning** of patients in their own blood.

(a) Insertion of a **double-lumen tube** to maintain ventilation on the sound side, and use of the other lumen for aspiration of blood.

(b) Introduction of a **Fogarty balloon embolectomy catheter** through a ventilating bronchoscope, and use of it as a blocker. The bronchoscope is then withdrawn, and a cuffed endotracheal tube is inserted.

(c) **Endobronchial intubation** of the sound side with an uncuffed endotracheal tube that has an aperture located opposite the beveled end of the tube, which will obviate the complications from occlusion of the beveled end against the tracheal wall (Murphy endotracheal tube). The tube is inserted through the larynx and then turned so that the concavity of the natural curve of the tube is facing the bronchus to be entered. Observation and auscultation confirm endobronchial intubation. Another, smaller endotracheal tube (6 mm ID or less) may be inserted into the bleeding side beside the first one for aspiration of blood.

J. **Anesthesia for bronchoscopy**

1. **A satisfactory anesthesia** for bronchoscopy presents many difficult problems, and the outcome depends in part on the disease.

a. Chronic lung disease, respiratory obstruction, bronchial spasm, coughing, expectoration of large amounts of blood or pus, and hypoventilation are all factors that require special management.

b. During bronchoscopy, the anesthesiologist and surgeon are in competition for control of the patient's airway.

2. There are many anesthesia methods for bronchoscopy, but no single technique is satisfactory for all patients. The choice of the anesthesia technique depends on the skill and experience of the anesthesiologist and the bronchoscopist.

a. **Topical anesthesia** under sedative drugs is the technique of choice. But when the patient is not cooperative, has dyspnea, or is apprehensive, **general anesthesia** is indicated.

b. The electrical activity of the heart must be **monitored** continuously during bronchoscopy performed under topical or general anesthesia.

3. **Topical anesthesia**

a. The **premedication drugs** used are diazepam (Valium) or droperidol-fentanyl (Innovar). Additional doses may be given IV on the patient's arrival in the operating room.

b. The oropharynx and larynx are sprayed with 4% lidocaine.

c. With the patient in the **semi-Fowler's position,** 2.5 ml of 2% lidocaine or 4 ml of 0.5% tetracaine is injected through the cricothyroid membrane into the trachea. The patient must not cough until the needle is removed. To ensure that some of the topical anesthetic solution enters the **left bronchus,** the injection is repeated with the patient in the semi-Fowler's position and leaning to the left side.

d. Topical anesthesia may be complicated by **systemic reactions** resulting from fast absorption of large amounts of the drug into the circulation. Apnea, convulsions, severe hypotension, or cardiac arrest may occur. These toxic effects can be avoided by limiting the total amount of the topical anesthetic agent. An IV route for treatment should be available.

4. **General anesthesia**

a. The **premedication drugs** used are: droperidol, fentanyl, and atropine; morphine and atropine; medperidine and atropine; or diazepam and atropine.

b. **Maintenance of anesthesia** is accomplished by either of the following agents:

(1) Thiopental, fentanyl, nitrous oxide with oxygen, and succinylcholine.

(2) Nitrous oxide, oxygen with halothane or enflurane, and succinylcholine.

c. When bronchoscopy is performed under general anesthesia, it is important that the pharynx, larynx, and trachea be sprayed with a low-toxicity topical anesthetic agent, such as 4% lidocaine, before introduction of the bronchoscope. This will prevent severe coughing and laryngospasm following removal of the instrument.

d. **Control of ventilation** is carried out by the following methods:

(1) With an **endotracheal tube** 5.5–6 mm ID lying alongside the bronchoscope.

(2) With the **ventilating bronchoscope,** which includes a wide-bore sidearm through which anesthetic gases are administered and a removable glass window that can be placed over the external orifice of the bronchoscope to prevent leakage of gases when applying intermittent positive-pressure ventilation. During bronchoscopic examination, the glass disc is removed and respiration is interrupted for a few seconds. Coughing may be induced by briefly discontinuing the succinylcholine infusion.

(3) **Sanders Venturi system**

(a) The system consists of the Venturi adaptor and a vented collar with an attached jet (0.9-mm orifice) that fits over the observer's end of the bronchoscope.

(b) The Venturi is connected by plastic tubing to an on-off toggle valve that, in turn, is connected by tubing to a two-stage variable-pressure regulator for an oxygen source. A driving pressure of 3–4 atmospheres is required.

(c) The jet of oxygen blown into the observer's end of the bronchoscope creates a Venturi effect (that is, it draws in ambient air, so that sufficient pressure is generated within the chest to inflate the lungs).

(d) The jet must be precisely in line with the axis of the bronchoscope. The slightest lateral deviation of the jet will reduce its ventilating efficiency by generating turbulence.

(e) **The advantages** of this technique are that (1) it eliminates an endotracheal tube, and (2) there is no interruption of ventilation for instrumentation and suction (as is the case with the ventilating bronchoscope, which has a proximal window).

(f) **Management of anesthesia.** Anesthesia is induced with thiopental, and maintenance of anesthesia is carried out with oxygen, thiopental, and fentanyl. Complete muscle relaxation with continuous or intermittent administration of succinylcholine is necessary to increase the overall compliance.

(4) **The endotracheal tube is at least 8 mm ID,** with a right-angle connector. There is an opening at a right angle, occluded with a rubber cap through which a **fiberoptic bronchoscope** (outside diameter 6.2 mm) can be passed.

Bibliography

Borg, U., Eriksson, I., and Sjostrand, U. High-frequency positive-pressure ventilation (HFPPV). A review based upon its use during bronchoscopy and for laryngoscopy and microlaryngeal surgery under general anesthesia. *Anesth. Analg.* (Cleve.) 59:594, 1980.

Eriksson, I., and Sjostrand, U. Effects of high-frequency positive-pressure ventilation (HFPPV) and general anesthesia on intrapulmonary gas distribution in patients undergoing diagnostic bronchoscopy. *Anesth. Analg.* (Cleve.) 59:585, 1980.

Heifetz, M., De Myttenaere, S., and Lemer, J. Intermittent positive pressure inflation during fiberoptic bronchoscopy. *Chest* 72:480, 1977.

Johnson, N. M., Hodson, M. E., and Clarke, S. W. Acceptability of fiberoptic bronchoscopy under local anaesthesia. *Practitioner* 221:113, 1978.

Lindholm, C. E., Ollman, B., Snyder, J. V., et al. Cardiorespiratory effects of flexible fiberoptic bronchoscopy in critically ill patients. *Chest* 74:362, 1978.

Malina, J.R., Nordstrom, S. G., Sjostrand, U. H., et al. Clinical evaluation of high-frequency positive-pressure ventilation (HFPPV) in patients scheduled for open-chest surgery. *Anesth. Analg.* (Cleve.) 60:324, 1981.

Satyanarayna, T., Capan, L., Ramanathan, S., et al. Bronchofiberscopic jet ventilation. *Anesth. Analg.* (Cleve.) 59:350, 1980.

Sjostrand, U. Review of the physiological rational for and development of high-frequency positive-pressure ventilation - HFPPV. *Acta Anaesthesiol. Scand.* [Suppl] 64:7, 1977.

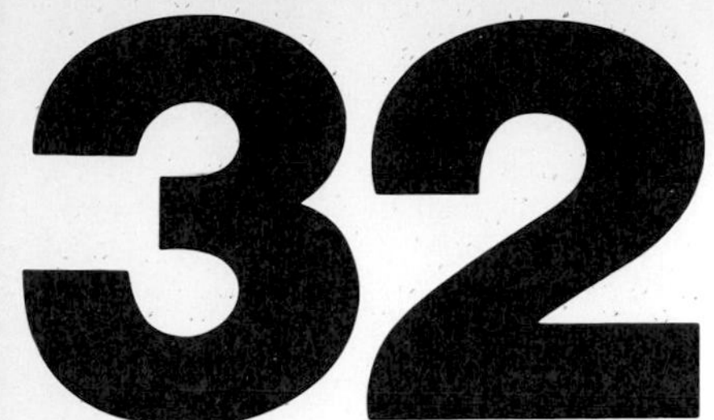

Anesthesia in Cardiac Surgery

I. General comments. Cardiac surgical patients present a complex problem to the anesthesiologist. Hemodynamic alterations induced by anesthesia and operation may further increase the burden placed on the diseased heart. **All anesthetics alter cardiovascular function.** An understanding of the hemodynamic consequences imposed by the cardiac lesion and knowledge of the effects of the anesthetics on the cardiovascular system are basic requirements for operating room management of these patients.

II. Preoperative evaluation and management

A. Preoperative evaluation of the patient's status is done to determine the degree and severity of cardiovascular disease and associated organ involvement. Information can be gathered from:

1. The history. Careful questioning about the onset of symptoms, including chest pain, dyspnea, syncope, palpitation, wheezing, hemoptysis, cough, and peripheral edema.

2. The physical examination must be performed carefully and should include the following:

a. Inspection of the patient

(1) Cyanosis indicates an excess of deoxyhemoglobin due either to increased tissue oxygen extraction in a low-output state (peripheral cyanosis) or the presence of intracardiac right-to-left shunts (central cyanosis).

(2) Jugular venous distention or pulsation will be apparent in right ventricular failure with tricuspid regurgitation.

(3) Respiratory effort can be substantial in congestive heart failure.

(4) An apical cardiac impulse may be visible in left ventricular hypertrophy.

(5) Peripheral edema is a late manifestation of congestive heart failure.

b. Auscultation of the heart to establish clearly the timing and characteristics of the heart sounds and to detect murmurs.

c. Examination of the arteries for heartbeat rate, rhythm, amplitude, and waveform. The main peripheral arteries are palpated to determine the pulsation, condition, and patency of the vessel.

d. Measurement of systemic arterial pressure in both arms. In coarctation, arterial pressure is lower in the lower extremities.

e. Examination of the lungs to disclose the presence of pleural effusion. Rales may be present in left heart failure and with chronic lung disease. The presence of pulmonary edema should be determined also.

3. An **ECG** is required to confirm the nature of any cardiac arrhythmias and to detect changes due to myocardial ischemia, altered conduction, the presence

of a digitalis effect, and electrolyte disturbances. A baseline preoperative tracing is useful for comparison during surgery.

4. **Cardiac catheterization and angiography** are performed to confirm the clinical diagnosis and to provide a basis for medical or surgical treatment. Understanding of the catheterization data is essential for proper patient management before, during, and after surgery.

5. A **chest x-ray** is needed to evaluate the degree of cardiac enlargement, to detect interstitial pulmonary edema, to examine the lung fields for gross parenchymal changes, and to examine the pulmonary vasculature for signs of vascular hypertension.

6. **Examination of the blood.** Serial blood tests are performed to obtain information on hemoglobin concentration, clotting factors, electrolytes, sugar, enzymes, and other constituents, depending on the patient's disease. Anemia may not be tolerated by patients with heart disease. Blood urea, nitrogen level and serum creatinine should be determined, especially if renal disease, hypertension, or congestive heart failure complicates the cardiac disease. Recording the serum electrolyte levels (particularly potassium), hematocrit, and daily urine output is necessary to provide guidelines for the administration of intravenous fluids.

7. **Examination of the urine** may reveal albumin, glucose, ketones, red and white blood cells, and electrolyte abnormalities.

B. Drug therapy

1. **Digoxin or other cardiac glycosides** are used in congestive heart failure and in atrial fibrillation or flutter to control the rapid ventricular response. Evidence of digitalis toxicity usually can be found in almost 20% of patients on digitalis. Cardiac arrhythmias produced by digitalis include premature ventricular contractions, atrioventricular block of varying degree, atrial tachycardia, and even ventricular fibrillation. **Hypokalemia** accentuates digitalis-induced arrhythmias and should be corrected. Premature ventricular contractions from digitalis toxicity respond to IV phenytoin sodium (Dilantin).

2. **Administration of diuretics** may cause:

   a. **Potassium depletion.** Serum potassium may be within normal limits when total body potassium is decreased. Potassium depletion should be corrected by potassium chloride administration. Spironolactones usually produce potassium retention.

   b. **Volume depletion.** Vigorous diuresis may cause a decrease in blood volume, which leads to low cardiac output, tissue underperfusion, and lactic acidosis. Depleted blood volume should be restored before anesthesia, because severe hypotension may occur during anesthetic drug administration. Diuretics are generally stopped 2 days before the operation.

   c. **Metabolic alkalosis** with a normal pH and increased PCO_2.

3. **Propranolol,** a beta-adrenergic blocker, is used to treat refractory or frequent angina pectoris, arrhythmias of ventricular origin, and occasionally essential hypertension. In most cases propranolol is discontinued 1–2 days preoperatively. However, the drug may be continued until shortly before the operation if the patient has recurrent angina. Bradycardia and hypotension may occur with propranolol. **Anesthetic drugs potentiate the myocardial depressant effect of propranolol** and should be administered cautiously. Isoproterenol and calcium chloride can be used to treat both complications.

4. **Procainamide** (Pronestyl) and **phenytoin sodium** (Dilantin) are myocardial depressants.

5. **Aspirin and clofibrate** (Atromid-S) may cause platelet dysfunction and should be discontinued a few days prior to surgery.

6. **Nitroglycerin and isosorbide dinitrate** (Isordil) need not be discontinued.

7. **Insulin and anticonvulsive therapy** should be continued up to the time of the operation.

8. A number of patients in heart failure may be **on vasopressor therapy** (epinephrine, isoproterenol) on arrival in the operating room.

C. **A thorough knowledge of the patient's medical history** and the proposed surgical procedure is essential. Information about drug allergies, previous operations, and anesthetic experience should be elicited.

D. Finally, it is important to **discuss with the patient** the preanesthesia preparation, the preoperative insertion of intravascular cannulae, and the problems of the immediate postoperative period. A carefully conducted preoperative visit that is sympathetic, unhurried, and informative will alleviate much of the patient's preoperative anxiety.

III. Preanesthetic medication

A. **Effective preanesthetic medication,** without circulatory or respiratory depression, relieves the patient's great preoperative anxiety. Many combinations of drugs (barbiturates, opiates, belladonna drugs, and sedatives) have been used for premedication in adult cardiac surgical patients. The doses administered to patients with valvular heart disease should be smaller than those administered to noncardiac patients, because severe cardiorespiratory depression is more likely to occur in the former patients than in patients with coronary artery disease and normal ventricular contractility.

B. **Morphine** 0.08 mg/kg and **scopolamine** 0.4 mg administered IM is a safe and satisfactory combination for most adult patients with valvular heart disease. Doses are reduced by half in patients with severe cachexia, cyanosis, congestive heart failure, and critical valvular stenosis. Higher doses of morphine (0.1 mg/kg) or additional sedation with diazepam 5–10 mg) or droperidol (2.5–5 mg) may be required for patients with coronary artery disease who are known to have normal ventricular contractility and in whom apprehension with elevated BP or tachycardia may elicit the symptoms of myocardial ischemia. On the other hand, **premedication should be omitted** in patients in severe cardiogenic shock, in emergency cases, and in patients with severe cardiorespiratory abnormalities until adequate hemodynamic monitoring and respiratory control are available. Morphine may occasionally cause respiratory depression with a rise in arterial PCO_2 and a decrease in arterial PO_2. Therefore oxygen supplementation with a face mask should be given after premedication in patients with low arterial PO_2 and respiratory problems. Furthermore, **following premedication,** all patients should be kept in bed to avoid orthostatic hypotension.

C. **Atropine is probably best omitted** from premedication because of the resulting tachycardia (particularly hazardous with mitral stenosis or coronary artery disease) and occasional temperature elevation in children.

D. **Infants** need not be premedicated. Older children are premedicated with scopolamine 0.01 mg/kg, morphine 0.1 mg/kg, and pentobarbital 1 mg/kg IM, given in an attempt to produce light sleep.

IV. Preparation for cardiac surgical anesthesia

A. **A cart containing all the drugs** required for support and/or resuscitation of the cardiac patient should be ready for immediate use. It must include vasopressors (epinephrine, norepinephrine, phenylephrine, isoproterenol), atropine, digoxin, propranolol, lidocaine, calcium chloride, nitroglycerin, and sodium bicarbonate.

B. **A source of oxygen,** as well as **suction and monitoring equipment,** including a defibrillator, should be available.

C. Anesthesia should not be started without proper **hemodynamic monitoring,** which is of paramount importance for successful anesthetic management.

1. **A radial artery cannula** (18-gauge) is inserted to record systemic arterial pressure continuously.
2. **A central venous line** is used for right atrial or superior vena cava pressure measurement and for drug administration.
3. **Pulmonary arterial and pulmonary capillary wedge pressure** can be obtained from a **pulmonary artery balloon (Swan-Ganz) catheter** inserted percutaneously, preferably via an internal jugular vein or an antecubital vein.
4. **Leads II and V_4 of the ECG** are used for continuous monitoring of heart rate, rhythm, and S–T segment changes.
5. **Continuous pressure recording** with an appropriate write-out system provides important information on hemodynamic trends and permits early detection of changes and assessment of the effectiveness of therapy.
6. **Arterial blood gases,** pH, electrolytes, hematocrit, and other laboratory variables can be determined from arterial blood samples drawn from the arterial cannula.
7. **Body temperature** must be measured continuously via an esophageal, nasopharyngeal, or tympanic membrane thermistor probe.
8. **Urine** is collected and measured via a catheter introduced prior to operation.

V. Anesthetic drugs and techniques

A. **Support of circulation** in a patient with cardiac disease should be the first priority for the anesthesiologist. All anesthetic drugs possess some myocardial depressant properties and must be administered carefully and slowly under continuous monitoring of vascular pressure and the ECG.

B. **A large variety of anesthetic drugs** have been used for cardiac surgery. It is beyond the scope of this chapter to describe them all, except in a general way (see **D–K**). Since all are effective, the choice depends largely on the anesthesiologist's personal preference and experience. However, a number of important considerations should be taken into account when the choice of anesthetic is made.

1. **Heart rate.** An increase in heart rate may be desirable for certain patients (aortic valve regurgitation) but should be avoided in others (coronary artery disease, mitral stenosis).
2. **Arterial BP.** An acute increase in arterial pressure can lead to acute hemodynamic derangements in patients with critical aortic stenosis or severe coronary artery disease.
3. **Myocardial "depression"** is desirable in the patient with idiopathic hypertrophic subaortic stenosis.
4. **A decrease in peripheral vascular resistance,** with or without changes in arterial pressure, can benefit patients with aortic valve regurgitation or coronary artery disease.
5. **Light levels of anesthesia** are required during cardiac surgey; a minimal level of anesthesia is needed once the incision and sternotomy are completed.
6. **The effect of vagal and sympathetic reflexes** on the heart and circulation may require treatment.
7. **Following intubation,** minimal muscle paralysis is required.

8. **Incomplete amnesia** may cause great emotional distress if it is unexpected. The possibility of its occurrence in the absence of pain perception should be explained to the patient preoperatively.

C. **Administration of ultrashort-acting intravenous barbiturates** (thiopental, 25–50 mg IV, repeated as needed) speeds induction, minimizes emotional stress, and may attenuate the hypertensive response to oral or laryngeal stimulation. They must be administered slowly and in small doses, since they are potent myocardial depressants.

D. **Halothane** (Fluothane) is widely used for cardiac surgery. It is still the anesthetic of choice for **pediatric patients.** Severe myocardial depression, as evidenced by a significant decrease in cardiac output and arterial pressure, may occur with halothane in concentrations exceeding 0.5%. The ECG should be carefully monitored when catecholamines are infused in the presence of halothane, because ventricular irritability may occur. This has not proved bothersome in our experience. Bradycardia and nodal arrhythmias are common during halothane anesthesia.

E. **Methoxyflurane** (Penthrane) is also used for cardiac surgery; its analgesic property makes it the agent of choice in some institutions. Methoxyflurane is also a myocardial depressant and is particularly likely to be nephrotoxic.

F. **Enflurane** (Ethrane) **and isoflurane** (Forane) also depress myocardial contractility. There is evidence that enflurane may contribute to deterioration of renal function in patients with severe renal disease.

G. **Nitrous oxide** is widely used in cardiac surgical patients. A decrease in arterial pressure with nitrous oxide frequently follows its administration in an inspired concentration of 50%. Myocardial depression and an increase in pulmonary and systemic vascular resistance have been noted following its administration. The increase in pulmonary vascular resistance may have serious hemodynamic consequences in the presence of pulmonary hypertension and right ventricular failure.

H. **Intravenous morphine in large doses** (1–3 mg/kg) has been used widely as a primary or supplementary anesthetic drug because of its minor hemodynamic side effects. Hypotension with morphine "anesthesia" is the major side effect. Morphine has been shown to be a safe drug that causes no, or minimal, myocardial depression and does not potentiate ventricular irritability. It should be administered IV in quantities of 5 mg/min or less.

I. **Succinylcholine,** a depolarizing muscle relaxant, is used mainly to facilitate endotracheal intubation. A single bolus (1–1.5 mg/kg) or an infusion of succinylcholine solution (1 g in 500 ml of 5% D/W) is administered IV. **Bradycardia or sinus arrest,** due to vagotonic action, may occur with succinylcholine. Bradycardia is more pronounced in pediatric patients, particularly cyanotic infants. Pressure changes are not seen with succinylcholine, whereas an acute increase in serum potassium may lead to cardiac arrhythmias. This occurs most often in patients with a history of diabetes; it can be minimized if these patients are pretreated with 3–6 mg of tubocurarine IV or 20 mg of gallamine IV.

J. **Tubocurarine** (curare), a nondepolarizing muscle relaxant, causes ganglionic blockade, which may result in arterial hypotension. Incremental administration of 3–6 mg of tubocurarine will minimize this effect. It has been suggested that the myocardial depression that follows tubocurarine is caused by the preservative rather than by the drug. However, recent evidence supports the direct myocardial depression effect. It is advisable not to use tubocurarine in patients with evidence of severely impaired myocardial function.

k. **Gallamine** (Flaxedil) and **pancuronium** (Pavulon) are both nondepolarizing drugs that may cause severe tachycardia. Their use should be avoided in the presence of a fast heart rate, rapid atrial fibrillation, severe aortic valve stenosis, or coronary artery disease. If either of these muscle relaxants is to be used, small incremental doses and slow administration are recommended.

VI. Specific considerations for anesthesia in various cardiac diseases

A. Aortic valve disease

1. Aortic stenosis

a. **Stenosis of the aortic valve** produces hypertrophy of the left ventricle. As the lesion progresses, the pressure gradient across the valve increases. Cardiac reserve is diminished.

b. **Patients with mild or moderate aortic stenosis** tolerate anesthesia well, provided it is administered carefully. A sudden fall in systemic arterial pressure and cardiac output may occur at any time during anesthesia and operation. In patients with chronic heart failure, arterial BP is maintained with increased peripheral vascular resistance and a lower cardiac output. Vasodilatation and myocardial depression produced by an anesthetic may severely compromise cardiac function. Therefore these drugs must be administered with great care and in smaller doses than usual. Acute hypotension and hypoxemia are of particular importance whenever coronary artery disease complicates aortic valve lesions.

c. **Severe arterial hypertension** may occur during tracheal intubation and surgical stimulation as a result of a massive autonomic discharge that may lead to transient left ventricular failure or circulatory collapse. It is particularly important to maintain an adequate level of anesthesia to attenuate sympathetic responses.

d. **Nodal rhythm** may impair left ventricular function by preventing the atrial contribution to ventricular filling, causing an acute decrease in cardiac output and BP. Severe tachycardia also may impair cardiac function.

2. **Aortic insufficiency.** Patients with free aortic regurgitation and a low diastolic pressure are very vulnerable both to a drop in arterial BP and to rhythm changes. Coronary filling may be sharply decreased as the result of a reduction in diastolic pressure. Volume replacement should be prompt to avoid relative hypovolemia and hypotension secondary to vasodilatation consequent to anesthesia.

3. **Sudden transient hypotension** during surgical manipulation may be due to interference with venous return, acute arrhythmias, or mechanical impairment of ventricular performance. This state of affairs usually can be rapidly reversed if the cause is removed. If hypotension persists, prompt treatment should be started, as follows:

a. **Transfusion with colloid or crystalloid solutions** to restore ventricular filling pressures (i.e., left and right atrial pressures) if they are low. Central venous pressure should be kept at 8–10 torr.

b. **Administration of inhalation anesthetic drugs** should be discontinued and the patient ventilated with 100% oxygen.

c. **Administration of peripheral vasoconstrictors** (e.g., phenylephrine, norepinephrine) should be considered only when systemic arterial pressure is low and there is risk of reduced coronary perfusion. A drug combining a peripheral vasoconstrictor with an inotropic effect should be used if vasodilatation is the cause of hypotension; isoproterenol is indicated in the presence of hypotension and bradycardia.

d. **Arterial pressure** may be restored rapidly by the administration of calcium chloride (3 mg/kg) IV, particularly in patients who have been on long-term propranolol therapy. In any case, the vasopressor should be carefully administered to avoid complications from overdosage.

e. **The following drugs or procedures** are used if a cardiac arrhythmia is present:

(1) **Lidocaine** 1 mg/kg should be given IV as a bolus to treat premature ventricular contractions. If the arrhythmia persists, a lidocaine infusion must be started (infusion rate, 1–4 mg/min).

(2) If atrioventricular nodal rhythm is present and the chest is open, **atrial pacing** may cause reversion to sinus rhythm.

(3) **Atropine,** 0.25–0.5 mg, is recommended to increase heart rate if bradycardia occurs. **Cardioversion** is indicated if atrial fibrillation or flutter develops suddenly.

(4) Hypokalemia should be corrected by **potassium chloride** administration.

(5) Repeated bouts of nodal tachycardia or premature ventricular contractions that are unresponsive to a continuous infusion of lidocaine may require the administration of **propranolol** (0.25 mg per bolus at 3-min intervals for a total dose not to exceed 2 mg). The drug should not be given if hypotension is present.

4. **Patients with idiopathic hypertrophic subaortic stenosis** need special consideration during surgery, because the pressure gradient across the aortic valve may worsen suddenly when myocardial contractility is enhanced. Intraoperative hypotension must be treated with a vasopressor that is effective on the peripheral vascular bed, e.g., phenylephrine.

B. **Mitral valve disease**

1. **Mitral stenosis**

a. **General considerations.** Mitral stenosis impedes blood flow from the left atrium into the left ventricle. As the lesion progresses, left atrial pressure increases, and the left atrium dilates progressively, with resulting increased pulmonary venous pressure and pulmonary vascular congestion (pulmonary edema), as well as an obligatory increase in pulmonary arterial pressure. Ultimately the function of the right ventricle will be affected as the low-output state develops. The left ventricle is not primarily affected in pure mitral stenosis. Dyspnea is the main symptom of pulmonary congestion. Pulmonary infection, fibrosis, and systemic and pulmonary emboli may complicate the course of the disease. Atrial fibrillation is common.

b. **Digitalis and diuretics** are usually stopped 48 hr before anesthesia. Patients in rapid atrial fibrillation should not have their preoperative digitalis stopped. **IV potassium** administration should be prompt, to prevent arrhythmias secondary to digitalis overdosage.

c. **Anesthesia management**

(1) **Volume** should be cautiously replaced in patients undergoing vigorous diuretic treatment, because severe hypotension may occur during induction of anesthesia.

(2) **Atrial fibrillation** with a rapid ventricular response can be treated with a supplemental dose of digoxin as indicated.

(3) **If severe bradycardia** is present, careful administration of small increments of atropine (0.05–0.1 mg) may be given.

(4) **Vasodilatation** and myocardial depression due to anesthetic drugs (thiopental, halothane) may severely reduce the already low cardiac output.

(5) **Nitrous oxide** should not be administered to patients with severe pulmonary hypertension, because it has been shown to increase pul-

monary vascular resistance, accentuate pulmonary hypertension, and produce systemic hypotension and a further decrease in cardiac ouptut due to impaired right ventricular function.

(6) **Care to avoid fluid overloading** is important, particularly in the presence of pulmonary congestion.

(7) **Induction of anesthesia** should be slow. In general, the same principles apply for the treatment of hypotension as in patients with aortic valve disease.

2. **Mitral insufficiency.** Cardiac failure may develop, but the low-output state is not as prominent as in mitral stenosis. However, left ventricular involvement complicates the disease. Acute mitral regurgitation due to ruptured chordae tendineae or papillary muscles presents serious problems because of the associated severe cardiac failure. It often requires inotropic support before and during anesthesia and surgery.

C. Coronary artery disease

1. **General considerations.** Patients with coronary artery disease have an inadequate coronary blood flow relative to their myocardial oxygen demand. An increase in demand may produce myocardial ischemia or even infarction. Hypertension and tachycardia enhance myocardial oxygen consumption, whereas severe hypotension with a drop in diastolic pressure jeopardizes coronary artery perfusion.

2. **Premedication** should ensure sedation and relaxation without undue cardiovascular or respiratory depression. A combination of morphine 5–8 mg, scopolamine 0.3–0.4 mg, and diazepam 5–10 mg IM is usually satisfactory when left ventricular function is not impaired. Smaller doses should be used if the patient is in left ventricular failure. Premedication should be avoided if severe cardiac failure accompanies recent acute myocardial infarction.

3. **Choice of anesthesia**

a. In general, **patients with normal ventricular function** tolerate anesthesia well. Almost all anesthetic drugs are used for patients with coronary artery disease. Proper and careful administration of anesthesia under continuous BP monitoring can do much to provide hemodynamic stability.

b. **The choice of anesthetic drugs and techniques** may be important for patients with impaired ventricular function or in a low-cardiac-output state, or both, such as following a recent myocardial infarction.

(1) **Preoperative insertion** of the intraaortic balloon pumping device for diastolic unloading of the left ventricle is often indicated to support the failing heart.

(2) **Anesthesia must be administered with extreme care.** Small increments of morphine—2.5–5 mg/min or a lesser rate as indicated, up to 1 mg/kg IV—are usually tolerated well. Diazepam, 1.25–2.5 mg, can be used to supplement morphine and aids in achieving amnesia. Succinylcholine infusion, properly regulated (1 g in 500 ml), is recommended to produce relaxation and facilitate endotracheal intubation. Nitrous oxide 50% in oxygen can be administered, provided the patient's arterial BP is normal. Tubocurarine may severely depress myocardial function, whereas gallamine or pancuronium is apt to produce tachycardia. These drugs should be avoided until hemodynamic stability is achieved. Halothane and methoxyflurane have a negative inotropic effect on the myocardium and may impair cardiac function.

4. **Hypertension** during anesthesia and surgery is usually the result of increased sympathetic activity. In most instances it can be treated by deepen-

ing the level of anesthesia. However, in a large number of patients, hypertension occurs in spite of an "adequate" level of anesthesia. In such a case, cautious infusion of a vasodilator (sodium nitroprusside, 15–20 micrograms/min) will restore arterial BP to the desired level. Vasodilator therapy should not be started if direct BP monitoring is not available, if ventricular filling pressures are low, or if the hypertension is caused by inadequate anesthesia.

5. **Hypotension** is a complicated problem. If mild hypotension is present and filling pressures are low, administration of 200–300 ml of crystalloid, colloid, packed red cells, or whole blood and temporary discontinuation of the inhalation anesthetic will restore arterial BP. If hypotension is pronounced, vasopressors may be considered. Alpha-adrenergic drugs (phenylephrine or methoxamine) causing peripheral vasoconstriction have been used with success in small increments to avoid overdose and an acute hypertensive response. On the other hand, small doses of a catecholamine (e.g., epinephrine) can be used successfully to restore arterial BP and improve both coronary blood flow and myocardial contractility.

6. **Patients with angina pectoris** are frequently receiving chronic propranolol therapy. Administration of the drug is generally discontinued 1 to 2 days before surgery. Occasionally, continuation until the day of the operation is necessary. In these patients, hypotension may be present as a complication during the induction of anesthesia. Infusion of isoproterenol, atropine 0.25–0.5 mg, and calcium chloride 200–300 mg IV has been effective in restoring arterial BP.

7. **Bradycardia** is usually present in patients who have received long-term propranolol therapy. Heart rates as low as 54–58 beats/min are generally tolerated well and require no treatment. Bradycardia below 50 beats/min may respond to atropine administration (0.3–0.5 mg). Atrial pacing is the treatment of choice to increase heart rate once the chest is open.

8. **Tachycardia** should be treated, because it increases myocardial oxygen consumption. If tachycardia persists after a deeper anesthesia level is achieved, careful administration of small doses of propranolol (0.25 mg IV up to a dose of 2 mg) may be helpful.

D. **Cardiac tamponade and cardiac constriction.** In both these conditions, diastolic expansion of the heart is impeded. Pulmonary arterial and venous pressures rise, whereas stroke volume and systemic arterial pressure fall. Because of the decline in cardiac output and arterial BP, syncope or cardiac standstill is common. The condition can be acute (e.g., tamponade following cardiac surgery) or chronic. Anesthesia should be administered cautiously for this condition, with reduced doses, under continuous hemodynamic monitoring.

E. **Pulmonary embolism.** An emergency operation for pulmonary embolism carries a high mortality risk. Major problems include a low cardiac output, arrhythmias, massive right ventricular failure with a high central venous pressure, and metabolic acidosis. Hypoxemia during ventilation with a high concentration of oxygen may be a problem but is not invariably present. Partial right heart bypass following femoral artery and vein cannulation under local anesthesia is usually indicated before general anesthesia. Right ventricular failure is the principal hemodynamic problem; it may persist following extracorporeal bypass and embolectomy.

F. **Congenital heart diseases**

1. **Coarctation of the aorta**

a. **General considerations.** Increased resistance to aortic flow is present. The obstruction is commonly located distal to the origin of the left subclavian artery, proximal (preductal coarctation) or distal (postductal coarctation) to the ligament of the ductus arteriosus. In preductal coarctation, the ductus is usually patent, and blood is shunted from the aorta into the pulmonary artery. If pulmonary hypertension develops secondary to increased pulmonary vascular resistance, the shunt may change direction and flow from the pulmonary artery to the aorta. In this case the left arm and lower body are perfused with venous blood. The persistent obstruction causes congestive heart failure. In postductal stenosis (adult coarctation), the ductus is usually closed, the resistance to the left ventricular output is increased, and hypertension is present in the upper limbs, while arterial BP is low in the lower limbs. Because of increased left ventricular effort, the ventricle hypertrophies, and cardiac failure may result if the disease remains untreated.

b. Anesthetic management. The aspects of chief concern to the anesthesiologist include:

(1) Hypertension of the upper body, which may result in cerebral hemorrhage.

(2) Left ventricular stress or failure.

(3) Excessive intraoperative bleeding due to enlarged collateral vessels.

(4) Hypotension on completion of the anastomosis following clamp removal.

(5) Spinal cord injury and renal failure if hypotension is produced in the distal aorta by cross-clamping of the aorta.

2. Patent ductus arteriosus

a. General considerations

(1) The ductus arteriosus normally closes completely within the first 4 months of life. If closure does not occur, blood flows from the aorta to the pulmonary artery.

(2) Pulmonary arterial hypertension and biventricular hypertrophy will develop.

(3) Blood flow is reversed from the pulmonary artery to the aorta when severe pulmonary hypertension exceeding aortic pressure or other congenital abnormalities are present.

(4) The diastolic BP is low, and the blood volume passing down the aorta is small. Left ventricular failure occurs as a result of the large left-to-right shunt.

b. Anesthesia management. Patients with uncomplicated patent ductus arteriosus and mild pulmonary hypertension tolerate anesthesia well. Administration of anesthetics should be cautious once blood flow is from right to left (i.e., pulmonary artery to aorta) or in the presence of left ventricular failure. Peripheral vascular resistance should remain high to minimize the right-to-left shunting volume. Ligation of the ductus increases systemic or forward blood, with an increase in the diastolic BP due to a redistribution of blood volume away from the lungs.

3. Tetralogy of Fallot

a. General considerations. The anatomic lesion is characterized by biventricular origin of the aorta above a large ventricular septal defect, pulmonary valve stenosis, and right ventricular hypertrophy. Obstruction of the right ventricular outflow tract may be severe enough to elevate right ventricular pressures to systemic levels. A right-to-left shunt is usually, but not invariably, present. Its magnitude depends on the obstruction to pulmonary outflow and on the systemic vascular resistance. The principal problems to consider are:

(1) An increase in **pulmonary vascular resistance** will increase the magnitude of the right-to-left shunt.

(2) A decrease in **systemic vascular resistance** will increase the magnitude of the right-to-left shunt. Vasopressors (e.g., phenylephrine or metaraminol) should be used to restore systemic vascular resistance if necessary.

(3) **Metabolic acidosis** is often the result of an inadequate cardiac output.

b. **Anesthesia management.** Hypoxemia presents a serious problem to the anesthesiologist. The severity of arterial hypoxemia will depend on the magnitude of the right-to-left shunt, which may not be relieved with high oxygen concentration. Because of the diminished pulmonary blood flow, induction with inhalation anesthetic drugs is very slow.

(1) **The red cell volume (hematocrit)** is higher than normal. As a result, blood viscosity is elevated, and spontaneous thrombosis may occur, particularly in dehydrated patients. Careful volume replacement is mandatory to avoid dehydration.

(2) **Coagulation difficulties,** common in these patients, may lead to increased intraoperative and postoperative blood loss.

(3) **Bradycardia** may develop during manipulation of the heart.

(4) **In infants** up to 1 year of age, a palliative operation may be required, with creation of a side-to-side anastomosis either between the ascending aorta and the right pulmonary artery (Blalock procedure) or between the upper descending aorta and the left pulmonary artery (Pott's operation). Early complete repair is now performed due to improved experience. **Open intracardiac repair** of the tetralogy of Fallot usually is performed any time after 6 months of age. Intubation can be performed easily, preferably following increments of gallamine (2–4 mg/kg) and ventilation with 100% oxygen.

(5) **Older children** tolerate halothane. Nitrous oxide–oxygen induction with gallamine or pancuronium (to prevent bradycardia) can be administered for muscle relaxation. The same general rule calling for cautious administration is applicable here also.

4. **Transposition of the great vessels.** These are complex malformations. At one end of the spectrum are children with total separation of the pulmonary and systemic circulation. Survival beyond a few hours post partum is possible only with emergency palliative surgery. Problems (atrial, ventricular, or both) include metabolic acidosis, poor oxygenation, cardiac arrhythmias, and very slow uptake of gaseous anesthetic drugs.

5. **Atrial and ventricular septal defects.** In both conditions, an intracardiac communication exists that leads to an increased pulmonary blood flow because of left-to-right shunt. These patients are well oxygenated. Anesthesia presents no problem and is tolerated remarkably well. Pulmonary hypertension secondary to increased pulmonary vascular resistance may lead to reversal of the shunt (right-to-left). In this setting, corrective surgery carries a very high risk because of intractable right ventricular failure.

VII. Cardiopulmonary bypass

A. **Understanding the physiology** of cardiopulmonary bypass is essential in the management of the patient.

1. **Hypothermia** is employed frequently in adults and invariably in children (28°–30° C or 32°–34° C in adults; 20°–32° C in children).

2. **Minimal flow rates** generally employed for adults are 40–50 ml/kg/min at 32° C.

3. **In children** the flow delivered is on the order of 2.5 L/min/m^2.

4. **Arterial pressure and bypass flows** should be monitored and regulated as indicated to prevent damage of vital organs during this period.

   a. **In adults,** arterial perfusion pressure should be adequate to avoid organ damage caused by tissue underperfusion. The main concern is cerebral function. Mean pressures of 65–85 torr are generally adequate.

   b. **If arterial pressure exceeds 100 torr** at the calculated flow, peripheral vasoconstriction is usually present. Vasoconstriction causes metabolic acidosis and tissue underperfusion. A vasodilator (droperidol, nitroprusside, or phentolamine) can be used in these circumstances.

   c. **Low arterial pressure** may result from an inadequate blood flow and/or excessive vasodilatation. Increase of the perfusion flow often restores good perfusion pressure. If the low pressure persists despite a high pump flow, administration of a peripheral vasoconstrictor (phenylephrine) may be considered.

   d. **High pump flows** and vasoconstriction drugs may not succeed in maintaining an adequate arterial pressure if functional aortic regurgitation or a high pulmonary venous drainage (e.g., high bronchial blood flow in cyanotic children) is present.

   e. **A precipitous decrease in arterial and venous pressures,** an acute rise in resistance in the arterial perfusion line, and cessation of venous return to the pump are classic signs of retrograde aortic dissection, which may occur from retrograde femoral artery perfusion. Prompt discontinuance of retrograde perfusion bypass is essential. Aortic arch cannulation eliminates these hazards, although antegrade dissection has been known to occur.

5. **Central venous pressure monitoring** is essential to ensure adequate venous drainage.

6. **Arterial samples** for blood gases and serum electrolyte determination should be performed during bypass.

   a. **Mild metabolic acidosis** is almost always present with hypothermia. It probably requires no treatment.

   b. **Severe metabolic acidosis** due to tissue hypoxia should be treated by:

      (1) Increasing blood flow.

      (2) Administration of vasodilators.

      (3) Improving perfusion pressure, if low.

      (4) Administration of sodium bicarbonate; if the base excess persists and exceeds −7 despite the previous measures, then $NaHCO_3$ is indicated.

   c. **Arterial PO_2 may occasionally decrease** during extracorporeal bypass. This may be corrected by an increase in oxygen flow through the oxygenator or a reduction of muscle oxygen consumption with a nondepolarizing muscle relaxant.

   d. **Arterial PCO_2 is regulated** either by:

      (1) Adding carbon dioxide to the gas mixture if a bubble oxygenator is used.

      (2) Changing oxygen flow through the disc oxygenator.

7. **The lungs need not be ventilated** during extracorporeal bypass, but they may be inflated with oxygen at a static pressure of 10 cm H_2O. Intermittent deflation of the lung may be required when the pleura is open.

8. **The hematocrit** is maintained between 15–22%.
9. **Serum potassium and calcium** concentrations decrease during bypass, depending on the quality of the perfusate.
   a. **Potassium** is administered to avoid hypokalemia and cardiac arrhythmias in the immediate postbypass period.
   b. **$CaCl_2$** as a single injection (3 mg/kg) usually may be used during separation from bypass as indicated. There is no need for additional general anesthesia during bypass, particularly when hypothermia is used.
10. Slow administration of 15–21 mg of **tubocurarine** provides satisfactory muscle relaxation and prevents respiration movements.
11. **Urine output** provides an index of renal blood status and function. Absence of flow is not necessarily indicative of trouble. Temperature should be allowed to rise and stay at 37.5° C for awhile, before bypass discontinuance, to achieve better equilibrium between blood and tissue temperature.

B. Following **electrical defibrillation of the ventricles,** the heart should be allowed to beat for a few minutes before the pump perfusion is slowly discontinued.
   1. **Gradual separation from bypass** allows the heart to resume the entire circulatory burden slowly.
   2. **As soon as the heart starts to eject,** the patient should be ventilated with 100% oxygen and continued in this way for some time.
   3. **Right and left atrial pressures** should be maintained within "normal" levels while the patient is on bypass. However, higher atrial pressures may be required to achieve satisfactory arterial pressure following bypass.
   4. Again, the decision should be made **on an individual basis,** because ventricular filling pressure requirements may vary from one patient to another and with the cardiac lesion. In general, patients with left ventricular failure or mitral or aortic valve disease require higher left atrial pressure. On the other hand, if right ventricular failure is present, higher right atrial pressure is required.
   5. **Systolic arterial BP** above 95–100 torr is adequate in most cases.
   6. **Inotropic support** may be required to increase arterial pressure. The choice of drugs should be directed by hemodynamic conditions.
   7. **Heart rate or rhythm abnormalities** are often encountered during separation from bypass.
      a. **Atrial pacing** is used to increase heart rate as indicated.
      b. **Atrioventricular pacing** is employed if atrioventricular dissociation is present.
      c. **Lidocaine 100 mg** is administered before defibrillation on bypass, while an infusion of lidocaine 1–4 mg/min is given at a rate adjusted to prevent or treat premature ventricular contractions.
      d. **Cardioversion** of long-standing atrial fibrillation is generally unsuccessful and unrewarding. However, digitalization may be required to control a rapid ventricular rate.

Bibliography

Dhadphale, P. R., Jackson, A. P. F., and Alseri, S. Comparison of anesthesia with diazepam and ketamine vs. morphine in patients undergoing heart-valve replacement. *Anesthesiology* 51:200, 1979.

Estefanous, F. G., Tarazi, R. C., Buckley, S., et al. Arterial hypertension in immediate postoperative period after valve replacement. *Br. Heart J.* 40:718, 1978.

Gale, G. D., Teasdale, S. J., Sanders, D. E., et al. Pulmonary atelectasis and other respiratory complications after cardiopulmonary bypass and investigation of aetiological factors. *Can. Anaesth. Soc. J.* 26:15, 1979.

Heiner, M., Teasdale, S. J., David, T., et al. Aorto-coronary bypass in a patient with sickle cell trait. *Can. Anaesth. Soc. J.* 26:428, 1979.

Jackson, A. P. F., Dhadphale, P. R., Callaghan, M. L., et al. Hemodynamic studies during induction of anesthesia for open-heart surgery using diazepam and ketamine. *Br. J. Anaesth.* 50:375, 1978.

Lappas, D. G., Lowenstein, E., Waller, J., et al. Hemodynamic effects of sodium nitroprusside during coronary operation in man. *Circulation* 54 [Suppl. III] 4, 1976.

Lappas, D. G., Ohtaka, M., and Buckley, M. J. Systemic and pulmonary effects of nitroprusside during mitral valve replacement in patients with mitral regurgitation. *Circulation* 58:118, 1978.

Noback, C. R., and Tinker, J. H. Hypothermia after cardiopulmonary bypass in man. Amelioration by nitroprusside-induced vasodilation during rewarming. *Anesthesiology* 53:277, 1980.

Panday, S., Mandke, N. V., Parulkar, G. B., et al. Bloodless open heart surgery. *Indian Heart J.* 30:104, 1978.

Quintin, L., Whalley, D. G., Wynands, J. E., et al. Oxygen-high dose fentanyl-droperidol anesthesia for aortocoronary bypass surgery. *Anesth. Analg* (Cleve.) 60:412, 1981.

Slogoff, S., Keats, A. S., and Ott, E. Preoperative propranolol therapy and aortocoronary bypass operation. *J.A.M.A.* 240:1487, 1978.

Stephenson, L. W., Vaugh, H. M., and Edmunds, L. H. Surgery using cardiopulmonary bypass in the elderly. *Circulation* 58:250, 1978.

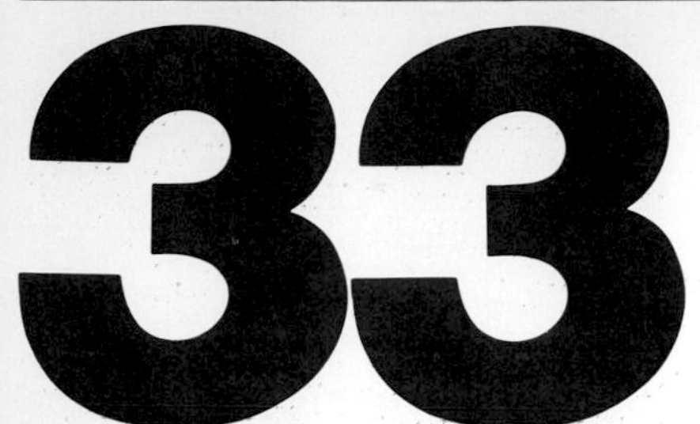

Anesthesia in Neurosurgery

I. **Principle.** To perform most effectively in administering anesthesia for neurologic surgery, the anesthesiologist must have, beyond technical proficiency, some background information about the patient's disease and about the neurologic procedure to be done—its rationale, major steps, and desired outcome.

II. **Approach to the patient with a brain lesion**

A. **Preoperative evaluation.** See Chapter 1.

1. **The preoperative evaluation includes** a physical examination and review of the history, laboratory findings, radiologic examinations, and consultants' reports.

2. **Study of the level of consciousness** and mental activity is important in determining the doses of drugs and the postoperative status.

B. **Factors in circulation**

1. **Changes in the pulse rate and BP** can be caused by damage to structures that lie in the floor of the third ventricle, in the hypothalamus, or in the floor of the fourth ventricle.

2. **Treatment of hypotension** due to surgical manipulation must include temporary cessation of the surgical procedure.

III. **Preoperative medication.** See Chapter 3.

A. **Light premedication**

1. **For the adult** who is conscious and alert: 10 mg of diazepam IM and 0.4 mg of atropine SQ, injected 1 hr before anesthesia.

2. **For children:** 2 mg/kg of pentobarbital IM and 0.1–0.4 mg of atropine SQ, injected 1 hr before anesthesia.

B. **Narcotics** are not recommended.

1. **Consideration of the use of narcotics** must be balanced with the knowledge that they increase intracranial pressure by decreasing the rate and depth of respiration, which increases the PCO_2, leading to a dilation of cerebral blood vessels and consequent reduction of reflex activity and level of consciousness in the postoperative period.

2. **The small, unreactive pupil** caused by the administration of opiates is a disadvantage in attempting to assess the patient.

IV. **Anesthesia management**

A. **Anesthetics and techniques**

1. **Thiopental** 2.5%, 4 mg/kg (200–300 mg in adults), is the dose, related directly to the level of consciousness; less thiopental is required for lower states of consciousness. **The patient in a coma** must first be oxygenated for 5 min with 100% oxygen.

2. **Succinylcholine,** 80–100 mg IV, is administered to an adult to facilitate a smooth, nontraumatic intubation. If an unusual position is to be used, it may be necessary to utilize an unkinkable endotracheal tube. It is extremely important to have the patient as relaxed as possible during intubation to avoid increased intracranial pressure due to bucking or straining.

3. **Succinylcholine drip 0.2% solution** (2 mg/ml), tubocurarine 0.2 mg/kg, or pancuronium 0.1 mg/kg is administered.

4. **Intracranial pressure** may increase to 200–400 mm H_2O even when the patient is completely relaxed, and it could be elevated to 800 mm H_2O during intubation if bucking or straining occurs.

5. **Hyperventilation** for 10 min is indicated before adding volatile agents, such as halothane or enflurane. Decreasing the PCO_2 first means that the intracranial pressure will tend to remain more constant.

6. **Oxygen lack and carbon dioxide retention** act directly to cause cerebral vascular engorgement and enlargement in the size of the brain substance. Hypoxia leads to an increase in capillary permeability and probably to an increase in the fluid content of brain cells. Therefore, for most operations, especially when deep anesthesia is not necessary, muscle paralysis and efficient controlled respiration are very desirable.

7. If the patient has **chronic pulmonary disease** with a PCO_2 of 60 torr, hyperventilation is indicated until the PCO_2 reaches 40 torr. If it is normally 40 torr, hyperventilation is indicated until it reaches 20 torr.

8. **If BP and pulse rate are normal,** maintenance of anesthesia is carried out with (a) 1% halothane, (b) 0.5% halothane with a 50% nitrous oxide and 50% oxygen mixture, or (c) 1% enflurane, or 1% isofluorane with a 50% nitrous oxide and 50% oxygen mixture. Volatile anesthetic agents should not be used to attain deeper anesthesia, since they lead to increased intracranial pressure. Rather, thiopental, fentanyl, or droperidol should be used. Low concentrations of halothane help to keep the intracranial pressure down.

9. **An adequate airway** is mandatory. Resistance to expiration leads to a rise in pressure in the cerebral veins and also in the vertebral plexus of veins. Further, increased intraabdominal pressure from the work of the abdominal muscles during forced expiration contributes to compression of the inferior vena cava.

B. Hypotensive techniques and induced hypothermia. See Chapter 19.

V. Fluids

A. Sodium. The distribution of fluids in the body depends on whether they contain sodium. The sodium governs the movement of the water. Fluids may be given on the basis of 15 ml/kg of body weight.

B. Do not use 5% D/W alone. This is potentially dangerous if it is given more quickly than water is lost. **Saline solutions** are preferable during intracranial surgery because sodium does not easily penetrate cells and is distributed, along with the administered water, equally throughout the extracellular fluid. The use of **5% dextrose in lactated Ringer's solution** or 5% dextrose in normal saline moves water out of the cells and CNS and produces shrinkage of the brain substance and decreased CNS pressure.

VI. Special techniques to reduce intracranial pressure

A. Intravenous infusion of hypertonic agents

1. **The value of hypertonic solutions** is primarily their effect of dehydrating normal brain tissue.

2. **Mannitol,** because it has a large molecular weight, is less likely to cause a secondary increase in intracranial pressure.

a. **The duration** of reduction of intracranial pressure and brain mass is longer with mannitol (4½ hr) than with urea (2½ hr).

b. **The amount** of decreased brain mass is greater with urea administered as 30% solution, 0.5–1.5 g per kilogram of body weight.

c. **Mannitol 20% solution** (with osmotic activity one-third that of urea) is given in doses of 1.5–4.5 g/kg. Starting with a large bolus, with the total dose given in 30–60 min and completed by the time the bone flap is turned, is recommended.

3. **The site of infusion** should be a large vein in the upper extremity, because there is the possibility of producing venous thrombosis with tissue necrosis at the site of infusion.

4. **An indwelling urinary catheter** should be used.

5. **Side effects**

a. Increased bleeding tendency.

b. Sludging and thrombosis.

c. Electrolyte disturbances.

d. Hemolysis.

6. **Contraindications.** The osmotic agents are relatively contraindicated in patients with impaired renal function, and they should be used with much caution in patients with decreased myocardial reserves.

B. **Cortisone therapy.** The main action of cortisone is to restore and preserve the blood-brain barrier in the presence of tumors and after injury or surgery. A breakdown in the integrity of the blood-brain barrier is perhaps the most important basic mechanism for the development of cerebral edema. Initial therapy is an IV dose of 50 mg of prednisolone, 40 mg of methylprednisolone, or 7.5 mg of dexamethasone. Maintenance doses of one-third to one-half the initial dose are given at 4–8 hr intervals for several days, with gradual reduction of the daily dose.

C. **Controlled hyperventilation** is a common practice and should not be considered a special technique. It helps relax brain tissue, which is conducive to hemostasis, and also allows better exposure of deep cerebral structures with less bleeding.

1. Controlled hyperventilation should be used with a ventilator.

2. **Potentially harmful effects**

a. Tetany.

b. Shift of the hemoglobin dissociation curve to the left (Bohr effect).

c. Cerebral vasoconstriction with possible cerebral hypoxia.

d. Decrease in cardiac output.

e. Increase in fixed acids.

f. Decrease in arterial oxygen tension.

VII. Positions for anesthesia and surgery

A. Sitting position

1. Air embolism is the greatest danger.

2. This position is used in operations on the cervical spine, posterior fossa, gasserian ganglion, and for ventriculography.

3. Venous drainage is improved, and better exposure is possible.

4. The legs should be wrapped in elastic bandages and placed at the level of the heart to facilitate venous return from the lower extremities.
5. The patient should be placed in the sitting position slowly, with frequent measurement of BP. Severe hypotension can develop.

B. Supine position

1. Most craniotomies are done with the patient in this position, with the head elevated 10 to 15 degrees for cerebral venous drainage.
2. Venous pooling in the lower extremities is minimized by correct wrapping of the legs with elastic bandages before the induction of anesthesia.
3. Venous drainage and respiration are not embarrassed when this position is used.

C. Lateral position

1. This position is used primarily for temporoparietal craniotomy.
2. Mean arterial pressure and systemic resistance may be decreased.
3. Little, if any, venous engorgement occurs.

D. Prone position

1. The prone position interferes with respiratory mechanics and predisposes the patient to atelectasis.
2. Marked venous congestion occurs frequently.
3. Obstruction of the inferior vena cava can cause a marked fall in BP and increased pressure in vertebral veins.

E. Improper positioning

1. Incorrect positioning may result in injury to peripheral nerves.
2. **Ocular complications** may be caused, such as retinal artery thrombosis from pressure over the eyeballs, especially in the presence of arterial hypotension. The use of eye ointment and closure of the eyelids before surgery usually prevents corneal injury.

VIII. Monitoring. See Chapter 6.

A. Central venous pressure must be monitored to determine proper fluid and blood replacement.

B. Arterial blood pressure

1. The indirect method includes a manometer, cuff, and stethoscope.
2. The direct method is called for under certain circumstances—in the very high-risk patient or when hypothermic or hypotensive techniques are utilized.

C. Electrocardiogram

1. **Intracranial surgical manipulation** may at any time produce sudden changes in cardiac rhythm or rate.
2. The most common disturbances, and those of greatest significance, occur in **posterior fossa surgery** and are due to pressure, distortion, or traction on the brainstem and cranial nerves. If this happens, the surgeon must be advised immediately and the source of the stimulus identified and removed.
3. Unless the **arrhythmia** is considered life-threatening, it should not be treated with antiarrhythmic drugs, since this will prevent subsequent detection of such untoward stimulation and increase the likelihood of unrecognized surgical trauma to vital brainstem centers.

4. **Sudden changes in cardiac rhythm or rate** may be associated with other neurologic procedures or complications, including:
   a. Orbital decompression.
   b. Carotid artery surgery.
   c. Sudden intracranial decompression.
   d. Trigeminal nerve surgery.
   e. Tonsillar herniation.
   f. Air embolism.
5. **Stimulation of the trigeminal nerve** is a common cause of ventricular arrhythmia and is frequently associated with hypertension. Most likely it represents a response to painful stimuli under light anesthesia rather than a true reflex arrhythmia.
6. **Further indications for electrocardiography** in neurosurgery include:
   a. Induced hypothermia for recognition of arrhythmias.
   b. Induced hypotension.
   c. Procedures associated with massive transfusions.
   d. Procedures for localization of right atrial catheters or ventriculoatrial shunts.

D. **Right atrial catheterization** is used for monitoring central venous oxygen levels and for aspiration of intracardiac air.

E. **Esophageal or precordial** stethoscope.

F. **The esophageal, rectal, or tympanic probes** for temperature monitoring are especially valuable in children; however, the temperature should be monitored in all neurosurgical patients. Severe hyperpyrexia is frequently due to thrombosis in the region of the brainstem or thalamus.

IX. The concept of "cerebral steal"

A. **Intracranial steal phenomenon** refers to a situation in which blood is drained from one area because of lowered cerebrovascular resistance in another. The term has been used to describe loss of blood flow from an area of ischemia to an area of relatively normal brain in which vascular resistance has been markedly decreased by carbon dioxide, anesthesia, or some other agent that impairs the autoregulation phenomenon.

B. **The mechanism** of the intracerebral steal phenomenon is as follows:

1. **Prior to the onset of the steal,** there is autoregulation of flow in the normal brain and a normal vascular resistance. The high resistance to flow in the normal areas of the brain increases the total resistance in the intracranial vessels, which in turn increases both the pressure in the intracranial vessels and, consequently, the perfusion pressure.
2. **The increased perfusion pressure** assists flow in the ischemic area. When the autoregulation phenomenon is lost or impaired in the normal brain, the decreased resistance in the vessels in the normal tissue decreases the perfusion pressure and permits a relative shift of flow from the ischemic area to the normal areas.

X. Postoperative care

A. Close observation of **ventilation and circulation** is mandatory. As soon as consciousness is regained and the systolic BP is over 100 torr, the patient is placed in a head-up position at an angle of 10 to 15 degrees, which will reduce the risk of cerebral edema and reactionary hemorrhage.

B. The vital signs are recorded every 15 min until the patient awakens; then every hour for 6 hr; then every 2 hr for the remainder of the operative day and night; then every 4 hr.

XI. Summary

Vital to optimal neurosurgical anesthesia are:

1. A good airway.
2. Adequate oxygenation.
3. Avoidance of coughing and straining.
4. Adequate removal of carbon dioxide.
5. Proper IV therapy.
6. Adequate cerebral perfusion.
7. Correct positioning of the patient and proper selection and use of anesthetics.

Bibliography

Chestnut, J. S., Albin, M. S., Gonzalez-Abola, E., et al. Clinical evaluation of intravenous nitroglycerin for neurosurgery. *J. Neurosurg* 48:704, 1978.

Dalrymple, D. G., MacGowan, S. W., and MacLeod, G. F. Cardiopulmonary effects of the sitting position in neurosurgery. *Br. J. Anaesth.* 51:1079, 1979.

Johnson, G. N., Palahniuk, R. J., Tweed, W. A., et al. Regional cerebral blood flow changes during severe fetal asphyxia produced by slow partial umbilical cord compression. *Am. J. Obstet. Gynecol.* 135:48, 1979.

Lassen, N. A., and Christensen, M. S. Physiology of cerebral blood flow. *Br. J. Anaesth.* 48:719, 1976.

Marsh, M. L., Marshall, L. F., and Shapiro, H. M. Neurosurgical intensive care. *Anesthesiology* 48:149, 1977.

Moss, E., Powell, D., Gibson, R. M., et al. Effects of tracheal intubation on intracranial pressure following induction of anesthesia with thiopentone or Althesin in patients undergoing neurosurgery. *Br. J. Anaesth.* 50:353, 1978.

Shapiro, H. M. Intracranial hypertension. Therapeutic and anesthetic considerations. *Anesthesiology* 43:445, 1975.

Vourc'h, G., and Tannieres, M. L. Cardiac arrhythmia induced by pneumoencephalography. *Br. J. Anaesth.* 50:833, 1978.

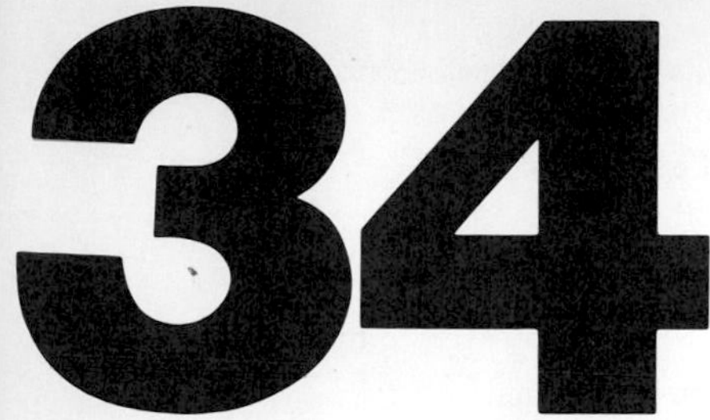

Anesthesia in Surgery for Endocrine Disorders

I. Thyroidectomy

A. General considerations. Generally, **euthyroid patients** tolerate anesthesia and surgery well. However, even in patients with normal thyroid function, **respiratory obstruction** may be present before or after surgery.

1. **Retrosternal goiter** may compress the trachea and cause respiratory obstruction. Careful examination of the chest x-ray may reveal the magnitude of the compression and deviation of the trachea. Endotracheal intubation and intraoperative ventilation may present a problem if the obstruction is severe. In the presence of **tracheal deviation,** intubation may be required in the awake patient under topical anesthesia.

2. **Reactive hemorrhage.** Postoperative hematoma at the site of the operation may require immediate evacuation to relieve pressure on the trachea.

3. **Recurrent laryngeal nerve injury.** Temporary damage from mechanical bruising of the nerve will heal within 2–4 weeks postoperatively. Permanent damage may occur from nerve dissection. **Unilateral injury** usually does not cause respiratory difficulties. **Bilateral damage requires tracheostomy.** Intubation or tracheostomy is indicated if respiratory obstruction occurs in a severely ill patient.

4. **Edema of the larynx** usually appears within 1–3 postoperative days and may require endotracheal intubation or tracheostomy if respiratory obstruction and stridor are apparent.

5. **Tracheal collapse** is a rare complication. If it appears, intubation or tracheostomy is indicated.

B. Special considerations

1. **Hyperthyroidism.** Severe circulatory and metabolic changes complicate the management of the thyrotoxic patient. Proper preoperative control of thyrotoxicosis is mandatory for safe anesthesia and operation. An uncontrolled thyrotoxic patient presents a serious problem that may evolve into a **thyroid storm.**

   a. **Manifestations** of the disease

      (1) **Changes in heart rhythm and rate.** Tachycardia, atrial fibrillation, and ventricular irritability.

      (2) **Hyperdynamic circulation.** High cardiac output state, cardiac enlargement or hypertrophy, moderately elevated systolic BP, and congestive heart failure.

      (3) **Metabolic changes.** Increased temperature and metabolic rate with increased oxygen consumption, weight loss, vomiting, and diarrhea.

      (4) **Tremor,** anxiety, and nervousness.

      (5) **Exophthalmos.**

(6) General **enlargement of the gland,** occasionally associated with respiratory obstruction and distress.

b. Measures required for **control of thyrotoxicosis**

(1) **Bed rest.**

(2) **Antithyroid drugs,** such as:

(a) Methimazole (Tapazole), 10–15 mg every 6 hr.

(b) Propylthiouracil or methylthiouracil.

(c) Iodine, as Lugol's solution (an aqueous solution of 5% iodine in 10% potassium iodide).

(3) **Digitalization,** diuretic therapy, and sodium restriction are indicated for treatment of congestive heart failure and atrial fibrillation. Drug requirements are greater in hyperthyroid than in euthyroid patients.

(4) Use of **reserpine** to reduce the cardiovascular hyperdynamic state.

(5) **Adequate preoperative sedation.** Sedatives, such as phenobarbital (30–60 mg every 6 hr), may be started several days before the expected time of surgery to control excitability and anxiety. Phenothiazine drugs and other sedatives also may be used preoperatively.

(6) **Propranolol.** In patients with severe tachycardia, resulting in congestive heart failure, with resistance to digitalis, administration of propranolol, 10–20 mg PO every 8 hr may be indicated.

c. **Anesthetic management**

(1) **Preanesthetic medication.** Sedation must be begun the day before the operation (e.g., phenobarbital, 30–60 mg every 6 hr). For preanesthetic medication, a combination barbiturate and narcotic has proved satisfactory. Full doses may be required in nervous and excitable patients to produce adequate sedation. Atropine should not be administered if tachycardia is present.

(2) **Preparation for anesthesia.** The following are essential: ECG and direct arterial BP monitoring; cart with drugs needed for cardiac resuscitation and a defibrillator; insertion of a central and a peripheral venous line; and monitoring of temperature during surgery.

(3) **Conduct of anesthesia.** Careful administration of adequate anesthesia to minimize sympathetic responses is mandatory under continuous monitoring, particularly in patients with severe heart failure.

(a) **Endotracheal intubation** is recommended for patients undergoing thyroidectomy, and it is essential if (1) the trachea is compressed or deviated, (2) respiratory obstruction is present or anticipated, (3) the goiter is retrosternal, (4) malignancy is suspected, or (5) in complicated cases. In general, endotracheal intubation is performed under anesthesia; however, if there is severe respiratory obstruction because of tracheal deviation or obstruction, intubation should be performed under topical laryngeal anesthesia. A smaller endotracheal tube than that used for patients with normal tracheas should be used for intubation.

(b) **Choice of anesthetic.** Induction of anesthesia can be performed with thiopental 150–250 mg and subsequent inhalation of nitrous oxide and oxygen. An inhalation agent also can be used during induction to supplement nitrous oxide–oxygen. Intubation of the trachea is facilitated with succinylcholine 100 mg (preceded by pancuronium, 1 mg IV), following spraying of the glottis and trachea with 4% lidocaine. Heart rate and BP may increase during intubation and following the skin incision. **Maintenance of anesthesia** can be achieved with nitrous oxide–oxygen supplemented with an inhalation agent (0.5–1% halothane, 1–2% enflurane). Ventilation is initially controlled and then assisted throughout the operation. Controlled respiration throughout the procedure with a nondepolarizing muscle relaxant, to avoid the use of an inhalation agent, is possible.

(c) The following points should be noted: (1) Hyperextension of the head should be avoided, because it may cause occipital headache postoperatively. (2) The eyes should be carefully protected during the operation. (3) Vigorous coughing immediately following the operation should be avoided because it may enhance reactive hemorrhage. (4) The vocal cords should be observed carefully at the time of extubation to assess the integrity of the recurrent laryngeal nerves.

d. Postoperative care. The patient should be observed carefully in the immediate postoperative period for thyroid crisis or early respiratory obstruction.

(1) The patient should remain in a Fowler's (semisitting) position.

(2) Sedation is essential, and administration of morphine may be indicated for pain.

(3) The patient should be kept moderately cool.

(4) Respiratory obstruction requires urgent treatment (intubation if necessary). Arterial blood gases should be determined.

(5) Thyroid crisis is now a rare postoperative complication that usually manifests itself within 24 hr postoperatively. Predominant signs of a crisis are:

(a) Rapid pulse rate and atrial fibrillation.

(b) Restlessness, delirium, and prostration.

(c) Pyrexia, sweating, vomiting, and dehydration.

(d) Hypertension followed by hypotension.

(e) Cardiac failure.

(6) Therapy of thyroid crisis consists of the following:

(a) Sedation with full doses of narcotics, barbiturates, or other sedative drugs to minimize restlessness and excitability.

(b) Sodium iodide 2–3 g IV and propylthiouracil 200 mg every 4–6 hr to prevent further synthesis of thyroid hormone.

(c) Digitalization if cardiac failure is present.

(d) Corticosteroids (hydrocortisone, 300 mg/day).

(e) Reduction of body temperature.

(f) Adequate hydration.

(g) Ventilation with added inspired oxygen.

(h) Propranolol, 0.25–0.5 mg IV, in repeated increments to treat tachycardia.

(7) Hypocalcemic tetany may occur if the parathyroids are injured or removed.

II. Parathyroidectomy

A. General considerations. Parathyroidectomy is performed for hyperparathyroidism that results from **adenoma of the gland.** Blood levels of the parathyroid hormone are elevated in this condition. **Hyperparathyroidism is characterized by:**

1. Hypercalcemia due to excessive bone resorption and enhanced gastrointestinal absorption of calcium.
2. Hypercalciuria leading to recurrent kidney stone formation and ultimate kidney damage.
3. Hypertension, in 50% of patients, that is related to the degree of renal function impairment.
4. Congestive heart failure.
5. ECG abnormalities, namely, prolonged P–R interval and short Q–T interval.
6. Hypovolemia as a result of vomiting, polyuria, and anorexia.
7. Hypercalcemic crisis leading to lethargy, confusion, and coma.

B. Anesthetic management

1. **Preanesthetic medication.** Small doses of barbiturates or narcotics can be used for premedication. Anticholinergic agents, such as scopolamine or atropine, are also used in average doses. The patient should remain in bed following premedication, because the presence of hypovolemia may predispose to orthostatic hypotension.
2. **Choice of anesthetic**
   - a. There is no apparent indication for a particular anesthetic agent. However, a nonflammable anesthetic is indicated if cautery will be used.
   - b. Although there has been no evidence of prolonged apnea following administration of muscle relaxants in these patients, their use requires care. Gallamine should be avoided if renal function is impaired.
   - c. **Endotracheal intubation** is essential to provide a patent airway during an operation.
   - d. **The head-up position** is used to provide a blood-free operating field. Air embolization is always a possibility, and appropriate monitoring should be included.
   - e. Hypovolemia, if present, may accentuate the hypotensive effect of anesthesia. Volume loss should be promptly replaced. Hypotension and bradycardia also may occur during intraoperative manipulation near the carotid sinus. Atropine and a vasopressor drug may be required.
   - f. **Pneumothorax** may develop during exploration of the mediastinum for adenoma of the gland.

III. Pheochromocytoma

A. General considerations. Pheochromocytoma is a tumor arising from chromaffin cells of the sympathoadrenal system. The tumor originates mostly from the adrenal medulla, but it may occur from chromaffin tissue in the paravertebral space, the aortic bifurcation, and the celiac plexus.

1. The tumor causes excessive secretion of **epinephrine** and **norepinephrine.**
2. **Severe hypertension,** paroxysmal or continuous, is the cardinal sign of pheochromocytoma.

3. Pounding headaches, sweating, palpitations, apprehension, flushing or pallor of the face, precordial pain, and paresthesia in the extremities are additional signs and symptoms of the disease.

4. **Ventricular arrhythmias** are common (multifocal, bigeminy, and ventricular fibrillation).

B. **Preoperative management.** Successful anesthetic and surgical management of patients with pheochromocytoma is dependent on preoperative evaluation and preparation.

1. **Alpha-blocking drugs** are used to control hypertension and restore BP toward normal levels.

   a. Phenoxybenzamine (Dibenzyline) is administered 20–80 mg PO daily for 5–8 days before the operation.

   b. Phentolamine (Regitine) is also used (10–100 mg PO every 4 hr) for 3–8 days preoperatively.

2. **Beta-blocking drugs.** Propranolol, 10–30 mg PO every 4–6 hr, may be added to control ventricular arrhythmias.

3. **Sedatives.** Adequate preoperative sedation is important.

4. **Hypovolemia** is usually present and results from a persistent preoperative elevation of BP and vasoconstriction. Preoperative treatment for a week with alpha-blocking drugs will help restore the BP, alleviate vasoconstriction, and restore blood volume toward normal.

C. **Anesthetic management**

1. **Premedication.** Atropine is generally omitted from the premedication regimen. Narcotics sometimes are used. Droperidol, 0.1–0.2 mg/kg IM, can provide adequate sedation.

2. **Continuous monitoring** of intraarterial pressure and the ECG should be established before induction of anesthesia. Central venous pressure monitoring also is desirable. A defibrillator should be immediately available.

3. **A peripheral venous line** is essential for volume transfusion, while a long central venous line should be used for intraoperative drug administration.

4. **Drugs** such as propranolol, phentolamine, atropine, vasopressors, hydrocortisone, calcium chloride, and lidocaine should be at hand.

5. **Choice of anesthetic.** Several anesthetic combinations have been used successfully. An essential prerequisite is smooth induction and maintenance of anesthesia and avoidance of straining, hypoxia, or carbon dioxide retention.

   a. **Induction of anesthesia** with **thiopental** is common. Careful administration to prevent hypotension is essential.

   b. **Nitrous oxide** is added to the inspired oxygen to supplement thiopental during induction of anesthesia.

   c. **Endotracheal intubation** is performed following IV administration of 1.5 mg/kg of succinylcholine IV.

   d. **Tubocurarine** is used to provide muscle relaxation during surgery. Gallamine may cause tachycardia and perhaps arrhythmia. On the other hand, pancuronium has been used satisfactorily for muscle relaxation.

   e. **A nonflammable inhalation agent** is often added to nitrous oxide–oxygen. Halothane tends to potentiate ventricular arrhythmias. Methoxyflurane is often preferred because it does not enhance ventricular arrhythmias. Fluroxene (Fluoromar) also has been used with success. Enflurane is the inhalation agent of choice.

f. **Neuroleptanalgesia** with fentanyl–droperidol (Innovar), supplemented with nitrous oxide, has been advocated by some anesthesiologists. However, this combination is thought to enhance epinephrine secretion.

D. Intraoperative problems

1. **Hypertension.** A marked and dangerous elevation in arterial BP may occur during induction of anesthesia, tracheal intubation, positioning of the patient on the operating table, surgical incision, and manipulation of the tumor. Hypertension can be controlled during anesthesia and operation with:

   a. **Phentolamine,** which has a shorter duration than phenoxybenzamine:

      (1) An IV infusion beginning at 2 micrograms/kg/min may control the hypertension.

      (2) Tachycardia is common following phentolamine administration.

      (3) The drug should be discontinued 30–40 min before the tumor is excised, to prevent accentuation of the hypotension that follows tumor removal.

   b. **Nitroprusside** (Nipride). Nitroprusside infusion in concentrations of 40 micrograms/ml effectively controls intraoperative hypertension. This drug has the advantages of rapid onset and short duration of action. Tachycardia usually does not follow nitroprusside use. Hypotension that occurs during nitroprusside administration can be controlled easily by reducing the rate of infusion and volume transfusion. If hypotension persists, the infusion should be stopped. The BP returns to normal levels a few minutes following discontinuation of the drug.

2. **Hypotension**

   a. Ligation of venous drainage of the tumor and tumor resection cause a rapid fall of catecholamine concentration in the blood. Hypotension can be treated with:

      (1) Vasoconstrictor drugs, such as phenylephrine or metaraminol infusion, regulated to restore BP toward normal.

      (2) Expansion of intravascular volume with blood, plasma, albumin, or crystalloid solutions.

      (3) Calcium chloride, 3 mg/kg IV, also has been used.

   b. Deep anesthesia may depress the cardiovascular system.

   c. Hemorrhage and hypovolemia may occur intraoperatively. Volume loss and blood loss should be promptly replaced.

   d. Hypotension may occur from overdosage of any drug used to control hypotension.

3. **Heart rate and rhythm abnormalities.** Continuous ECG monitoring is essential to detect and treat cardiac arrhythmias. Tachycardia and ventricular arrhythmias are frequent during anesthesia and surgery.

   a. **Propranolol** has been used successfully in doses of 0.25–0.5 mg IV to a total of 1–5 mg during operation. Relative contraindications to the use of propranolol are cardiac failure and bronchial asthma.

   b. **Lidocaine,** 50–100 mg IV as a bolus, followed by a lidocaine infusion (1 g in 250 ml of 5% D/W), 1–4 mg/min, also may be used to control ventricular arrhythmia.

E. Postoperative course. Continuous monitoring of the BP and ECG should be carried out in the immediate postoperative period. Intravascular volume expansion should be performed carefully to avoid overload, and hypotension should be treated with volume replacement and vasopressor drugs. Arterial blood gases and serum electrolyte determination are mandatory. If adrenalectomy also was performed, prophylactic administration of hydrocortisone is indicated.

IV. **Adrenalectomy** is performed for adrenocortical tumors, metastatic breast carcinomas, and other diseases. These clinical entities share common problems and complications that resection of the adrenal glands causes. However, the pathogenesis of these diseases differ.

A. **Primary aldosteronism**

1. **General considerations.** Primary aldosteronism usually is due to an adrenal adenoma but occasionally is associated with adrenal hyperplasia. Clinical and chemical abnormalities result from aldosterone hypersecretion. **Aldosterone promotes conservation of sodium and excretion of potassium by the kidneys.**

a. Excessive excretion of potassium results in potassium depletion, leading to:

(1) Hypokalemic alkalosis.

(2) Muscle weakness, areflexia, paresthesia, and tetany.

(3) ECG abnormalities, namely, S–T segment depression, flattening of the T wave, appearance of U waves, and atrial and ventricular arrhythmias.

(4) Kaliopenic nephropathy with progressive impairment of renal function.

b. Excessive conservation of sodium and extracellular volume expansion.

c. Malignant hypertension. These hypertensive cardiovascular complications may develop:

(1) Cardiac hypertrophy.

(2) Congestive heart failure.

(3) Strokes.

(4) Retinopathy.

(5) Renal function impairment.

2. **Preoperative preparation.** Correction of hypertension and hypokalemia is essential to reduce intraoperative and postoperative complications.

a. Spironolactone (Aldactone) has been used preoperatively to replenish the body stores of potassium and control hypertension.

b. Sodium restriction and oral administration of potassium chloride, 2–6 g/day, may be used in the immediate preoperative period to replenish serum potassium.

c. Diuretics and digitalis may be indicated to control cardiac failure.

3. **Anesthetic management**

a. **Premedication.** Barbiturates and narcotics have been administered satisfactorily as preanesthetic medication. An anticholinergic drug can be added to the premedication regimen.

b. **Choice of anesthetic**

(1) BP and ECG are monitored continuously (electrolytes and arterial blood gases also are determined).

(2) Cardiac resuscitation drugs and a defibrillator should be immediately available.

(3) Thiopental and succinylcholine can be used for induction of anesthesia and intubation.

(4) Nitrous oxide–oxygen with an inhalation anesthetic or narcotic are administered in a semiclosed system for maintenance of anesthesia.

(5) A nondepolarizing muscle relaxant can be used without difficulty.

c. **Intraoperative complications**

(1) Hypertension may occur during induction and surgical manipulation of the tumor. A vasodilator drug is indicated.

(2) Hypotension responds promptly to volume replacement administration. Vasopressors are rarely required.

4. **Postoperative care.** Serum electrolytes rapidly return to normal after the tumor resection. Therapy with corticosteroids will be necessary if a total adrenalectomy is performed.

B. **Cushing's syndrome**

1. **General considerations.** Cushing's syndrome (hyperadrenocorticism) is caused by a disorder in the regulation of cortisol (hydrocortisone) or ACTH secretion. Cortisol excess may be caused by hyperplasia of the adrenal cortex, adrenal adenoma, or carcinoma. ACTH excess may be the result of an ectopic malignancy. **Abnormally high levels of cortisol** will result in:

a. Hypertension.

b. Retention of sodium and water.

c. Enhanced potassium excretion, resulting in severe hypokalemia.

d. Impaired glucose tolerance.

e. Attenuated reaction to injury and infection.

f. Metabolic changes.

g. Osteoporosis.

h. Pleural effusion.

i. Psychological abnormalities.

2. **Preoperative management**

a. Dietary sodium restriction and potassium chloride administration are necessary to replenish body potassium.

b. Hypertension or congestive heart failure should be treated with cardiac glycosides, diuretics, and antihypertensive medication as indicated.

c. If diabetes is present, it should be controlled with insulin.

d. Hydrocortisone can be used if indicated.

3. **Anesthesia management**

a. **Preanesthetic visit and medication.** Because psychological abnormalities and personality changes may be present, it is important to approach these patients with optimism and understanding. Sedation may be required to control aberrant behavior. Morphine, a short-acting barbiturate, and an anticholinergic drug can be combined for premedication.

b. **Choice of anesthetic.** Most anesthetic agents cause an increase in secretion of cortisol. **Thiopental** is the exception; it attenuates the rise in plasma cortisol that follows the administration of inhalation anesthetics. Halothane, enflurane, and methoxyflurane cause an increase in plasma cortisol concentrations.

4. **Intraoperative management**
   a. **Diabetes.** Preoperative control of diabetes is essential. Insulin should be given on the morning of surgery. IV glucose should be administered intraoperatively and continued in the postoperative period. Blood and urine sugar levels should be determined during and after the operation.
   b. **Hypokalemia** must be corrected with potassium chloride infusion as indicated.
   c. Hypertension should be treated.
   d. Pleural effusions should be aspirated.
5. **Postoperative care.** Following adrenalectomy, the cortisol level may drop sharply. Substitution therapy with glucocorticosteroids is indicated. Potassium should be given as needed to restore serum potassium levels.

Bibliography

Brock, L. Hypovolemia and pheochromocytoma. *Ann. R. Coll. Surg. Engl.* 56:218, 1975.

Dagget, P., Verner, I., and Carruthers, M. Intraoperative management of pheochromocytoma with sodium nitroprusside. *Br. Med. J.* 2:311, 1978.

Desmonts, J. M., LeHouelleur, J., Remond, P., et al. Anesthetic management of patients with pheochromocytoma. A review of 102 cases. *Br. J. Anaesth.* 49:991, 1977.

Janeczko, G. G., Ivankovich, A. D., et al. Enflurane anesthesia for surgical removal of pheochromocytoma. *Anesth. Analg.* (Cleve.) 56:62, 1977.

Kopriva, C. J., and Eltringham, R. The use of enflurane during resection of pheochromocytoma. *Anesthesiology* 41:399, 1974.

Kruel, J. F., Dachot, P. J., and Anton, A. H. Hemodynamic and catecholamine studies during pheochromocytoma resection under enflurane anesthesia. *Anesthesiology* 44:265, 1976.

Mackin, J. F., Canary, J. J., and Pittman, C. S. Thyroid storm and its management. *N. Engl. J. Med.* 291:1396, 1974.

Ortiz, F. T., and Diaz, P. M. Use of enflurane for pheochromocytoma removal. *Anesthesiology* 42:495, 1975.

Oyama, T., Taniguchi, K., Ishihara, H., et al. Effects of enflurane anesthesia and surgery on endocrine function in man. *Br. J. Anaesth.* 51:141, 1979.

Pratilas, V., and Pratila, M. G. Anesthetic management of pheochromocytoma. *Can. Anaesth. Soc. J.* 26:253, 1979.

Stehling, L. C. Anesthetic management of the patient with hyperthyroidism. *Anesthesiology* 41:585, 1974.

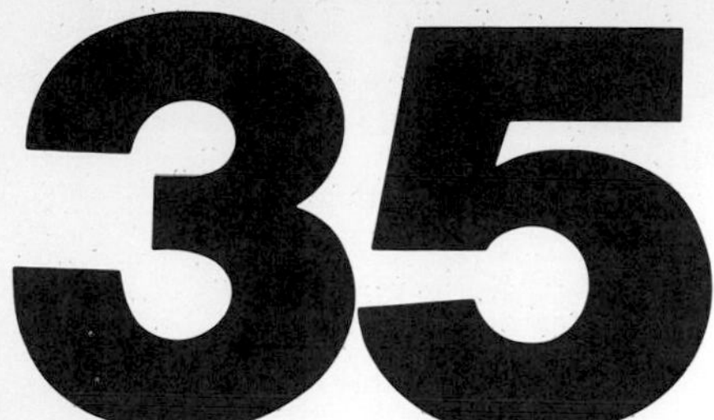

35 Anesthesia and Analgesia in Obstetrics and Gynecology

I. Anesthesia and analgesia in obstetrics

A. Obstetric anesthesia and analgesia are different from surgical anesthesia in the following ways:

1. **The mother may enter the hospital** at any time of the day or night and from minutes to hours before delivery.
2. **There are two persons** to consider, the mother and the unborn baby. The condition of both should be monitored carefully.
3. **Physiologic changes** occurring in the pregnant patient during the last 3 months are:
   - a. Increased cardiac output.
   - b. Increased blood volume.
   - c. Increased oxygen consumption.
   - d. Decreased vital capacity and pulmonary resistance.
   - e. Decreased liver function.
   - f. Decreased glomerular filtration and renal plasma flow.
   - g. Decreased serum cholinesterase activity.
   - h. Possible development of **supine hypotensive syndrome;** this is a function of decreased venous return through the large abdominal vessels, caused by compression of the enlarged uterus.
4. **There is an increased risk of emesis,** regurgitation, and aspiration at all times.
5. **Analgesia** is often required for a period of hours.
6. **All drugs** used for the relief of apprehension and pain during labor and delivery **cross the placenta** and affect the baby, who is markedly susceptible to the depressant effects of drugs used in labor. **Nitrous oxide with 50% oxygen** produces analgesia with minimal effects on the fetus. **The skeletal muscle relaxant** drugs do not cross the placenta and therefore do not affect the infant (with the exception of gallamine, which crosses the placenta).

B. Analgesia during labor

1. **Labor** is divided into three stages. **The first stage** is from the onset of labor until full cervical dilation. **The second stage** lasts from full dilation to delivery. **The third stage** lasts from the time of delivery of the fetus until the placenta has been delivered.
2. **Natural childbirth.** The prenatal education and instructions that compose this approach to labor and delivery are intended to alleviate fear and apprehension, so that the mother can relax properly during labor. However, if labor is prolonged and the mother seems exhausted, sedation or regional anesthesia may be indicated.

3. **Medical hypnosis** is a technique that can be used to alleviate anxiety and produce physical and mental relaxation. **Disadvantages** include (a) the prolonged period necessary to establish rapport between the therapist and the patient, (b) the need for the hypnotist to be present during childbirth, and (c) the problems that may arise if cesarean section or major manipulations become necessary.

4. **Acupuncture** presently is under investigation, but it is not yet accepted as a standard practice.

5. **Drugs**

   a. **Barbiturates** depress respiration in the infant, and are contraindicated in labor.

   b. **Tranquilizers** are administered IV and/or IM to treat apprehension early in labor: promazine 25–50 mg, promethazine 25–50 mg, propiomazine 10–20 mg, and hydroxyzine 25–50 mg. These drugs should be administered carefully when combined with narcotics or sedatives, because they cause ventilatory and cardiovascular depression in the mother and in the baby.

   c. **Narcotics** are helpful for pain relief at the end of the first stage of labor and during the second stage. IM or IV injections of narcotics are used. For IM injection, meperidine 50 mg or alphaprodine 20 mg may be administered. These drugs cross the placenta and may cause respiratory depression in the newborn. If this occurs, a narcotic antagonist, e.g., naloxone, is administered via the umbilical vein.

   d. **Inhalation analgesia** can be administered for pain relief at the end of the first stage of labor and during the second stage. Low concentrations of anesthetics, either alone or in conjunction with local or pudendal nerve block, are used. Properly administered, this procedure provides pain relief without abolishing laryngeal reflexes or decreasing the ability of the parturient patient to bear down during the second stage of labor. There is no neonatal depression, but there is a risk of aspiration of vomitus. **Late in the second stage of labor** and during delivery, 50% nitrous oxide–oxygen mixture is very useful, particularly in combination with pudendal nerve block.

C. Selection of anesthesia

1. **Regional anesthesia** is generally superior to general anesthesia. Local infiltration of the episiotomy field, transvaginal pudendal nerve block, paracervical block, low spinal anesthesia, continuous lumbar epidural anesthesia, and continuous caudal anesthesia are all satisfactory, acceptable methods.

2. **When regional anesthesia is contraindicated,** or when general anesthesia must be used due to imminent delivery, nitrous oxide with a minimum of 33% oxygen is very useful. Also suitable is 50% nitrous oxide–oxygen mixture preceded by thiopental.

3. **When general anesthesia is indicated,** succinylcholine can be administered for tracheal intubation.

   a. **The lighter and shorter** the general anesthesia, the less quantity of anesthetic there will be to reach and depress the newborn.

   b. **For cesarean section,** anesthesia with thiopental, succinylcholine, a 50% nitrous oxide–oxygen mixture, and tracheal intubation is safe and effective.

II. Regional anesthesia in obstetrics

A. Anatomy and physiology

1. **During the first stage of labor,** pain is due to dilation of the cervix and lower uterine segment and, to a lesser degree, to the contractions of the uterus. **The pain impulses** travel through sensory nerves that accompany the sympathetic chain. The pain from the uterus travels via the uterine plexus, pelvic ganglia and plexus, hypogastric nerve, superior hypogastric plexus, and lumbar and lower thoracic sympathetic chain and enters the spinal cord through the posterior roots of spinal nerves T_{10} and T_{12}. Thus continuous epidural, caudal, or paracervical block can relieve the pain of the first stage of labor when properly applied to include T_{10} and L_1 segments.
2. **During the second stage of labor,** the expulsive stage, the pain impulses are due to uterine contractions and stretching of the lower part of the birth canal by the presenting part. The impulses travel via the pudendal nerve and enter the spinal cord through the $S_{3\text{-}4\text{-}5}$ nerves. Thus pudendal nerve block, low spinal block, or caudal block directed only at $S_{3\text{-}4\text{-}5}$ segments will relieve the pain of the second stage of labor.
3. **Only continuous spinal,** continuous epidural, or continuous caudal block that reaches segments T_{10} through S_5 will relieve the pain of both the first and second stages of labor.

B. Paracervical block

1. **Indication.** Relief of pain during the first stage of labor.
2. **Anatomy.** The paracervical block anesthetizes the pain pathways at the pelvic (inferior hypogastric) ganglia and plexus, located on both sides of the cervix at a depth of 1–1.5 cm and under the vaginal mucosa of the lateral fornices.
3. Paracervical block **anesthetizes sensory nerves** from the fundus and cervix but does not affect the areas innervated by the pudendal nerve (vagina and perineum).
4. **Technique**
   a. The woman in labor lies supine with her legs in the **lithotomy position.**
   b. **A guide** is used to allow the 20-gauge, 15-cm needle to protrude no more than 1–1.5 cm. The injection is made by the obstetrician into the paracervical tissues at the 4 and 8 o'clock positions.
   c. **Following a careful aspiration of blood,** 5–10 ml of 1% lidocaine or 1% mepivacaine is injected into each side, 200 mg is the total maximal dose. Epinephrine is contraindicated. The needle is repositioned if blood is aspirated.
5. **Complications**
   a. Intravascular injection.
   b. **Fetal bradycardia** (incidence ranging up to 30%) and even fetal death may be caused by excessive amounts of injected local anesthetic solution, direct injection into the uterine artery, or injection into the myometrium.
   c. Injection into the fetal head.

C. Pudendal nerve block (usually done by the obstetrician).

1. **Indication.** For anesthesia of the vagina and perineum during delivery.
2. **Anatomy.** The pudendal nerve derives from the $S_{3\text{-}4\text{-}5}$ nerves. It leaves the pelvis through the lower part of the greater sciatic foramen, passes behind

the spine of the ischium, and reenters the pelvis through the lesser sciatic foramen.

3. **Technique.** Next to local infiltration, pudendal nerve block is the simplest method of regional anesthesia for vaginal delivery. The block is performed through the transvaginal or transperineal approach and is usually carried out by the obstetrician. **The transvaginal approach** is the simplest and most effective. The block, done on each side, anesthetizes the posterior area of the perineum.

   a. **The ischial spine** is located, and the sacrospinal ligament is palpated. A 20-gauge spinal needle is inserted through this ligament 1 cm posterior and medial to the spine and to a depth of 1 cm.

   b. **Following aspiration,** 5–10 ml of 1% lidocaine or 1% mepivacaine is injected on each side.

4. **Complications**

   a. Intravascular injections.

   b. Puncture of the maternal rectum.

D. **Continuous lumbar epidural anesthesia.** See Chapter 16, section **I.**

1. **Indication.** Total relief of pain during the first and second stages of labor and delivery or during cesarean section.

2. **Contraindications**

   a. Refusal by the patient.

   b. Infection at the site of injection.

   c. Uterine bleeding.

   d. Anticoagulant therapy.

   e. Extreme obesity.

   f. Hypovolemia, shock, or severe anemia.

   g. Preexisting spinal cord disease or back pain.

3. **Advantages of the lumbar epidural over the caudal route**

   a. **Reduction** of the anesthetic drug dosage by 50%. With the lumbar epidural approach, the hazards of toxicity and overdosage to the mother and baby are decreased.

   b. **Due to anomalies,** with the caudal approach, 20% of attempts to accomplish an adequate block fail.

   c. Rarely, puncture of the maternal rectum or **injection into the fetal presenting parts** has occurred with attempted caudal block.

   d. There is **decreased risk of infection** to the mother with lumbar epidural as compared with caudal block.

4. **Pelvic congestion increases** as pregnancy progresses. The veins in the peridural space become enlarged, resulting in **decreased epidural space.** Thus the average dose that would be administered to the nonparturient patient must be reduced for lumbar epidural, caudal, or spinal anesthesia performed in the obstetric patient.

5. **Technique**

   a. **Lumbar epidural anesthesia** is accomplished with the patient in the left lateral position. A plastic catheter is inserted into the epidural space at the level of the $L_{3\text{-}4}$ or $L_{4\text{-}5}$ vertebral interspace through an 18-gauge epidural needle, followed by injection of a 2-ml test dose of the local anesthetic solution.

b. **Following aspiration** and ruling out subarachnoid puncture, an additional 10–12 ml is injected through the catheter into the epidural space.

c. **The anesthetic solution** used is 1–1.5% lidocaine with epinephrine 1:200,000, 1% mepivacaine, or 0.25–0.5% bupivacaine.

6. **During uterine contractions,** the pressure within the spinal canal is elevated. For this reason, no injections are made during uterine contractions.

7. **Complications**

a. Hypotension (supine hypotensive syndrome).

b. **High epidural anesthesia** may be caused by extensive spread of the anesthetic solution into the epidural space or by accidental administration of a large amount of anesthetic solution into the subarachnoid space, resulting in total spinal anesthesia.

c. **Total spinal anesthesia** may occur. If anesthesia is established above the C_4 dermatome, the patient stops breathing. **Treatment** includes immediate ventilation with oxygen, insertion of an endotracheal tube, turning the patient on her left side, vasoconstrictors, and rapid IV administration of fluids. **Total spinal anesthesia is a life-threatening emergency.**

E. **Continuous caudal anesthesia.** See Chapter 16, section **II.**

1. **Indications and contraindications** are similar to those of continuous lumbar epidural anesthesia (see sec. **II.D**). The caudal approach of epidural anesthesia is preferable for analgesia when delivery is imminent.

2. **The sacral hiatus** is close to the anus and therefore is much more vulnerable to contamination than is the lumbar area.

3. **The probability** of puncture of the dura, postlumbar puncture headache, and total spinal anesthesia is much lower than with lumbar epidural anesthesia.

4. **The dose** of anesthetic solution should be smaller than the dose for the nonpregnant woman. Administration of 12–18 ml of anesthetic solution is adequate.

5. **Technique**

a. **When the pelvis,** fetus, and presentation are normal and labor is well established, a plastic catheter is inserted through an 18-gauge epidural needle into the epidural space through the sacral hiatus and caudal canal.

b. **A test dose** of 3 ml of 1–1.5% lidocaine with epinephrine 1:200,000 is administered through the catheter, and the patient is monitored carefully for evidence of a subarachnoid injection. Following aspiration, an additional 12-ml dose is injected.

c. **Due to anesthesia of the lower vagina and perineum,** the patient does not feel the urgency to bear down; she must be encouraged and taught to do so.

6. **Complications**

a. Intravascular injections.

b. Hypotension.

c. Puncture of the maternal rectum.

d. **Insertion of the needle** into the fetal head. **Diagnosis:** Caudal anesthesia is not successful; the child is born in a depressed condition; there is gastric aspiration; and convulsions follow the baby's resuscitation. The diagnosis is confirmed by examining the scalp. **Therapy** includes (1) intubation of the newborn and ventilation with oxygen and (2) exchange transfusion.

F. Spinal anesthesia. See Chapter 15.

1. **Indications.** In the primipara, spinal anesthesia is indicated when the presenting fetal part is on the perineal floor. If spinal anesthesia is indicated in a multipara, it should be carried out when the cervix is dilated to about 8 cm.

2. **Technique.** The patient is placed in the left lateral or sitting position. A 25- or 26-gauge spinal needle is inserted at the $L_{3\text{-}4}$ or $L_{4\text{-}5}$ interspace via an 18-gauge IV needle, which is used as an introducer.

3. **The anesthetic solution** used is lidocaine 40–50 mg of a 5% solution in 7.5% D/W or tetracaine 4–5 mg of a 0.4% solution in 10% D/W. Do not inject during uterine contractions. The patient is advised not to bear down for 5 min following the administration of the local anesthetic solution, to prevent a higher spread of spinal anesthesia.

4. **Complications**

   a. **Hypotension** (supine hypotensive syndrome).

      (1) The decreased subarachnoid space in the pregnant woman should be kept in mind, so that unnecessarily high levels of anesthesia and the associated hypotension are avoided.

      (2) **Therapy**

         (a) IV administration of lactated Ringer's solution with 5% D/W.

         (b) Left uterine deviation is achieved manually, using a mechanical device, by tilting the table into a left lateral position or by raising the patient's right side and hip with a folded blanket or pillow.

         (c) Ephedrine, 25 mg IV.

   b. **Postlumbar puncture headache** occurs twice as frequently in parturient patients as in nonpregnant patients of equivalent ages.

      (1) **The incidence** of headache is related to the size of the needle used: A 25- or 26-gauge needle reduces the incidence and severity of headache.

      (2) **The headache** is moderate to severe—more severe in pregnant women. It is relieved when the patient is in the horizontal position and is associated with neck pain and stiffness.

      (3) The **cause** is loss of cerebrospinal fluid via the punctured dura.

      (4) **Therapy** consists of hydration and analgesic drugs. If headache is extremely severe, homologous blood can be injected at the site of the dural puncture in the epidural space.

III. General anesthesia in obstetrics. General anesthesia is indicated for many obstetric emergencies for two reasons: rapid induction of anesthesia time and avoidance of the expanded vascular space that follows sympathetic blockade.

A. Indications

1. **Hypovolemia** associated with hemorrhagic conditions. Patients with placenta previa or abruptio placentae would be aggravated much more by major blocks than by general anesthesia.

2. **Acute fetal distress** (cord prolapse, cord compression) requires immediate, rapid delivery; therefore time prohibits regional blocks.

3. **Patients who refuse regional anesthesia** and, at times, patients with a language or other communications barrier.

B. Problems associated with general anesthesia

1. Depression of the newborn.
2. Emesis and pulmonary aspiration of gastric contents.
3. **When general anesthesia is administered,** the degree of depression of the infant is directly proportional to the depth and duration of anesthesia.
4. **If regional anesthesia is contraindicated,** nitrous oxide with a minimum of 33–50% oxygen is the best choice until the fetus is delivered. If more potent anesthetics are indicated, the depth and duration of anesthesia before childbirth should be kept to a minimum, since all general inhalation anesthetics cross the placenta to enter the blood of the fetus immediately following inhalation by the mother.

C. Anesthetic agents

1. **Nitrous oxide.** Little or no depression of the newborn is observed when nitrous oxide with a minimum of 20% oxygen is administered for a period of less than 20 min. There is no significant depression of the newborn when nitrous oxide is administered in analgesic concentrations of 40–50% before delivery.
2. **Halothane** in anesthetic concentrations causes (a) atony of the uterus and postpartum bleeding and (b) respiratory depression in the infant. It is administered for (a) analgesia and (b) anesthesia to achieve relaxation of the uterus, which allows manipulations within the uterus. Halothane is rarely used today.
   a. **Indications for uterine relaxation only**
      (1) Tetanic contractions of the uterus.
      (2) Internal or external versions.
      (3) Manual removal of retained placenta.
      (4) Uterine inversion.
      (5) Breech delivery.
      (6) Multiple births.
      (7) Bandl's ring.

D. Thiopental in less than a 250-mg dose does not produce an important degree of depression of the infant. A safe method is administration of oxygen followed by IV injection of thiopental less than 250 mg and succinylcholine 80 mg, endotracheal intubation, and maintenance of anesthesia with 50% nitrous oxide–oxygen mixture. The following are **indications for thiopental and nitrous oxide anesthesia** with or without succinylcholine:

1. Vaginal delivery (when regional anesthesia is contraindicated and inhalation analgesia is not satisfactory).
2. Cesarean section (when regional anesthesia is contraindicated).

E. Muscle relaxant drugs are very useful in obstetrics because they are the only agents that do not cross the placenta (gallamine excepted). Anesthetic drugs administered in analgesic concentrations with muscle relaxants for prolonged periods have no depressant effects on the baby.

IV. Anesthesia management with specific indications

A. General considerations

1. **Every woman in labor** is a person under stress. Labor and delivery are normally painful experiences, but no mother has died from the pain of childbirth.

2. For anesthesia purposes, **all obstetric patients** are considered to have full stomachs.

3. **Appropriate facilities and physicians** should be available for the management of respiratory and circulatory problems. Every patient coming for delivery should have an IV infusion with a plastic catheter, and vital signs must be monitored constantly. **Hemorrhage** is one of the leading causes of obstetric mortality, and it can occur quickly and unexpectedly at any time during labor and childbirth.

4. All techniques of anesthesia in obstetrics should be considered **emergency procedures** except anesthesia techniques performed for elective inductions and elective cesarean sections.

B. Anesthesia for vaginal delivery

1. **Local infiltration of the perineum,** with or without **pudendal block,** is a satisfactory approach for spontaneous and for most outlet forceps deliveries. This method, combined with **inhalation analgesia** with nitrous oxide–oxygen, will offer further comfort to the mother.

2. **Regional anesthesia** accomplishes a more profound analgesia than local infiltration.

3. **Lumbar epidural** or caudal anesthesia.

4. **A low spinal anesthesia** (saddle block) is excellent for vaginal delivery.

5. **When general anesthesia is indicated,** there is always the risk of aspiration of gastric contents. Thus an oral antacid liquid is given before anesthesia.

   a. **Induction of anesthesia** is carried out with thiopental, and succinylcholine is injected to facilitate endotracheal intubation. Injection of 1 mg of pancuronium (or 3 mg of tubocurarine) before thiopental administration will decrease or abolish the fasciculations due to succinylcholine and also will prevent increased intragastric pressure. The external cricoid pressure is a great help.

   b. **Maintenance** of general endotracheal anesthesia is carried out with nitrous oxide, oxygen, and succinylcholine drip. On completion of anesthesia, the pharynx is suctioned, and a nasogastric catheter is introduced into the stomach. Extubation is performed when the patient is awake.

C. Breech presentation

1. **Heavy sedation** is contraindicated because of the high incidence of premature births associated with this condition.

2. **The second stage of labor** is managed with regional anesthesia or inhalation analgesia and pudendal nerve block. If necessary, general anesthesia is administered.

D. Multiple births. The first and early second stages of labor can be managed under regional anesthesia, and birth of **the first twin** ordinarily is accomplished without difficulty.

E. Tetanic contractions of the uterus are controlled by administration of oxygen and halothane.

F. Fetal distress. Delivery is achieved under emergency conditions using regional anesthesia or pudendal nerve block and inhalation analgesia.

G. Antepartum hemorrhage results in hypotension and hypovolemia in the mother, which seriously threatens both mother and fetus; blood transfusion should be carried out right away. In the absence of available blood, albumin or lactated Ringer's solution with 5% D/W should be given immediately. Oxygen is administered, the mother is placed in the Trendelenburg position, and ephedrine is injected IV or IM.

H. **Postpartum hemorrhage.** The hypovolemia and hypotension are treated by administration of fluids, blood, and vasopressors.

I. **Toxemia of pregnancy** occurs in 7% of all pregnancies. Seizures are not common, but the liver and kidney are affected. Toxemia of pregnancy is often associated with severe hypertension, and the baby is born prematurely. Continuous caudal or lumbar epidural anesthesia is the method of choice.

J. **Prematurity.** Prematures are at the highest risk of all delivery situations. For those with birth weights below 1000 g, mortality is about 98%. The choice of anesthesia for the mother does not make a difference in the baby's prognosis. Continuous caudal or lumbar epidural anesthesia is the method of choice during the first and second stages of labor. **For emergency delivery,** a low spinal anesthesia or pudendal nerve block may be instituted immediately.

K. **Anesthesia for cesarean section**

1. **For elective cesarean section,** the technique of choice is regional anesthesia: lumbar epidural anesthesia, spinal anesthesia, or caudal anesthesia. If regional anesthesia is not applicable, general anesthesia or local infiltration can be used.

    a. **Spinal anesthesia** should be accomplished by injection of tetracaine, 6–10 mg of 0.4% solution in 10% D/W, or lidocaine, 60–80 mg of 5% solution in 7.5% D/W. The sensory level should be fixed at the T_6 dermatome.

    b. **Hypotension** is a major complication, usually due to supine hypotensive syndrome. Prophylactically, the Trendelenburg position is assumed, and up to 1000 ml of fluids is given IV 10–15 min before spinal anesthesia is begun. If hypotension develops, the uterus is lifted upward and displaced to the left. If this is not adequate and BP is below 100 torr, 25–50 mg of ephedrine or 15–30 mg of mephentermine (Wyamine) is injected IV.

2. **For emergency cesarean section**

    a. A balanced combination of **magnesium and aluminum** hydroxides, 15 ml, is given orally.

    b. The patient is brought to the delivery room in the **lateral position** and remains so until she is placed on the delivery table.

    c. **The uterus** is displaced to the left and sustained with a mechanical displacement device.

    d. **An IV infusion** using a 16-gauge plastic catheter is started.

    e. The patient breathes **oxygen** from the anesthesia machine for at least 5–8 min. The mask can be retained on the face with head straps.

    f. **Tubocurarine, 3 mg** (or pancuronium, 1 mg) is injected IV 2–3 min before induction of anesthesia.

    g. The patient is draped and the obstetrician is ready to incise, after which 4 mg/kg of **thiopental** is injected IV, followed by 100 mg of **succinylcholine.**

    h. External **cricoid pressure** is applied and maintained.

    i. **Laryngoscopy** is performed, the endotracheal tube is inserted, and the cuff is inflated. Cricoid pressure may then be released.

    j. **Maintenance of anesthesia** is accomplished with nitrous oxide and 30% oxygen. Increasing the dose and duration of nitrous oxide anesthesia before delivery carries with it the risk of producing diffusion hypoxia in the neonate. If the induction-delivery period exceeds 20 min, nitrous oxide should be discontinued.

k. An IV drip of 0.1–0.2% **succinylcholine** or a single IV dose of 18–24 mg of **tubocurarine** (or 6 mg of pancuronium) is given when muscle activity begins to reappear following intubation.

l. After the **umbilical cord** has been clamped, anesthesia may be deepened by using a moderately increased concentration of inhalation agents or narcotics, such as fentanyl, meperidine, or morphine.

L. Anesthesia for the parturient patient with heart disease

1. **Heart disease** is one of the leading causes of maternal mortality. A woman in labor with heart disease, and particularly with dyspnea, should not be permitted to make strong expulsive efforts.
2. **Continuous caudal** or lumbar peridural anesthesia should be instituted as early as possible.
3. **The postpartum period** is especially dangerous for patients with heart disease because of suddenly increased venous pressure.

V. Complications

A. The five leading causes of maternal mortality are:

1. Hemorrhage.
2. Infection.
3. Toxemia.
4. Heart disease.
5. **Anesthesia.** These anesthetic deaths are related to pulmonary aspiration of gastric contents, hypotension, or respiratory failure; 98% of them are preventable.

B. Aspiration of gastric contents

1. **Aspiration of vomitus** due to vomiting (active process) or regurgitation (passive process) is one of the main causes of obstetric anesthesia mortality. It may cause death from respiratory obstruction, or it may be followed by development of aspiration pneumonia. If the pH of the aspirated liquid is below 2.5, a chemical pneumonia will follow within a few hours, with dyspnea, cyanosis, tachypnea, tachycardia, and development of expiratory wheezing due to bronchoconstriction.
2. **The patient in labor** should always be considered for anesthesia purposes to have a full stomach, since (a) the onset of labor delays emptying of the stomach; (b) during labor, gastric secretions accumulate in the stomach; and (c) the patient under the stress of labor often does not remember the time of her last meal.
3. **Preventive measures.** Often the obstetric patient will have eaten shortly before the onset of labor. Measures should be taken to prevent aspiration of gastrointestinal contents.

   a. **When anesthesia is indicated,** the safest techniques are regional anesthesia or inhalation analgesia. If both these methods are contraindicated, general anesthesia should be undertaken, but only with a cuffed endotracheal tube in place.

   b. **Intubation of the trachea with the patient awake** is one of the more effective and safe ways in which to avoid aspiration in the obstetric patient who is liable to vomit or regurgitate. The most secure approach is to insert the tube under topical anesthesia before induction of general anesthesia.

   c. **General anesthesia.** If intubation of the trachea with the patient awake is not feasible, oral antacids are administered and induction of general anesthesia is carried out by IV injection of 1 mg of pancuronium to minimize fasciculations and the accompanying increased intragastric pressure following injection of succinylcholine. This is followed a few minutes later by 250 mg of thiopental and 100 mg of succinylcholine. External digital pressure is maintained against the cricoid cartilage, and tracheal intubation with a cuffed tube is performed rapidly. Anesthesia is maintained with nitrous oxide, oxygen, and succinylcholine drip.

4. **Treatment** of pulmonary aspiration of stomach contents includes endotracheal intubation, oxygenation, suctioning of the trachea and bronchi, large doses of corticosteroids (hydrocortisone 500 mg), aminophylline, and antibiotics. Respiration is assisted or controlled. If indicated, a bronchoscopy is performed. A chest x-ray must be obtained as soon as possible. Bronchospasm is reduced by isoproterenol given IV.

C. **Hypotension in the patient in labor** is caused by:

1. Inferior vena cava compression (supine hypotensive syndrome).
2. Sympathetic blockade following spinal, peridural, or caudal anesthesia.
3. Toxicity of the local anesthetic agents.
4. Hemorrhage (atony of the uterus).
5. Amniotic fluid embolism.
6. Acute congestive heart failure.
7. Any hypotension less than 100 torr systolic has ill effects on the newborn and should be treated.

D. **Supine hypotensive syndrome**

1. **The supine hypotensive syndrome** can occur during routine delivery conditions, natural childbirth, regional anesthesia, or general anesthesia.
2. **During late pregnancy** and when the mother lies on her back, venous return to the right heart is decreased, and cardiac output is 20% less than when she is in a lateral position. This is caused by pressure of the enlarged uterus on the inferior vena cava, which produces symptoms of hypotension, dyspnea, apprehension, and vomiting.
   a. **Under normal conditions** the increased sympathetic action on the vessels of the legs and pelvis increases venous return through the paravertebral collateral circulation to enter the azygos or superior vena cava, resulting in maintenance of a normal cardiac output.
   b. **The compensatory sympathetic mechanism** is inactivated during regional anesthesia or deep general anesthesia.
3. **Therapy**
   a. Hypotension 25% below initial recordings, or less than 100 torr systolic, is a threat to the fetus, and treatment should be begun immediately.
   b. The patient is turned on her left side. If she is in the lithotomy position for delivery, the gravid uterus is displaced to the left.
   c. Oxygen is administered.
   d. If hypotension persists, efforts are made to increase the circulating volume by rapid IV administration of lactated Ringer's solution or 5% dextrose in normal saline.
   e. Ephedrine 15–25 mg is injected IV. The use of stronger vasoconstrictors (methoxamine, phenylephrine) with uterine artery vasoconstriction will certainly interfere further with the blood flow of the placenta and with fetal oxygenation.

E. **Respiratory failure** following spinal anesthesia, one of the leading causes of mortality in obstetric anesthesia, should be treated immediately by endotracheal intubation with assisted or controlled ventilation.

F. **Toxic reactions to local anesthetic drugs**

1. **During the last trimester** of pregnancy, the size of the peridural venous plexus is increased, while that of the peridural space is decreased by 50%. Thus intravascular administration of a local anesthetic solution carries with it increased risk of toxic reactions.

2. **Symptoms** include drowsiness, slurred speech, and loss of coordination. These may be followed by convulsions, loss of consciousness, and/or cardiovascular collapse.

3. **Therapy**

   a. Maintenance of the airway and oxygenation.

   b. The cardiovascular system is supported by IV injection of lactated Ringer's solution with 5% D/W, together with 15–25 mg of ephedrine.

   c. The convulsions are controlled by IV administration of 50–100 mg of thiopental or 100 mg of pentobarbital.

G. **Uterine relaxation**

1. **Halothane** is a powerful relaxant of the uterus. The degree of relaxation is related to the depth of anesthesia.

2. **Thiopental and nitrous oxide** have no effect on the uterus.

3. **Muscle relaxant drugs** have no effect on uterine activity.

4. **Spinal,** lumbar peridural, and caudal anesthesia do not alter uterine contractions but may interfere with the extrauterine forces during labor.

H. **Puncture of the fetal scalp or skull** can occur by accident during caudal anesthesia, and in this manner the local anesthetic solution may be injected into the fetus. When this happens, the fetal heart shows bradycardia, and the newborn is depressed at birth. In spite of artificial respiration and oxygenation, bradycardia persists and convulsions ensue. **Therapy** includes exchange transfusion and gastric lavage.

I. **Postpartum hypertension** is a potentially dangerous condition that may be due to (1) oxytocic agents, (2) vasoconstrictor drugs, (3) hypoxia, (4) hypervolemia, and/or (5) toxemia of pregnancy.

1. **Ergot alkaloids and vasopressors,** administered together or following one another, may lead to severe hypertension and a cerebrovascular accident.

2. **Therapy** for severe headache and potential cerebrovascular rupture includes continuous diluted IV administration of 0.1% trimethaphan or chlorpromazine IV in doses of 2.5 mg every minute until the BP falls.

VI. Resuscitation of the newborn

A. **The Apgar scoring method** is a numerical index of the viability of a newborn baby at 1 and 5 min after completion of childbirth (disregarding the umbilical cord and placenta).

1. **The newborn infant is evaluated** for heart rate, respiratory effort, muscle tone, reflex response to stimulation, and color. A score of 0, 1, or 2 is assigned for each of these five evaluations.

2. **The neonate scoring 7 or above** is considered in good condition; if the score is 4 to 6, the infant is moderately depressed; if the score is less than 4, the infant is considered seriously depressed.

3. **The Apgar rating at 5 min** reflects the results of the resuscitative efforts and provides an index of the value of further efforts.

B. **Following birth,** the infant is kept head down until the posterior pharynx and nose are cleared by suction. The airway is maintained by extension of the head. **Respirations,** if not already started, are initiated by slapping the soles of the feet or rubbing the back. Administration of oxygen helps vasodilation of the pulmonary vessels.

1. **Equipment for infant resuscitation** should be readily available at all times: suction apparatus and oxygen to be delivered under intermittent positive pressure by mask, oral airways, laryngoscopes, and endotracheal tubes.

2. **The depressed infant** may respond to clearing of the airway, stimulation, and oxygen administration. If the infant does not improve rapidly, tracheal intubation is performed using a 2.5-, 3-, or 3.5-mm ID tube, and oxygen is administered.

3. **Any newborn** who does not establish spontaneous respirations should be assisted immediately or hypoxia and acidosis will ensue. About 35% of all deaths during the first year of life occur within the first 24 hr, and half of these are related to anoxia and pulmonary pathology.

VII. Anesthesia and surgery during pregnancy

A. Surgery and anesthesia in pregnant women **should be avoided** if possible. If surgery cannot be avoided, attempt to postpone it until the second half of pregnancy.

B. **If major surgery** is necessary, skillfully managed **regional anesthesia** (spinal, epidural, or peripheral nerve block) should be utilized whenever applicable. If general anesthesia is necessary, the potent inhalation agents should be avoided if possible, and IV agents, which have not been highly suspect as teratogens, should be employed. **Thiopental, muscle relaxants, narcotics,** and endotracheal anesthesia with minimal use of nitrous oxide might be considered to be satisfactory. Nitrous oxide itself is a teratogen and a well-known antimitotic agent.

VIII. Anesthesia for gynecology

A. General considerations

1. **Gynecologic surgery** includes procedures involving the lower abdomen or perineum. These operations are performed with the patient in the supine, lithotomy, or Trendelenburg position.

2. The **duration** of a gynecologic procedure varies from the 10-min pelvic examination to an 8-hr pelvic exenteration.

3. To place the patient in the **lithotomy position,** both legs should be raised together when the legs are placed in the stirrups. Raising one leg at a time when the patient is under anesthesia is comparable to manipulation of the sacroiliac joint, and this can be the cause of backache. When surgery is completed, restoration to the supine position should be made slowly; otherwise, the BP may fall.

4. **A steep head-down position** is hazardous to ventilation in the anesthetized patient. When surgery is carried out under general anesthesia, respiration should be controlled via a tracheal tube in place.

5. **Pelvic surgery** performed through the abdomen or vagina incurs an increased risk of thrombophlebitis. The leg veins should be supported at all times with elastic stockings.

B. Anesthetic management

1. **Preanesthetic preparation.** See Chapter 1.

2. **Preanesthesia medication.** See Chapter 3.

3. **Monitoring.** See Chapter 6.

4. **Anesthetic techniques**

   a. **For short procedures** performed with the patient in the lithotomy position, such as dilatation and curettage, general anesthesia is induced with IV thiopental. Maintenance of anesthesia is carried out with nitrous oxide and oxygen by mask, supplemented by IV injections of thiopental. Succinylcholine drip may be added. Anesthesia by mask always risks the possibility of aspiration of stomach contents.

      (1) **Alternate methods** are (a) nitrous oxide, oxygen, and narcotics or (b) nitrous oxide, oxygen, and halothane, enflurane, or isoflurane. Ventilation is assisted or controlled.

      (2) **Spinal,** lumbar peridural, and caudal anesthesia methods are not recommended for short procedures. In the young female, spinal anesthesia more frequently causes postlumbar-puncture headache.

   b. **For longer vaginal procedures** performed with the patient in the lithotomy position, such as vaginal hysterectomy, general endotracheal or regional anesthesia is indicated.

   c. **For extensive gynecologic procedures,** such as exenteration, general endotracheal anesthesia is recommended. This type of surgery is accompanied by a great loss of blood and therefore adequate monitoring is mandatory: BP cuff, esophageal stethoscope, central venous pressure ECG, CVP, arterial BP readings by means of a cannulated radial artery, temperature probe, and measurement of urine output and blood loss.

   d. **For laparoscopy.** This procedure includes (1) a steep Trendelenburg position to displace the abdominal contents toward the diaphragm and (2) insufflation of the peritoneal cavity with carbon dioxide. These procedures permit the gynecologist to insert the laparoscope through the lower abdominal wall with a trocar. The insufflated carbon dioxide has little effect on the arterial PCO_2. The general endotracheal anesthesia includes nitrous oxide and oxygen with narcotics, halothane, enflurane, or isoflurane, and controlled ventilation. The procedure is short, and muscle relaxation can be provided by continuous infusion of 0.2% succinylcholine.

Bibliography

Abboud, T. K., Shnider, S. M., Wright, R. G., et al. Enflurane analgesia in obstetrics. Anesth. Analg. (Cleve.) 60:133, 1981.

Baraka, A., et al. Control of gastric acidity by glycopyrrolate premedication in the parturient. *Anesth. Analg.* (Cleve.) 56:642, 1977.

Bleyaert, A., Soetens, M., Laes, L., et al. Bupivacaine, 0.125 per cent, in obstetric epidural analgesia. Experience in three thousand cases. *Anesthesiology* 51:435, 1979.

Brock-Utne, J. G., Barclay, A. J., and Houlton, P. J. C. Gastric volume and acidity at cesarean section. *S Afr. Med. J.* 52:182, 1977.

Coombs, D. W., Hooper, D., and Colton, T. Prenanesthetic cimetidine alteration of gastric fluid volume and pH. *Anesth. Analg.* (Cleve.) 58:183, 1979.

Crawford, J. S. Experience with spinal analgesia in a British obstetric unit. *Br. J. Anaesth.* 51:531, 1979.

Cusick, J. F., Myklebust, J. B., and Abram, S. E. Differential neural effects of epidural anesthetics. *Anesthesiology* 53:299, 1980.

Datta, S., and Apler, M. H. Anesthesia for cesarean section. *Anesthesiology* 53:142, 1980.

Donchin, Y., Amirav, B., Sahar, A., et al. Sodium nitroprusside for aneurysm surgery in pregnancy. *Br. J. Anaesth.* 50:849, 1978.

Downing, J. W., Buley, J. R., Brock-Utne, J. G., et al. Etomidate for induction of anaesthesia at caesarean section. Comparison with thiopentone. *Br. J. Anaesth.* 51:135, 1979.

Downing, J. W., Houlton, P. C., and Barclay, A. Extradural analgesia for caesarean section. A comparison with general anaesthesia. *Br. J. Anaesth.* 51:367, 1979.

Drummond, G. B., and Martin, L. V. H. Pressure-volume relationship in the lung during laparoscopy. *Br. J. Anaesth.* 50:261, 1978.

Duffy, B. L. Regurgitation during pelvic laparoscopy. *Br. J. Anaesth.* 51:1089, 1979.

Fishburne, J. I. Anesthesia for laparoscopy. Considerations, complications and techniques. *J. Reprod. Med.* 21:37, 1978.

Grundy, E. M., Ramamurthy, S., Patel, K. P., et al. Extradural analgesia revisited. *Br. J. Anaesth.* 50:805, 1978.

Holdsworth, J. D. Relationship between stomach contents and analgesia in labor. *Br. J. Anaesth.* 50:1145, 1978.

Hunt, T. M., Plantevin, O. M., and Gilbert, J. R. Morbidity in gynecological day-case surgery. A comparison of two anesthetic techniques. *Br. J. Anaesth.* 51:785, 1979.

Jouppila, R., Jouppila, P., Kuikka, J., et al. Placental blood flow during cesarean section under lumbar extradural analgesia. *Br. J. Anaesth.* 50:275, 1978.

Morishima, H. O., Pedersen, H., and Finster, M. Influence of maternal psychologic stress on the fetus. *Am. J. Obstet. Gynecol.* 131:286, 1978.

Pedersen, H., and Finster, M. Anesthetic risk in the pregnant surgical patient. *Anesthesiology* 51:439, 1979.

Towey, R. M., Standford, B. J., Ballard, R. M., et al. Morbidity of day-case gynecological surgery. A comparison of thiopental and Althesin. *Br. J. Anaesth.* 51:453, 1979.

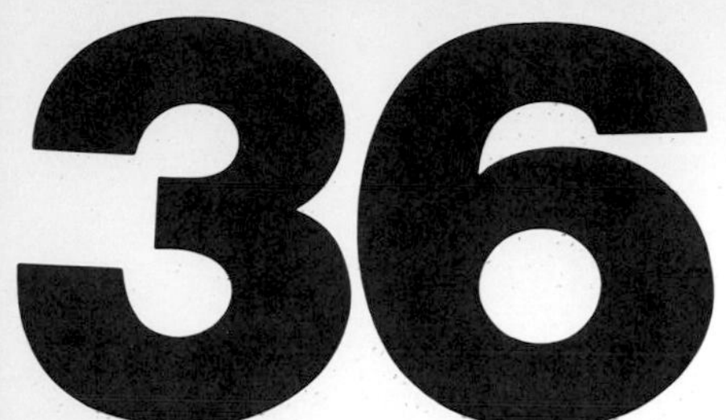

36 Pediatric Anesthesia

I. General considerations

A. In infants and children

1. **Definitions**

   Newborn (neonate). The first month of life.

   Infant. The first year of life.

   Child. The first 12 years of life.

2. **Size** is the most obvious distinction between children and adults. Less obvious are the differences in proportions, or relative sizes, of body structures.
3. **The infant's head** is large compared to the body, and the **neck muscles** are inadequately developed to maintain it in any position without support.
4. **The thoracic cage** is relatively small and weak, and its expansion is reduced by horizontally positioned ribs. Thus expansion of the thorax depends entirely on diaphragmatic contractions.
5. **The abdomen** is weak, and the legs are short and poorly developed.
6. **The body surface area** is one of the most significant measurements, since the curve of body surface area as related to body weight is very similar to the curve of basal metabolic activity measured in calories/m^2/hr.

B. Respiratory system

1. **In the infant** the **upper airway** is predisposed to obstruction because of the narrow passages of the nose, glottis, and trachea and the presence of lymphoid tissue and a comparatively large tongue.
2. **The infant larynx** is located more cephalad, with the larynx at the level of the fourth cervical vertebra, as compared with its location at the level of the sixth cervical vertebra in the adult.
   a. **The epiglottis** is stiff and U-shaped, in contrast to the flexible, flat epiglottis of the adult.
   b. **The cricoid ring** is the narrowest part of the larynx in children. Thus an endotracheal tube may be squeezed through the glottis but may stop at the cricoid ring, causing true trauma and edema. If this occurs, a smaller tube should be substituted.
   c. **Subglottic edema** due to infection or mechanical irritation may result in **croup** (resonant barking cough, hoarseness, and persistent stridor), which causes serious difficulties in breathing.
3. Infants and children require **larger amounts of oxygen** because of their increased metabolic rate.
4. **A negative pressure** is sometimes created in the stomach during inspiration, allowing air or anesthetic gases to be sucked in. A gastric tube should be used if the abdomen is distended or if breathing is labored.

5. **When there is airway obstruction,** substernal, suprasternal, and intercostal retractions are more marked both in older children and when dyspnea is severe. In the very young child, these signs must be looked for very carefully if obstruction is to be recognized early.

6. **Respiratory dead space** is equal to one-third of the tidal volume.

C. **Cardiovascular system**

1. **Congenital cardiovascular anomalies** are the anesthesiologist's most frequent cause of concern in relation to the cardiovascular system in children.

2. **The heart rate** of the infant is about 120 beats/min, and **BP** is 80/60 torr. After 5 years of age, the heart rate and BP approximate those of an adult.

3. **BP** in the infant and child can be **measured accurately** if a cuff with the proper width is used. The correct cuff width at any age is one-half to two-thirds the length of the patient's arm, or the width that encircles half the circumference of the patient's arm. A cuff that is too wide in relation to the diameter of the arm results in low values, and a too-narrow cuff results in high readings.

4. **A precordial or esophageal stethoscope** is very useful in monitoring heart sounds and respiration.

D. **Nervous system**

1. **The spinal cord** extends to the third lumbar vertebra at birth. When the child is 1 year old, the spinal cord takes its permanent position, ending at the first lumbar vertebra.

2. **The infant's nervous system** is immature. Sensory tracts are myelinated, but motor tracts are incompletely myelinated, as the infant's muscular activities demonstrate.

3. **Children are susceptible to convulsions.** This may be due to infants' lack of myelin, greater water content of the brain, a higher metabolic rate, or an immature inhibitory response pattern.

E. **Body temperature control**

1. **In infants** the temperature-regulating center in the hypothalamus is active but not well developed. This explains why infants are considered **poikilothermic** (body temperature tends to approach that of the environment).

2. **Body temperature** is increased by elevated heat production or increased heat retention.

3. **The development of hyperthermia** during pediatric anesthesia is a particular hazard. Predisposing factors are:

   a. Fever.

   b. Dehydration.

   c. Elevated room temperature.

   d. Drugs inhibiting sweating (atropine, scopolamine) or disturbing temperature regulation (general anesthetics).

   e. Excessive use of drapes.

4. **Malignant hyperthermia.** See Chapter 30, section **VI.**

5. **Hypothermia.** Heat loss may occur via convection of air, contact with a cooler object, evaporation of sweat, and radiation. Body heat is due to decreased heat production, vasodilatation, or a cold environment and when the viscera are exposed.

6. **For major surgery** the infant should be placed on a mattress with circulating water coils, so that rewarming can be done if necessary.

7. Continuous **monitoring of body temperature** with a rectal, esophageal, or tympanic thermistor probe should be routine for all children.

F. Fluid and electrolyte balance

1. **Throughout childhood** there is greater metabolism turnover and water turnover than in the fully grown adult.

2. **Blood volume** represents 7–8% of the child's weight. Replacement is necessary if there is loss of more than 10% of the circulating blood volume. **The margin of safety is very small.**

3. **Clinical signs of blood loss** include:

   a. BP.

   b. Color of the skin and mucous membranes.

   c. Volume of heart sounds.

   d. Central venous pressure.

   e. Urine output.

4. **Rapid transfusion of blood** can produce metabolic acidosis in the infant when the transfused blood is more than 50% of the estimated blood volume. Sodium bicarbonate minimizes acidosis if given in doses of 1–2 mEq/100 ml of blood transfused.

G. Sites of venipuncture

1. **Umbilical vein in the newborn.** This site is indicated only for short-term blood infusions in the operating room, since thrombophlebitis results very frequently when it is used.

2. **Scalp veins** in infants.

3. **Dorsum of the hand or foot** in older children.

4. **The anteoubital spaoe** is not recommended unless venipuncture can be done easily, because arterial and median nerve injury can result.

5. **Following induction of anesthesia,** venipuncture can be accomplished much easier due to increased central venous pressure and vasodilatation.

II. Preparation for surgery

A. Psychological aspects

1. It must be remembered that children do not realize the reasons for hospitalization and separation from home, family, and friends.

2. Inappropriate preparation for surgery can result in psychic trauma that may last for years.

3. All children must receive an abundance of attention at all times, and they should be segregated completely from diseased or ailing adults.

B. A preoperative evaluation by the anesthesiologist must include a preoperative visit, a physical examination, discussion with the parents, and study of the patient's records and laboratory data.

C. Restriction of food and fluids

1. **Infants** are given the regular formula up to 4 hr before anesthesia, and clear fluids (most often dextrose solutions) up to 2 hr before surgery.

2. **Children** over the age of 2 years are permitted clear fluids up to 4 hr prior to anesthesia.

3. **Gastric emptying** may be delayed for 12 hr by fear or in the presence of peritoneal irritation.

D. **Preanesthetic medication** See Chap. 3.

E. **Aspiration of gastric contents** during induction of anesthesia is a serious complication that can happen as a result of vomiting or regurgitation, especially in children with pyloric stenosis, tracheoesophageal fistula, intestinal obstruction, or food in the stomach. This complication can be minimized by inserting a gastric tube and aspirating the gastric fluids before induction of anesthesia.

III. **Equipment and techniques**

A. **Systems** most often used in children are bag-and-mask anesthesia, variations of Ayre's T-piece, and the semiclosed carbon dioxide absorption system with assisted or controlled ventilation (see Chaps. 9 and 10).

B. **Monitoring.** See Chapter 6.

IV. **Anesthesia management**

A. **In the operating room,** the records are reviewed, the child is identified positively, and the correct surgical procedure is verified.

B. **Induction of anesthesia.** Everything possible should be done to produce a smooth induction of anesthesia.

1. **Anesthesia is induced** by blowing gently over the patient's face a mixture of nitrous oxide and oxygen and increasing concentrations of halothane or enflurane, followed a few minutes later by a firm application of the face mask. **Halothane** is considered safe to use in children because very few cases of halothane hepatotoxicity have been reported.

2. **If the child accepts a needle** while awake, induction of anesthesia can be achieved by IV thiopental.

C. **Endotracheal intubation** is indicated in all intrathoracic, neurosurgical, intraabdominal, and head and neck operations, as well as in procedures performed with the patient in the prone position and in most emergency operations.

1. **The anatomy of the infant** is such that the laryngoscope with a straight blade is preferable. A straight laryngoscope blade better exposes and immobilizes the larynx of small infants and young children.

2. **Orotracheal intubation**

a. **Awake intubation** is indicated in neonates up to 2 weeks of age, in children who have a compromised airway, and in children who have retained gastric contents. **In neonates** it is safer to insert the tube while the baby is still conscious; this is easy, and it avoids the possibility of hypoxia due to laryngospasm or obstruction.

b. **Intubation under general anesthesia** is carried out with either (1) nitrous oxide, oxygen, and halothane or enflurane, with or without succinylcholine, or with (2) nitrous oxide, oxygen thiopental, and succinylcholine.

c. **To avoid trauma,** several tubes should be readily available before intubation.

3. **Nasotracheal intubation** is used when indicated. It should be limited to those cases in which the nasotracheal route offers marked advantages over the oral route. However, nasotracheal intubation introduces the added risks of (1) adenoidal bleeding, (2) introduction of foreign material into the trachea, and (3) transient bacteremia.

4. **Following intubation:**

   a. Both lungs should be examined for proper respiration and to exclude endobronchial intubation.

   b. The endotracheal tube should be immobilized securely to prevent accidental dislodging or advancement of the tube.

   c. A catheter should be inserted through the mouth into the stomach to aspirate any liquid or gas that might interfere with respiration.

D. **Maintenance of anesthesia** is carried out with (1) nitrous oxide, oxygen, halothane or enflurane, and spontaneous or assisted ventilation or (2) nitrous oxide, oxygen, halothane or narcotics with muscle relaxants, and controlled ventilation.

E. **Muscle relaxants**

1. **Tubocurarine.** The neonate is more sensitive to **tubocurarine** than the adult. This sensitivity gradually decreases over the first months of life. **Gallamine** is used less frequently. **Pancuronium** offers a number of advantages and is more popular than tubocurarine. When **nondepolarizing relaxants** are used for muscle relaxation, **reversal with atropine and neostigmine** should be carried out at the end of anesthesia; 1 mg of atropine is given IV, together with 2 mg of neostigmine.

2. **Succinylcholine**

   a. **Bradycardia** is elicited readily with repeated doses of succinylcholine. It is treated with IV atropine.

   b. **Muscular fasciculations** are not seen in infants.

3. **Prolonged apnea** may be induced with hypothermia, excessive concentrations of volatile agents, large doses of antibiotics, and respiratory acidosis.

F. **Extubation** is performed during light anesthesia with spontaneous respiration. If **laryngospasm** develops, it is generally treated by positive pressure and/or IV administration of succinylcholine.

G. **Basal anesthesia with rectal anesthetio agents**

1. **Rectal administration** of thiopental, thiamylal, or methohexital has the advantage of involving neither mask nor needle. **The dose** of thiopental is 10 mg/kg.

2. Most children under the age of 6 years have no objection to the **passage of a rectal tube,** and following the administration of the solution, they fall asleep rapidly, considerably decreasing the possibility of psychic trauma.

3. **The following disadvantages** have made this technique less popular:

   a. **Absorption rates** may vary so much that there is little control over the anesthetic effect.

   b. **It is time-consuming** and requires careful preoperative attention by the anesthesiologist or nurse-anesthetist.

   c. **In young children,** despite careful instillation, the anesthetic may act as an enema.

4. **Rectal thiopental** should be used carefully and where there are facilities for constant supervision, since complete elimination of rectal thiopental requires 48 hr.

H. **Local and regional techniques** are indicated in certain circumstances, such as lacerations and fractures in children with full stomachs or in the premature infant.

V. **Ketamine in children.** See Chapter 11, section **III.**

A. **Ketamine** is a useful IM or IV anesthetic in children.

B. **The indications** are superficial operations; multiple procedures, such as dressing of burns; long operations that do not require relaxation; and eye examination in mentally retarded children or adults. **Ketamine is advantageous** as a supplement to regional anesthesia and for quieting the uncooperative child.

C. **Induction of anesthesia** is achieved with an IV dose of 1–2 mg/kg, and **maintenance of anesthesia** is accomplished with a supplementary dose of 0.5 mg/kg. Nitrous oxide supplementation is useful.

D. **Disadvantages.** In children under 1–2 years old there may be a respiratory depression effect.

VI. **Recovery period**

A. **Recovery room facilities** must be available to provide special attention to the patency of the airway, adequacy of respiration, cardiovascular stability, and maintenance of body temperature.

1. Efforts should be made to ensure that **body temperature** stays above 35° C. Below this level there is a high incidence of respiratory depression, apnea, bradycardia, and hypotension.

2. The child should be placed in the **semiprone position,** with the head slightly lowered to prevent aspiration of gastric contents.

B. **Oxygen therapy.** The choice of a tent with mist and oxygen or an incubator and the degree of humidification and oxygen supplementation are very important in pediatric patients.

1. **Incubators** improve control of temperature, humidity, and oxygen concentration in the premature or the very ill newborn.

2. **Tents** cover the entire body of the patient and also allow control of humidity, temperature, and oxygen concentration. However, access to the patient without disturbing the environment is poor.

3. **Masks and nasal catheters** are not generally acceptable to children.

C. **Laryngeal or subglottic edema**

1. **Laryngeal edema** may occur within ½–1 hr following extubation when an acute infection is superimposed on a minimal trauma during intubation. This can lead to **respiratory obstruction.**

2. **The obstruction results** from development of an exudate in the areolar tissue just below the vocal cords.

3. **A croupy cough,** hoarseness, expiratory stridor, and, as edema increases, signs of respiratory obstruction develop. Progression of edema can be suspected if there is an inability to clear the airway by coughing and retraction of the intercostal spaces and sternum during quiet respiration. Restlessness, pallor, sweating, cyanosis, and other signs of hypoxia follow.

4. **Therapy**

a. The child is placed in an oxygen-enriched atmosphere in a tent or hood with ultrasonically generated mist.

b. Dexamethasone, 4–8 mg IV, is administered.

c. Racemic epinephrine, 0.25–0.5 ml in 5 ml saline, is given every hour by intermittent positive-pressure breathing.

d. Hydration.

e. Antibiotics are given.

f. Mild hypothermia, 35° C, is induced.

g. If the child is still restless and hypoxic, an **endotracheal reintubation** should be performed immediately, after which the necessity of a tracheotomy may be considered.

Bibliography

Boix-Ochoa, J., Peguero, G., Seijo, G., et al. Acid-base balance and blood gases in prognosis and therapy of congenital diaphragmatic hernia. *J. Pediatr. Surg.* 9:49, 1974.

Cook, D. R. Neonatal anesthetic pharmacology. A review. *Anesth. Analg.* (Cleve.) 53:544, 1974.

Cook, D. R. Paediatric Anesthesia. Pharmacological considerations. *Drugs* 12:212, 1976.

Cook, D. R., and Fischer, C. G. Neuromuscular blocking effects of succinylcholine in infants and children. *Anesthesiology* 42:662, 1975.

Dierdorf, S. F., and Krishna, G. Anesthetic management of neonatal surgical emergencies. *Anesth. Analg.* (Cleve.) 60:204, 1981.

Diaz, J. H., and Lockhart, C. H. Is halothane really safe in infancy? *Anesthesiology* 5:S313, 1979.

Furman, E. B., Roman, D. G., Lemmer, L. A. S., et al. Specific therapy in water, electrolyte and blood-volume replacement during pediatric surgery. *Anesthesiology* 42:187, 1975.

Goudsouzian, N. G., Donlon, J. V., Savarese, J. J., et al. Re-evaluation of dosage and duration of action of d-tubocurarine in the pediatric age group. *Anesthesiology* 43:416, 1975.

Lindgren, L., Saarnivaara, L., and Himberg, J. J. Comparison of I.M. pethidine, diazepam and flunitrazepam as premedicants in children undergoing otolaryngological surgery. *Br. J. Anaesth.* 51:321, 1979.

Tochen, M. L. Orotrachael intubation in the newborn infant. A method for determining depth of tube insertion. *J. Pediatr.* 95:1050, 1979.

37 Anesthesia for Orthopedic Procedures

I. Orthopedic surgery

A. General considerations

1. **Orthopedic operations** range in complexity from simple, short procedures, such as the closed reduction of fractures or dislocations, to very long procedures, such as total hip replacement.

2. **Some major orthopedic operations** include internal fixation of hip fracture, laminectomy, ankle fusions, excision of Dupuytren's contractures, total hip replacement, and prosthetic replacement.

3. **Preoperative evaluation**

   a. During evaluation of the patient **for elective surgery,** considerations are given to the (1) medical and anesthetic history, (2) complicating medical diseases, such as heart and lung illnesses, and (3) current medications.

   b. **For emergency surgery.** In addition to the preceding considerations, the patient must be questioned as to recent oral intake, and his blood volume status should be evaluated. Special attention should be given to breathing, bleeding, and bone fractures.

      (1) **Obstruction of the airway,** pneumothorax, and flail chest require immediate diagnosis and therapy. If orthopedic surgery is combined with a lower abdominal incision, the vital capacity is decreased by 30%; if combined with upper abdominal surgery or thoracotomy, the vital capacity is decreased by 50%.

      (2) **Large amounts of blood** may be lost in accident victims due to bleeding from open wounds or hematoma formation around the area of fractures, particularly in the thigh and pelvis. Blood loss should be replaced before anesthesia and surgery. Hematocrit and hemoglobin values are only gross guides to the extent of restoration of lost blood. **The best guides** are improved BP, decreased pulse rate, improvement in color and capillary refill time, and measurement of central venous pressure which, in addition, gives a warning of overloading of the circulatory system.

      (3) **Patients having emergency therapy of fractures** or dislocations may have **full stomachs** either from having eaten before the accident or from swallowing blood from injuries around the face. **For anesthesia,** the safest approach is regional nerve block or spinal anesthesia. The second choice is general anesthesia. Induction of anesthesia is accomplished by intubating the trachea while the patient is awake, using topical anesthesia and IV diazepam, 15–20 mg.

B. Evaluating the urgency of surgery

1. **The advantages of delaying surgery** to correct or decrease a complicating factor should be weighed against the disadvantages incurred by not performing surgery immediately. There is an element of urgency in many orthopedic

situations; however, immediate operation is rarely needed, except in open wounds.

2. **Reduction of a simple fracture** can be carried out on a semiemergency basis.

3. **Tendon and open fracture repairs** should be done within a few hours following injury. In the elderly, fracture of the hip is considered a semiemergency and is treated accordingly.

4. Fractures associated with **arterial obstruction** are **true emergencies,** and surgery should be performed immediately. Included in this category are fracture and/or dislocation of the elbow and posterior dislocation of the knee.

II. Anesthesia management

A. **Preanesthetic preparation.** See Chapter 1.

B. **Preanesthesia medication.** See Chapter 3.

C. **Monitoring.** See Chapter 6.

D. **Surgery on the extremities** is performed in the majority of operations with a **tourniquet** in place.

1. **Responsibility for the tourniquet** rests with the **surgeon** who requests and applies it. However, it is a common practice for **the anesthesiologist** or nurse-anesthetist to be asked to keep a record of the time that it has been inflated. When the anesthesiologist or nurse-anesthetist accepts this responsibility, he must write on the patient's anesthesia record the length of time that the tourniquet has been in use.

2. **A tourniquet can cause vascular injury** if left inflated too long, and nerves can be damaged if it is improperly applied or inflated to too high a pressure. Damage may occur sometimes even if properly applied.

3. **The pneumatic tourniquet** is inflated from a reservoir of liquid Freon. It is necessary to check from time to time the gauge supplied with the tourniquet against a standard manometer.

4. **The safe length of time** for ischemia to be permitted in the extremities is not settled, but it decreases with increase in age; generally **2 hr should not be exceeded.** Pressure is set on the upper limb at 275 torr and on the lower limb at 550 torr.

5. Application of a tourniquet is contraindicated in a patient with **sickle cell disease.**

E. **Rheumatoid arthritis.** Deformities of the hands and many other areas caused by rheumatoid arthritis are amenable to corrective surgery. However, it must be remembered that rheumatoid arthritis is a systemic disease affecting the cervical spine and the laryngeal, temporomandibular, and/or costovertebral joints, so endotracheal intubation and ventilation may be compromised. The situation may be complicated further by the use of corticosteroids.

F. **Simple fractures** and some dislocations can be reduced without anesthesia within a short time following injury. Morphine or meperidine may be administered for analgesia.

G. **Regional anesthesia.** See Chapter 17, sections **III, IV, and V.**

1. **Regional anesthesia of the upper or lower extremity** conveys the advantages of analgesia, muscle relaxation, and immobilization while having very little effect on respiration and circulation. Additional advantages, in the postoperative period, are (a) prolonged analgesia and (b) paralysis of the vasoconstrictor nerve fibers, which results in improved blood circulation in the extremity.

   a. **The upper extremity** can be anesthetized by brachial plexus block (using the supraclavicular, axillary, or interscalene route), elbow block, wrist block, digital block, or intravenous regional anesthesia. The choice of anesthesia depends on the location of the surgical area and the presence or absence of the pneumatic tourniquet.

b. During brachial plexus block using the **supraclavicular route.**

(1) **Pneumothorax** occurs at a rate of about 1 in 100 cases.

(2) The presence of a tourniquet high on the arm requires circumferential injection of a local anesthetic solution for relief of **tourniquet pain.**

2. Regional anesthesia of the lower extremity

a. **The lower extremity** can be anesthetized by subarachnoid spinal anesthesia, epidural (lumbar or caudal) block, sciatic and femoral peripheral nerve block, or intravenous regional anesthesia.

b. **The most common complication** of spinal anesthesia is **hypotension,** especially in patients with reduced circulating blood volume. This is a serious complication in **pregnant women** and in patients with aortic insufficiency or coronary heart disease. However, the extent of spinal anesthesia and the severity of hypotension can be limited by proper positioning of the patient and injection of small amounts of anesthetic solution.

c. The main **advantage of peridural anesthesia over spinal anesthesia** is the avoidance of postural headache in the postoperative period.

d. **Sciatic and femoral nerve blocks** are useful for surgery and manipulations below the knee. Open surgery often requires the additional anesthesia of the obturator and lateral femoral cutaneous nerves.

3. Intravenous regional anesthesia. See Chapter 17, section **VII.**

a. Local anesthetic solution occasionally **is injected intravenously** for production of analgesia of the upper or lower extremity. **Lidocaine 0.5%** is the drug used.

b. Indications

(1) For surgery and manipulations of the upper or lower extremity that last less than 1¾ hr.

(2) For soft tissue surgery less than 1¾ hr in duration, such as ganglionectomy and surgery of the hand.

4. Brachial plexus block. See Chapter 17, section **III.**

H. General anesthesia

1. **Regional anesthesia** usually is indicated, especially in an emergency case when the patient may have a full stomach. However, **general anesthesia** is preferable when regional anesthesia is contraindicated or positioning the patient for regional anesthesia is very painful.

2. **Induction of general anesthesia** is achieved with IV thiopental or thiamylal, and endotracheal intubation is facilitated with succinylcholine.

3. **Indications for a tracheal intubation** depend on (a) the patient's position on the operating table; (b) the difficulties the case may present in maintaining a free airway without an endotracheal tube; (c) the use of muscle relaxant drugs; and (d) the duration of surgery.

4. **Maintenance of anesthesia** is accomplished with (a) nitrous oxide, oxygen, and halothane or enflurane with assisted respiration or (b) nitrous oxide, oxygen, narcotics, and muscle relaxants with controlled respiration.

III. Special anesthesia and surgical problems

A. Surgery performed with the patient **on the orthopedic table.**

1. The orthopedic table allows traction on the extremities to hold a reduced hip fracture, a wider abduction of the legs to accommodate the x-ray machine for lateral x-ray films of the hip, and application of plaster casts.
2. Patients placed on the orthopedic table are often elderly. Because the tabletop is unpadded, during positioning of the patient, caution should be exercised to protect the patient from **pressure points and peripheral nerve injuries.**

B. Fractured hip

1. The usual **patient with a fractured hip** is elderly and suffers from lung or heart disease. Surgery is performed on an emergency or semiemergency basis immediately after complicating factors are corrected (dehydration, anemia, shock, pneumonia, or heart failure). This correction may require 1–2 days of intensive treatment or scheduling surgery for later on the day after chest physiotherapy has achieved the patient's maximal ventilatory function.
2. The patient with a hip fracture has **0.5–1 L less blood volume** than normal.
3. **Induction of anesthesia** is complicated when the patient is brought into the operating room with the injured limb in traction. **Spinal anesthesia** can be achieved by gently placing the patient in the lateral position, so that the fractured extremity is dependent.
4. **If the lateral position cannot be obtained** or is very painful, induction of general endotracheal anesthesia is accomplished with the patient still in bed and the fractured limb in traction. Then the anesthetized patient is moved onto the operating table. **Maintenance of anesthesia** is carried out with small amounts of narcotics, muscle relaxants, and controlled ventilation. During surgery, **hypotension,** most often due to blood loss, trauma of hammering the nail, or deep anesthesia, is the most common complication requiring therapy.
5. These patients are extremely vulnerable to **thrombophlebitis.** Pulmonary embolism is one of the main causes of death.

C. Total hip replacement

1. Removal of the head of the femur following subcapital fracture and replacement with a prosthesis is not accompanied by much blood loss. However, surgery for osteoarthritis or degenerative disorders of the hip joint is **prolonged** and is associated with **hemorrhage.**
2. During prosthetic hip surgery, an **acrylic bone cement** is used that consists of two components, a liquid and a powder. At the time of use, the powder and liquid are mixed, resulting in the exothermic polymeric formation of a soft, pliable, dough-like mass. As the reaction progresses, within a few minutes a hard, cement-like complex is formed.
3. **Hypotension** and even **cardiac arrest** may follow the application of the mixed methyl methacrylate cement to raw bone surfaces. A decrease in BP may occur within 2–3 min of implanting the acrylic cement into the **femoral shaft,** but there is no change in BP associated with implanting the acrylic cement in the acetabulum.
4. **The cause** of sudden severe cardiovascular depression may be the direct effect of the polymerizing agent on the myocardium.
5. **For prevention** of hypotension and cardiac arrest, adequate preoperative hydration and careful blood replacement during surgery should be carried out. **At the time of cementing,** meticulous attention should be given to the status of the circulation.
6. **Absolutely sterile technique** should be used at all times. Wound infection is a serious threat to the surgical result.

7. **Methods of anesthetic management** include spinal anesthesia, continuous peridural anesthesia, and general endotracheal anesthesia.

8. **In the immediate postoperative period,** any unstable BP (hematocrit may drop rapidly) must be treated carefully with blood or fluid replacement.

9. **Hip fracture patients** almost always belong to an advanced age group. When these patients are undergoing anesthesia, surgery, and extensive instrumentation of the bones, a physiologic change occurs that renders them especially vulnerable to the insult of trauma, hemorrhage, and acrylic bone cement implantation. Careful preoperative preparation, intraoperative monitoring, and postoperative followup will help to ensure an uncomplicated intraoperative and postoperative course.

D. Surgery on the vertebral column

1. **Surgery in the prone position.** Surgery on the cervical, thoracic, and lumbar spine is carried out with the patient in the prone position, either suspended on the sternum and pelvis or in the prone jackknife position, so that the width of the intervertebral spaces can be varied by changing the degree of flexion of the operating table.

2. **Induction of anesthesia** and intubation are best achieved with the patient on a stretcher. Special provision should be made for the secure positioning of the IV plastic catheter and endotracheal tube. The patient is then turned onto the operating table in the prone position. During turning of the patient, the head must be supported, and the position of the endotracheal tube must be protected. In addition, the eyes must be kept closed and protected from pressure.

3. **Methods for maintenance of anesthesia** include nitrous oxide and oxygen with enflurane, halothane, or narcotics with muscle relaxants and controlled respiration.

4. **In the prone position** the patient should be supported in a manner that allows space for abdominal ventilatory excursion.

5. **Any pressure on the anterior abdominal wall** will be reflected in the **epidural veins,** which anastomose with the lumbar and mesenteric veins. Increased pressure within the epidural veins will result in increased bleeding during surgery.

6. **When surgery is completed,** the patient is turned onto the stretcher in the supine position. Then the narcotics and muscle relaxants are reversed.

7. **Bleeding** during surgery on the spine is due to three sources.

   a. **From the bone surface.** This is persistent but small in volume.

   b. **From severed arteries,** which is easily controlled.

   c. **Retrograde bleeding** from epidural, spinal, and lumbar veins can be considerable.

      (1) **This hemorrhage is enhanced** by pressure exercised on the anterior abdominal wall that causes the venous return from the abdominal cavity to seek an alternate route through the lumbar and epidural veins to the azygos vein.

      (2) **Prevention** of this bleeding can be accomplished by proper positioning of the patient in the prone position.

Bibliography

Bolton, C. F., and McFarlane, R. M. Human pneumatic tourniquet paralysis. *Neurology* 28:787, 1978.

Giannestras, N. J., Crauley, J. J., and Lentz, M. Occlusion of the tibial artery after a foot operation under tourniquet. *J. Bone Joint Surg.* [Am.] 59:682, 1977.

Hazlett, J. W. Orthopedic outpatient surgery. *Can. J. Surg.* 21:446, 1978.

Knight, P. R., Lane, G. A., Nichols, M. G., et al. Hormonal and hemodynamic changes induced by pentolinium and propranolol during surgical correction of scoliosis. *Anesthesiology* 53:127, 1980.

Lund, P. C., Cwik, J. C., and Gannon, R. T. Extradural anesthesia. Choice of local anesthetic agent. *Br. J. Anaesth.* 47:313, 1975.

Modig, J. Respiration and circulation after total hip replacement surgery. *Acta Anaesthesiol. Scand.* 20:225, 1976.

Neill, R. S. Postoperative analgesia following brachial plexus block. *Br. J. Anaesth.* 50:379, 1978.

Sculco, T. P., and Ranawat, C. The use of spinal anesthesia for total hip replacement arthroplasty. *J. Bone Joint Surg.* [Am.] 59:173, 1975.

Thompson, G. E., Miller, R. D., Stevens, W. C., et al. Hypotensive anesthesia for total hip arthroplasty. Study of blood loss and organ function (brain, heart, liver and kidney). *Anesthesiology* 48:91, 1978.

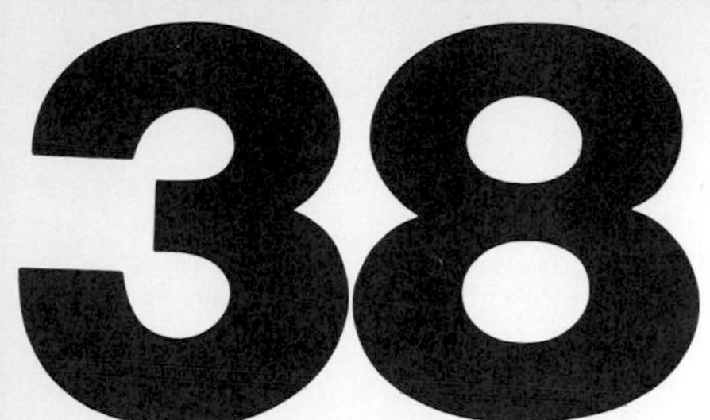

Dental Anesthesia

I. General considerations

A. Preanesthetic preparation. See Chapter 1.

B. Preanesthesia medication. See Chapter 3.

C. Monitoring. See Chapter 6.

D. Anesthesia problems encountered during dental surgery are similar to those mentioned in Chapter 40, sections **I.A.** and **B**.

1. **The airway,** shared with the dental surgeon, should be protected at all times from obstruction and aspiration of blood, saliva, operative debris, and water irrigating the dental drill.
2. **A suction apparatus** and packing of the pharynx are essential.
3. **A wide-open mouth and unobstructed airway** are of first priority during dental surgery.
4. Throughout the operation, **the eyes** should be covered with moist gauze to prevent injury from flying bits of dental debris and other objects.

II. Outpatient dental anesthesia

A. Anesthesia for outpatient surgery (see Chap. 42) includes local analgesia, IV anesthesia, inhalation anesthesia, inhalation analgesia, and IV sedation. Correct use of any of these techniques requires appropriate patient evaluation and preparation, together with knowledge of the anesthetic drugs and procedures indicated for ambulatory practice.

1. Dental outpatient anesthesia and/or sedation should be administered only by a **physician, dentist, or nurse-anesthetist** trained in ambulatory anesthesia, since these individuals possess the necessary knowledge and skill for this procedure.
2. **The sitting position, in the dental chair,** is used during anesthesia and surgery in the majority of procedures. However, the sitting position is stressful to the cardiovascular system, so it may produce adverse cardiovascular effects and consequent decreased cardiac output. When anxiety-produced vasovagal situations occur or vasodilatory anesthetics are administered with the patient in the sitting position, the cardiovascular depression produced may be more serious than it is when these events occur with the patient in the supine or semisupine position, in which cardiac output is increased by a greater venous return.
3. **The oxygen pressure of the brain** is determined by:
   - **a.** The arterial oxygen pressure reaching the brain. The most important factor in determining the arterial oxygen pressure under anesthesia is the partial pressure of oxygen in the inhaled gases.
   - **b. The rate of cerebral blood flow,** which depends on the mean arterial BP and cerebrovascular resistance. **In the sitting position,** the cerebrovascu-

lar resistance is minimal, and the cerebral blood flow varies directly with changes in the mean arterial BP.

4. **The contour dental chair.** A patient sitting in the semierect position in a contour dental chair is more stable than one in the sitting position. This chair can be used for both oral surgery and restorative dentistry. The contour dental chair allows the dentist to work comfortably, with full access to the patient's mouth, in either a sitting or a standing position.

   a. When the **dentist both performs the dental work and administers the sedative drugs,** the contour dental chair position is most desirable. This position is stable from a cardiovascular viewpoint, mechanically permits maintenance of the airway without tracheal intubation, and provides an adequate working position for the dentist.

   b. When the dentist is working **with another professional who is well trained in anesthesia,** having the patient in the supine position with a tracheal intubation is the preferred technique.

5. **Additional problems**

   a. **Silent regurgitation or vomiting** with aspiration of the stomach contents is a serious complication during anesthesia, whether the patient is in the sitting or the supine position. Every effort should be made to prevent this hazard or, if it occurs, to treat it immediately.

   b. **Aspiration of blood and debris** can be prevented by proper packing of the back of the mouth, reliable suction, and/or insertion of a cuffed endotracheal tube.

      (1) Soft, rounded cotton packs on strings placed to the back of the last molars and extending to the midline prevent aspiration of dental drillings, dust, tooth chips, and blood. We have found these packs more beneficial than gauze strips.

      (2) Another way to prevent aspiration of dental drillings is the use of the rubber dam, which isolates the tooth or teeth.

   c. **Airway control** under anesthesia can be accomplished by tracheal intubation regardless of the patient's position. However, this may not be practical for many outpatient procedures. A nasopharyngeal airway may be of value in this situation.

   d. **Anterior pressure on the mandible** will keep an airway open even without a nasal tracheal tube if one cannot be placed securely. In much office dentistry, the jaw is held as described above, and a nasal mask is placed over the nose to supply nitrous oxide, oxygen, and any of the halogens. This requires a strong arm.

B. Anesthesia management

1. **Indications for anesthesia.** A considerable amount of outpatient dental surgery—extraction and conservative work—is performed under local analgesia achieved by infiltration or nerve block. However, IV anesthesia, inhalation anesthesia, inhalation analgesia, or IV sedation is indicated in the following circumstances:

   a. Children (unable emotionally to accept local anesthesia).

   b. Patients with acute infective conditions; because of the low pH of the inflammatory tissues, solutions of local anesthetics will not relieve pain.

   c. Uncooperative, apprehensive, or mentally retarded patients.

   d. Patients requiring multiple extractions.

   e. Patients allergic to local anesthetic drugs.

2. Contraindications

- **a.** Recent intake of food or fluids.
- **b.** Congenital or acquired heart disease.
- **c.** Respiratory obstruction or disease.
- **d.** Edema of the floor of the mouth or swelling of the neck.
- **e.** Difficulty in opening the mouth.
- **f.** Cerebrovascular disease.
- **g.** Diabetes and/or obesity.
- **h.** Pregnancy.
- **i.** Anemia or hemorrhagic disorders.

3. Preparation of the patient

a. Prior to dental therapy

- **(1)** Written instructions should be given to the patient, particularly that no food or fluids can be taken for at least 6–8 hr prior to anesthesia.
- **(2)** Basic laboratory tests must be done.
- **(3)** The patient's records must be completed, including a medical history and physical examination.
- **(4)** The informed consent form must be signed and witnessed.

b. Prior to anesthesia

- **(1)** The stomach and bladder must be empty.
- **(2)** Dentures and contact lenses must be removed.
- **(3)** Premedication is not necessary for most patients and actually is disadvantageous because of its effect of increasing the recovery period and delaying the time of discharge; however, an IV dose of atropine is essential.

4. In the outpatient clinic

a. The monitors for BP, ECG, and respiration are placed on the patient, and an IV route is started in the hand with an 18-gauge plastic catheter running with 1000 ml lactated Ringer's solution in 5% D/W. The nasal mucosa is sprayed with 0.5% phenylephrine or 4% cocaine.

b. Position in the dental chair. The patient is seated comfortably in the dental chair, tilted slightly backward, and the headrest is adjusted to allow surgical access. The patient's hands rest on the abdomen, the knees are bent at right angles, and the feet are brought together. Lamps should not shine on the patient's face.

5. Intravenous anesthesia (methohexital)

a. Methohexital (see Chap. 11, sec. **I.B**) is 2½ times more potent than thiopental (or thiamylal) and is best suited for use as an anesthetic for induction rather than for maintenance of anesthesia during outpatient dental surgery. It is useful for short procedures because of its rapid onset, short duration, and rapid recovery time (when small doses are injected). For longer procedures, intermittent doses of methohexital are injected over the duration of the procedure.

b. Methohexital 1% is injected IV in doses of 1.5 mg/kg to a maximum of 200 mg. Its lack of analgesic properties makes it necessary to supplement it with local analgesia or nitrous oxide and oxygen.

c. **Anesthesia with methohexital can be supplemented** by inhalation agents (such as nitrous oxide, halothane, enflurane, or isoflurane) or other IV drugs (such as diazepam). **Induction of anesthesia** is carried out with methohexital. **Maintenance of anesthesia** is achieved with 50% nitrous oxide and 50% oxygen through a nasal mask. This mixture is satisfactory for the extraction of one or two teeth. If a longer operating time is necessary, or if it is difficult to open the mouth, 1% halothane, 2% enflurane, or 2% isoflurane is added to the mixture.

d. **Effects and side effects of methohexital**

(1) **Cardiorespiratory depressant effects** (hypotension, apnea) may occur when the procedure is prolonged and more than 200 mg of methohexital is administered.

(2) **Hiccups** occur often following rapid IV injection of large doses. There is no threat to the patient, but the hiccuping may make surgery difficult.

(3) **Involuntary movements** (muscle twitchings and tremors) may occur. Diazepam, 5–10 mg, injected IV prior to the induction dose of methohexital may decrease the incidence of such movements.

(4) The competence of the **protective laryngeal reflexes** is compromised.

(5) **Recovery** following methohexital anesthesia is rapid.

6. **Inhalation anesthesia**

a. The methods of administering inhalation anesthesia for dental outpatients are similar to those used in the hospital operating room.

b. The patient is placed in the supine or semisupine position in the contour dental chair. **Induction of anesthesia** is carried out with IV methohexital or with an inhalation anesthetic. Nasotracheal intubation is facilitated with succinylcholine (preceded by pancuronium, 1 mg IV). **Maintenance of anesthesia** is achieved with nitrous oxide, oxygen, and halothane, enflurane, or isoflurane. Ventilation is assisted or controlled.

c. **When the patient is adequately anesthetized,** the dentist puts in place a mouth prop and pharyngeal packs and then begins the procedure. On completion of the surgery and return of the patient's protective reflexes, the patient is extubated. He remains in the recovery area until fully recovered (at least 2 hr), after which he may be discharged to go home accompanied by a responsible person.

d. **Nitrous oxide–oxygen analgesia**

(1) The term **analgesia** implies the loss of pain sensation without loss of consciousness. The administration of nitrous oxide–oxygen analgesia involves the use of an anesthesia machine marked **analgesia machine.** This machine has continuous or demand flow and is connected to a nasal mask through which the nitrous oxide–oxygen mixture is administered to the patient.

(2) Nitrous oxide–oxygen anesthesia may be produced with **concentrations of nitrous oxide that vary between 30 and 80%.** A 20% minimum of oxygen is always used. For most restorative dental procedures, concentrations of nitrous oxide below 50% are adequate to relax the patient. When 45–65% concentrations of nitrous oxide are used, nausea and vomiting may occur. As the concentration of nitrous oxide approaches 80%, loss of consciousness can occur, bringing on all the hazards of general anesthesia.

(3) Nitrous oxide–oxygen analgesia is widely accepted in dental practice. However, it must be kept in mind that **nitrous oxide is an anesthetic**

and must always be administered in accordance with the basic principles of anesthesia, even when it is administered as an analgesic.

7. Intravenous sedation

a. Sedative drugs decrease the discomfort of dental therapy but also prolong the recovery time. When they are used, facilities should be available to permit patients to recover slowly and safely.

b. Sedatives can be given by mouth; however, this route of administration is unpredictable in timing and effectiveness. The **IV route** predictably produces a tranquil situation because the dose is adjustable to individual requirements with no ventilatory or cardiovascular depression.

c. One method of IV sedation (Jorgensen), which uses **pentobarbital, meperidine, and scopolamine,** provides sedation, analgesia, and amnesia. Pentobarbital, 5 mg, is given IV, and a few minutes later doses of 10 mg each are injected at 30-sec intervals until the patient begins to feel sleepy and the vision starts to blur. Up to 100 mg can be administered. This is followed by slow IV injection of a mixture of meperidine (25 mg) and scopolamine (0.4 mg). The patient, in a cooperative state of light sedation, can now receive the injections of the local anesthetic without discomfort. During this IV sedation procedure, respiratory depression and vomiting may occur. To prevent this, **the Jorgensen technique can be modified** by using smaller doses of pentobarbital and by replacing meperidine and scopolamine with methohexital.

d. Diazepam is a sedative and amnesic drug with good cardiovascular stability. The IV dose is up to 0.2 mg/kg; as the dose is increased, the respiratory depression is also increased.

(1) The patient should be in **the supine position.** Incremental doses of diazepam (2.5–5 mg) are injected slowly IV until the patient seems relaxed and in a sedated state—slurred speech and blepharoptosis to a midpupil level are indications of an adequate state of sedation. A maximum of 20 mg should be injected to achieve this state. Higher doses will induce general anesthesia.

(2) The IV injection of diazepam should be made slowly into a rapidly running IV solution and into a large vein; solid push will irritate the vein and often leaves a sore arm and vein postoperatively. Injections into small veins may be painful and may lead to venous thrombosis. The injection of the local anesthetic can be carried out immediately after diazepam has been injected. This method provides satisfactory surgical conditions even in the most nervous patient. For prolonged procedures, diazepam may be supplemented with methohexital.

(3) Recovery is prolonged, but most patients may be safely discharged, accompanied by a responsible person, within 2 hr of injection of the drug.

e. Neuroleptanalgesia (see Chap. 11, sec. **II**) is a state characterized by somnolence without total unconsciousness, psychological indifference to the environment, no voluntary movements, analgesia, and satisfactory amnesia.

(1) The technique of neuroleptanalgesia calls for the administration of a neuroleptic drug (tranquilizer) and a narcotic analgesic drug, injected IV either individually or in combination. **Droperidol** is the neuroleptic drug, and **fentanyl** is the synthetic narcotic analgesic drug. **Innovar** is a mixture of droperidol and fentanyl in a ratio of 50:1. Each milliliter contains 2.5 mg of droperidol and 0.05 mg of fentanyl. **Innovar is not recommended** for outpatient dental sedation.

(2) **Droperidol** is a long-acting tranquilizer and is administered IV in a dose up to 0.1 mg/kg. **Fentanyl** is then added in increments, with the total dose not exceeding 0.1 mg (2 ml). This dose of fentanyl is not adequate to accomplish analgesia for dental procedures; usually it is supplemented with nitrous oxide–oxygen inhalation and/or local anesthetic block.

(3) **Respiratory depression** may occur following the injection of fentanyl. This effect can be reversed by IV administration of a narcotic antagonist **(naloxone).**

(4) Satisfactory application of this technique, as with all the other sedation techniques, requires that it be carried out by one who is **well trained in anesthesia** and prepared to manage its complications.

III. Inpatient dental anesthesia

A. Indications for inpatient dental surgery

1. Patients requiring extensive dental surgery, such as extraction of impacted wisdom teeth.
2. Patients whose general health contraindicates outpatient dental therapy. Among these are patients with cardiovascular or lung disease, mental retardation, diabetes, and hemorrhagic disorders and pregnant patients.

B. Management of general anesthesia

1. The patient is **premedicated** with a sedative and atropine. **In the operating room,** the patient is placed in the **supine position,** and the monitors for BP, ECG, and respiration are attached. An IV route is started in the hand with an 18-gauge plastic catheter running with 1000 ml of lactated Ringer's solution in 5% D/W. The nasal mucosa is sprayed with 0.5% phenylephrine or 4% cocaine.
2. **Induction of anesthesia** is accomplished by IV injection of 1 mg of pancuronium. This is followed by IV administration of 250–300 mg of thiopental and 100 mg of succinylcholine.
3. **Nasotracheal intubation** with a cuffed tube with a 5–6.5 mm ID is performed following hyperventilation with oxygen. However, **nasal bleeding** may result, especially in a patient with a history of hypertension or hemorrhagic disorder. In addition, **infection** present in the nose may be transmitted to the lungs.
4. **Maintenance of anesthesia** is carried out with nitrous oxide, oxygen, and halothane, enflurane, or isoflurane. Respiration is assisted or controlled. Following extubation, the patient is placed on the side.
5. **During the recovery period,** respiratory obstruction, emergence excitement, or shivering may occur and must be managed.

IV. Major oral and maxillofacial surgery

A. Surgery for the correction of jaw deformities is performed on patients who usually are young and healthy. **Osteotomies of the mandible and/or maxilla** vary in complexity and may require bone grafts.

1. **Nasotracheal intubation** is performed using thiopental and succinylcholine, and a nasogastric tube is inserted. Anesthesia is maintained by (a) nitrous oxide, oxygen, and halothane, enflurane, or isoflurane or (b) nitrous oxide, oxygen, and narcotics with muscle relaxants. Ventilation is assisted or controlled.
2. **Blood loss** may be serious enough to require blood transfusion.
3. At the end of surgery, **the jaws are immobilized** with elastic bands or wires.

4. **In the recovery room,** the nasogastric tube is connected to the suction apparatus. Extubation is performed when the patient is fully recovered from the anesthetics, and a nasopharyngeal airway is inserted. During the recovery period, **wire cutters** should remain near the patient in case of an emergency, so that the elastic bands or wires may be cut if severe ventilatory obstruction occurs and cannot be relieved by simple measures.

5. **Postoperative vomiting** can be prevented by evacuation of the gastric contents with a continuously functioning nasogastric tube, and administration of antiemetic drugs. If vomiting occurs, the patient is placed on the side, which allows the vomitus to drain through the space between the molar teeth and cheek.

B. **Serious difficulties** may be encountered during insertion of the nasotracheal tube in patients with diseases for which hemimandibulectomy, hemiglossectomy, and maxillary resection, with or without neck dissection, are required.

1. Displacement of normal structures in these patients may require **awake or blind intubation,** which is best carried out with topical anesthesia, IV injection of sedatives and amnesic drugs, and spontaneous respiration.

2. These operations are of long duration, and large amounts of **blood loss** are to be expected.

3. **A hypotensive technique** may be indicated.

4. At the completion of surgery, a **tracheotomy** may be performed.

C. **Maxillofacial surgery**

1. **Acute trauma** may cause a variety of maxillofacial injuries, ranging from a fracture of the nasal bones, requiring simple reduction, to complicated injuries involving the facial bones, nose, maxilla, mandible, and considerable soft tissue damage. **Concomitant injuries** to the head, chest, abdomen, and/or extremities, with or without loss of consciousness, may be present.

2. **Immediate surgery** for repair of maxillofacial injuries is required in the presence of uncontrollable bleeding or an obstructed airway. **An obstructed airway** occurs often because blood, teeth, and/or dentures are lying in the pharynx. If the obstructed airway cannot be relieved, a **tracheotomy** is performed under local anesthesia.

3. **There may be bleeding** in the mouth and pharynx, so the stomach may contain swallowed blood; further, the patient may have had a recent meal. These factors must always be taken into account in managing anesthesia in these patients.

4. **Management of general anesthesia**

   a. **For premedication,** only atropine is given.

   b. **An awake tracheal intubation** is accomplished under topical anesthesia and sedative drugs. If the mouth can be opened adequately, intubation is carried out with thiopental and succinylcholine. The decision for nasal or oral intubation lies with the oral surgeon and anesthesiologist.

5. **A nasotracheal intubation is contraindicated** when cerebrospinal fluid is draining from the nose.

6. **Maintenance of anesthesia** is usually carried out by (a) nitrous oxide, oxygen, and halothane, enflurane, or isoflurane or (b) nitrous oxide, oxygen, and narcotics with muscle relaxants. Respiration is assisted or controlled.

7. **The recovery room.** When the jaws have been wired together, the patient should leave the operating room with the nasotracheal or orotracheal tube in place. In the recovery room, the nasogastric tube is connected to the suction apparatus, and a pair of **wire cutters** is placed near the patient so they can be

used in an emergency to free the jaws. **Extubation** is performed when the patient is fully awake.

D. **Craniofacial surgical (LeForte osteotomy) procedures** require tracheotomy; harvesting of rib and iliac crest grafts; LeForte III osteotomy in the facial bones to position them properly; LeForte I osteotomy in the bones of the upper jaw to position teeth properly after other facial bones are moved; application of a metal head frame around the head to aid in positioning of the bones; craniotomy as indicated to protect the brain while the facial bones are incised; application of intermaxillary fixation; and wiring together of jaws.

1. LeForte osteotomy procedures are **the longest** elective surgical and anesthetic procedures and require extensive soft tissue dissection, fracturing of bones, and blood replacement. Total expected time for the duration of anesthesia and surgery is 10–14 hr.

2. **Anesthetic considerations.** Craniofacial surgery is especially stressful for the patient because of the duration and location of the surgery, as well as the massive loss of blood, which is very difficult to measure. Thus in anesthesia management of craniofacial surgical patients, attention is directed to blood replacement and the cardiovascular, respiratory, thermoregulatory, and the central nervous systems.

3. **Management of anesthesia**

   a. **Premedication** includes a sedative and atropine.

   b. **Induction of anesthesia** and intubation are achieved with thiopental and succinylcholine. **A tracheotomy** is performed, and **maintenance of anesthesia** is carried out through a tracheotomy tube with (1) nitrous oxide, oxygen, and halothane, enflurane, or isoflurane or (2) nitrous oxide, oxygen, and narcotics with muscle relaxants. Respiration is assisted or controlled.

   c. **Arterial, central venous pressure, and Foley catheters** are placed, blood volume is determined, and a rectal probe for monitoring body temperature is inserted. The patient's head is shaved, and the needle electrodes for an electroencephalogram are sutured in the biparieto-occipital areas.

   d. **Monitoring the cardiovascular system.** The continuous **direct arterial pressure reading** is the most important monitor. In addition, the arterial line helps in the evaluation of blood gases values by giving information on PO_2, PCO_2, pH, and hematocrit.

   e. **Blood replacement.** Fresh blood and platelets are administered to replace clotting factors at the end of surgery unless their use is indicated earlier.

   f. The main considerations concerning **the respiratory system** are the humidification of the anesthetic gases and the establishment and maintenance of the airway.

   g. **Hypotensive anesthesia** is useful in shortening the length of surgery and in lessening the degree of blood loss and replacement. Use of the elective hypotensive state is limited to two separate periods: the first during the coronal flap and orbital osteotomies and the second during the LeForte I osteotomies. Anticipated time for the first stage is 1 hr and for the second stage, 2½ hr.

4. **Recovery period.** The patient is extubated when fully awake and vital signs are stable.

Bibliography

Alexander, J. P., and Murtagh, J. G. Arrhythmia during oral surgery. Fascicular blocks in the cardiac conducting system. *Br. J. Anaesth.* 51:149, 1979.

Brodsky, J. B., Cohen, E. N., Brown, B. W., et al. Exposure to nitrous oxide and neurologic disease among dental professionals. *Anesth. Analg.* (Cleve.) 60:297, 1981.

Cleaton-Jones, P., Austin, J. C., Moyes, D. G., et al. Nitrous oxide contamination in dental surgeries using relative analgesia. *Br. J. Anaesth.* 50:1091, 1978.

Cohen, E. N., Brown, B. W., Bruce, D. L., et al. A survey of anesthetic health hazards among dentists. *J. Am. Dent. Assoc.* 90:1291, 1975.

Cohen, E. N., Brown, B. W., Wu, M. L., et al. Occupational disease in dentistry and exposure to waste anesthetic gases. *J. Am. Dent. Assoc.* 101:21, 1980.

Gutmann, L., Farrell, B., Crosby, T. W., et al. Nitrous oxide-induced myeloneuropathy: Potential for chronic misuse by dentists. *J. Am. Dent. Assoc.* 98:58, 1979.

Layzer, R. B. Myeloneuropathy after prolonged exposure to nitrous oxide. *Lancet* 2:1227, 1978.

Layzer, R. B., Fishman, R. A., and Schafer, J. A. Neuropathy following abuse of nitrous oxide. *Neurology* (Minneap.) 28:504, 1978.

Michenfelder, J. D. Exposure to anesthetic gases and health problems in dental workers. *Anesthesiology* 53:1, 1980.

Spence, A. A., Cohen, E. N., Brown, B. W., et al. Occupational hazards for operating room-based physicians. *J.A.M.A.* 238:955, 1977.

Thompson, J. M., Barratt, R. S., Hutton, P., et al. Ambient air contamination in a dental outpatient theatre. *Br. J. Anaesth.* 51:845, 1979.

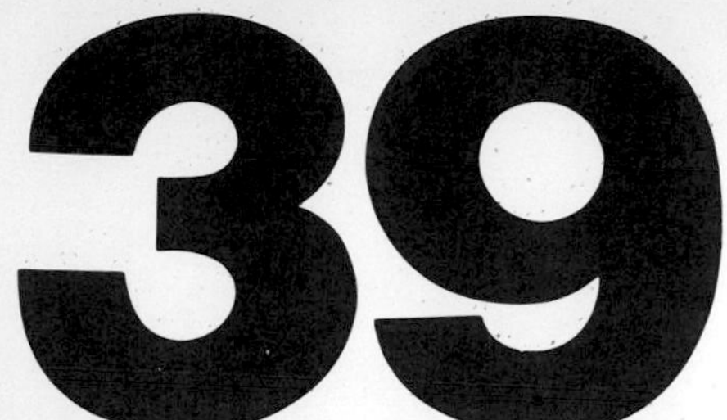

Anesthesia in Ophthalmology

I. General considerations

A. Anesthesia for ophthalmic surgery

1. **In children,** ophthalmic surgery is done under general endotracheal anesthesia. The most frequent indications for surgery are strabismus, blepharoptosis, congenital cataracts, congenital glaucoma, and eye injuries.

2. **In adults,** ophthalmic surgery is carried out under either local or general anesthesia. Major orbital procedures, extensive plastic repairs, and prolonged operations for detached retina require general endotracheal anesthesia.

3. The presence of the diathermy machine, photocoagulator, and other electrical instruments **precludes the use of flammable anesthetics.**

4. **Little muscle relaxation** is required. Muscle relaxants are used to facilitate endotracheal intubation and for maintenance of light anesthesia.

5. **Epinephrine** 1:200,000 is included in local anesthetic solutions for hemostasis or prolongation of local anesthesia. The use of **halothane is not precluded** by this use of small amounts of epinephrine.

6. **The oculocardiac reflex,** activated by pressure on the eyeball or by traction on the extraocular muscles, results in bradycardia and cardiac arrhythmias; it may even cause temporary or permanent cardiac arrest. The afferent limb of the reflex is the ophthalmic branch of the **trigeminal nerve,** and the efferent limb is the **vagus nerve** to the heart. The undesirable reflexes can be reduced or eliminated by IV injection of atropine before surgery and/or retrobulbar nerve block.

7. **Atropine and glaucoma**

    a. There is no danger in using atropine or scopolamine IM for preoperative medication in patients with open-angle glaucoma. A dose of atropine (up to 0.5 mg) or scopolamine (up to 0.5 mg) may be administered.

    b. **Topical application** of an anticholinergic drug (atropine, amprotropine, cyclopentolate, homatropine, or scopolamine) may induce narrow-angle glaucoma in 1 out of 4000 persons over 30 years of age. **Systemic administration** of the same drugs may produce similar effects in the eye, but the amount of drug reaching the eye is much smaller and the intensity of its effects is proportionately reduced.

8. **Abrasion of the cornea** may be caused by the anesthesia face mask or surgical drapes. The eyelids of the nonsurgical eye should be sealed with a bland ophthalmic ointment.

9. **During intraocular surgery,** every effort must be made to maintain the intraocular pressure at or below normal levels. **Succinylcholine is contraindicated.**

B. The anesthesiologist and the anesthesia machine are placed together at one side of the patient, preferably at the side opposite the surgical field. This will secure both a sterile surgical field and ample space for the ophthalmologist and assistants.

1. **Local anesthesia** is the responsibility of the ophthalmologist. However, the anesthesiologist or nurse-anesthetist may be asked to monitor the vital signs during surgery, to administer additional sedative or analgesic drugs, or to treat oversedation or toxic reactions produced by local anesthetics.

2. **One drop of 1% atropine** may contain 1 mg. One drop of epinephrine 1:1000 may contain 0.1 mg. One drop of 10% phenylephrine may contain 10 mg. These doses may have systemic effects.

II. Intraocular pressure

A. The normal intraocular pressure is up to 21 torr. Maintenance of the intraocular pressure at a normal level depends on the following factors:

1. **Aqueous humor.** The intraocular pressure is a function of the ratio between formation of the aqueous humor, produced by the ciliary epithelium, and the resistance to its outflow. An increase or decrease in either formation or absorption will result in a change in the intraocular pressure. The aqueous humor from the posterior chamber enters the anterior chamber through the pupillary opening. In the anterior chamber, the aqueous humor flows peripherally, and by the filtering process it enters Schlemm's canal, which leads to the venous systemic circulation.

2. **Blood pressure.** The intraocular pressure is increased when there is an increase in the venous pressure of the orbital veins.

3. **Other factors.** The intraocular pressure can be increased by (a) contraction of the orbicular muscles of the eye (squeezing of the eye) or of the extraocular muscles, digital pressure, or pressure caused by a poorly placed retractor and (b) coughing, sneezing, retching, vomiting, breath-holding, hypoxia, hypercapnia, or resistance to expiration. All increase the venous pressure and hence the intraocular pressure. In addition, venous congestion increases bleeding during surgery.

B. Control of intraocular pressure

1. When the intraocular pressure is intermittently or constantly increased, the condition is referred to as **glaucoma.** This condition can create degeneration of the optic nerve and atrophy of the retina.

2. **For treatment,** various methods are used. These include acetazolamide (Diamox), instillation of miotics (pilocarpine, physostigmine, or echothiophate). Recently, topical beta blockers (timolol) have been proved to be extremely effective. However, the topical administration of timolol may produce systemic beta blockade. For acute episodes, the administration of dehydrating agents (glycerin, urea, or mannitol) is indicated.

   a. **Miotics** increase the efficiency of the outflow channels and the elimination of aqueous humor. Some of the miotics are cholinesterase inhibitors, such as echothiophate (Phospholine).

   b. **Glaucoma and succinylcholine.** Instillation of echothiophate solution in the eyes of glaucoma patients markedly depresses both plasma and red cell pseudocholinesterase levels. **Prolonged apnea** may follow the administration of succinylcholine. **Echothiophate** is a long-acting miotic; after it is discontinued, it takes 4–6 weeks for the normal pseudocholinesterase action to return. Succinylcholine should be used carefully in patients who have received echothiophate eyedrops within 6 weeks before general anesthesia. These patients may have a decreased pseudocholinesterase effect that is sufficient to reduce the metabolism of succinylcholine and thus prolong its neuromuscular effect.

c. **Mannitol and urea** are osmotic diuretics and have the ability to move fluids from the extracellular space to the IV circulation. These agents should be administered cautiously, especially in patients with impaired heart or kidney function.

3. **Surgery is indicated** early in acute glaucoma and in the later stages of chronic glaucoma, if medical therapy is no longer adequate.

III. Influence of anesthetics and muscle relaxants on intraocular pressure

A. During general anesthesia

1. **A decrease in intraocular pressure** proportional to the depth of anesthesia occurs during general anesthesia with all general anesthetic drugs. This is partly the result of decreased tone of the extraocular muscles.

2. **An increase of intraocular pressure** may occur during general anesthesia due to an increase in central venous pressure caused by straining, coughing, retching, vomiting, breath-holding, obstruction of the upper respiratory airway, or tightness of the chest.

3. **Hyperventilation decreases** intraocular pressure, and **hypoventilation increases** it.

B. Ketamine is a nonbarbiturate, short-acting anesthetic drug. Unlike other anesthetic agents, ketamine increases intraocular pressure. There is no association between this change and either changes in BP or the patient's age.

C. All nerve blocks used in ophthalmic surgery decrease intraocular pressure by relaxing the extraocular muscles.

D. Muscle relaxants

1. **Tubocurarine** lowers intraocular pressure by relaxing the extraocular muscles. **It is safe to use** during ophthalmic surgery. It causes relaxation of eye muscles and limits eye movements, so it prevents vitreous prolapse during intraocular surgery.

2. **Gallamine** (Flaxedil) and **pancuronium** (Pavulon) have effects similar to those of tubocurarine.

3. **Succinylcholine** increases intraocular pressure and should be **used very carefully** during eye surgery.

   a. **It increases intraocular pressure** by causing a sustained contraction of the extraocular muscles. This increase is of short duration (3–5 min) and is not directly related to the duration of neuromuscular block.

   b. Succinylcholine can be used safely for tracheal intubation in ophthalmic surgery, since any elevation in intraocular pressure is dissipated by the time surgery is begun. However, **it should never be injected during intraocular surgery.**

   c. **Succinylcholine is contraindicated** during cataract extraction when the eye is open, repair of lacerated cornea, or other penetrating wounds of the eye. The sudden compression of the eye may lead to catastrophic expulsion of intraocular contents.

IV. Anesthesia management

A. Preanesthetic preparation. See Chapter 1.

B. Preanesthesia medication. See Chapter 3.

C. Monitoring. See Chapter 6.

V. Topical, infiltration, and nerve block anesthesia

A. Topical (surface) anesthesia of the eye is achieved with proparacaine (Ophthaine), benoxinate (Dorsacaine), or tetracaine (Pontocaine). These drugs are adequate for tonometry, minor procedures such as removal of superficially embedded foreign bodies, or irrigation of the eye following chemical irritation. **Cocaine should not be used** in ophthalmology, because it causes desiccation of the corneal epithelium and delays healing.

B. Any topical anesthetic delays healing, but there is no real problem if it is instilled only during surgery.

C. **Infiltration and nerve block anesthesia** for ophthalmic surgery can be accomplished with local anesthetics, such as 2% procaine, 2% lidocaine, 2% mepivacaine, or 0.5% bupivacaine. Epinephrine 1:200,000 may be added as indicated.

VI. **Surgery of the eyelids and lacrimal apparatus**

A. **Blepharoptosis** is characterized by drooping of the upper eyelid.

1. **Myasthenia gravis** should be suspected in every patient with blepharoptosis. It is gradual in onset, appearing in the evening with fatigue and improving during the night. A test with neostigmine or edrophonium will aid in the diagnosis.
2. **Surgery on the eyelids** in children requires general endotracheal anesthesia with nitrous oxide, oxygen, and halothane or enflurane. In adults it is usually performed under local anesthesia.

B. **The lacrimal apparatus** consists of the lacrimal gland, the lacrimal sac, and the nasolacrimal duct.

1. **Probing of the nasolacrimal duct** in infants is a short procedure carried out on an outpatient basis. For anesthesia, nitrous oxide, oxygen, and halothane are administered by mask.
2. **Excision of a lacrimal tumor** is done under general endotracheal anesthesia.
3. **Dacryocystectomy** (excision of the lacrimal sac) is performed under local or general endotracheal anesthesia.
4. **Dacryocystorhinostomy** (establishment of a communication through the bone between the lacrimal sac and the nasal cavity) is done under local or general endotracheal anesthesia.

VII. **Surgery on the conjunctiva, cornea, and lens**

A. **The pterygium** resembles a wing and extends from the conjunctiva to the center of the cornea. In adults, excision of the pterygium or transplantation of its head under the conjunctiva in the lower conjunctival sac is done under topical and local anesthesia.

B. **Corneal transplantation (keratoplasty)**

1. **A donor cornea** can be obtained from an enucleated eye with a normal cornea or from an eye removed after the death of the donor. Such removal is performed under sterile conditions immediately after death, and the transplantation surgery is performed as soon as possible.
2. A disc of clear cornea is separated **from the donor eye** with a trephine. The same trephine is used to remove the opaque portion of the cornea from the **recipient eye.** The donor cornea is then sutured into place.
3. **Surgery in children** is done under general endotracheal anesthesia and **in adults** under local or general endotracheal anesthesia. **Induction of anesthesia** and endotracheal intubation are accomplished with thiopental and succinylcholine. **For maintenance,** (a) nitrous oxide and oxygen with halothane or enflurane and assisted respiration or (b) nitrous oxide, oxygen, narcotics with muscle relaxants, and controlled respiration. During extubation and the recovery period, every effort must be made to avoid hypoxia, restlessness, and vomiting.

C. Cataract extraction

1. **Intracapsular extraction** of a cataract is the surgical removal of a cataractous lens with its capsule intact; in the United States it is usually performed in adults under local anesthesia. **Extracapsular extraction** includes the removal of a cataractous lens after rupturing the lens capsule; it is performed in children under general endotracheal anesthesia.

2. **Cataract extraction in adults** under **local anesthesia** is a safe practice provided the intraocular pressure is under control at all times.

   a. **When the eye is opened,** the intraocular pressure should be as low as possible. If the pressure is high at the time of incision, with a sudden loss of pressure, the iris, lens, vitreous, and retina may be expelled through the incision, resulting in severe visual impairment or even blindness.

   b. **For adequate local anesthesia and akinesia,** it is necessary to immobilize the orbicular and extraocular muscles and to anesthetize the ocular structures. Surface anesthesia is achieved with a few drops of 0.5% proparacaine instilled into the conjunctival sac. Paralysis of the orbicular muscle is done with 2% lidocaine with epinephrine 1:100,000, using the Van Lint, O'Brien, or Atkinson method. This is followed by a retrobulbar injection with 2% lidocaine into the muscle cone to anesthetize the ciliary ganglion and the nerves to the extraocular muscles.

3. **General anesthesia in adults**

   a. Following induction and intubation with thiopental and succinylcholine, anesthesia is maintained with nitrous oxide and oxygen with halothane or enflurane and assisted ventilation.

   b. Every effort should be made during anesthesia, extubation, the recovery period, and the first 24 hr to prevent coughing, straining, and vomiting.

   c. Succinylcholine causes a sharp increase in intraocular pressure for a very short time, which dissipates prior to surgery. **Succinylcholine should not be administered during surgery.**

D. Congenital cataracts associated with congenital heart disease may occur as a result of maternal rubella (German measles) during the first 2 months of pregnancy.

1. **Surgical treatment**

   a. Discission (needling) of the lens.

   b. Linear extraction.

   c. Aspiration.

2. General endotracheal anesthesia is accomplished with nitrous oxide and oxygen with halothane or enflurane and assisted respiration.

3. Coughing, straining, or vomiting will not endanger the successful removal of an extracapsular congenital or traumatic cataract.

VIII. Glaucoma

A. Glaucoma is a condition characterized by **increased intraocular pressure.** It is due to interference in the outflow mechanism of the aqueous humor, and it may cause impairment of vision that can progress to blindness.

B. Classification of glaucoma

1. **Primary glaucoma.**

   a. **In open-angle glaucoma,** there is increased resistance to the flow of the aqueous humor through the trabecular meshwork.

b. **In narrow-angle glaucoma,** the iris obstructs entrance of the aqueous humor into the trabecular meshwork.

2. **Congenital glaucoma.**

3. **Secondary glaucoma** results from the preexisting condition of the eye structures, such as uveitis, hemorrhage, tumor, trauma, or enlarged cataract.

C. **The diagnosis** is made by tonometry, gonioscopy, tonography, ophthalmoscopy, and perimetry.

D. **The medical treatment of glaucoma** includes administration of miotics: pilocarpine, physostigmine, echothiophate, isoflurophate, carbonic anhydrase inhibitors (acetazolamide), and dehydrating agents (glycerin, urea, or mannitol). **Echothiophate** may cause prolonged apnea in the postanesthesia recovery period following injection of succinylcholine.

E. **Surgical techniques** performed to control the intraocular pressure include peripheral iridectomy, iridencleisis, trephination with iridectomy, sclerectomy, trabeculectomy, cyclodialysis, and goniotomy.

F. **Anesthesia management. In adults** the surgical procedures are carried out under local anesthesia. **In children,** general endotracheal anesthesia is indicated, using nitrous oxide and oxygen with halothane or enflurane and assisted ventilation.

IX. Surgery of the retina

A. **Detachment of the retina.** A hole or tear in the retina permits vitreous fluid to enter behind the retina. An untreated detached retina may become total; when this happens, the patient may permanently lose vision in the affected eye.

1. **Contributing factors.** It is estimated that one out of every four adult patients requiring surgery for repair of a detached retina has, or has had, emphysema, bronchial asthma, obesity, hypertension, a myocardial infarct, coronary heart disease, or diabetes. Trauma (including cataract surgery) and myopia are important contributing factors.

2. **Management of anesthesia**

a. The surgical treatment of retinal detachment is an extensive procedure requiring general endotracheal anesthesia and lasting 1–5 hr. A reoperation lasts longer.

b. Induction of anesthesia and intubation are carried out with thiopental and succinylcholine. Anesthesia is maintained with (1) nitrous oxide and oxygen with halothane or enflurane and assisted respiration or (2) nitrous oxide and oxygen, narcotics with muscle relaxants, and controlled ventilation.

c. During this long period of general anesthesia, a very thin scleral layer remains. Under light anesthesia, the patient may start coughing, straining, or squeezing the eye, causing a sudden increase in intraocular pressure that may rupture the eye with serious complications.

3. **Surgical therapy** includes the following techniques:

a. Scleral buckling with a circling element.

b. Trap-door operation.

c. Retinopexy.

d. Photocoagulation with a xenon arc photocoagulator.

e. Cryosurgery.

f. Following the primary operation, reoperation may be done using a silicone implant with an encircling silicone band.

4. **In the recovery room,** nausea and vomiting may respond successfully to trimethobenzamide (Tigan), droperidol (Inapsine), or phenothiazines (Compazine, Trilafon, Phenergan).

B. Giant retinal breaks

1. In an occasional patient, retinal detachment is associated with a giant retinal break that extends 90 degrees or more over the circumference of the eye.
2. The surgical treatment of giant retinal breaks requires general endotracheal anesthesia lasting 5–7 hr.
3. The patient is placed in the supine position on a power-driven multipositional operating table and is secured by leather and heavy web canvas straps attached to the sides of the operating table and extending across the patient's legs, thighs, abdomen, and chest.
4. Anesthesia is induced with 2.5% thiopental IV. Endotracheal intubation is facilitated by administration of succinylcholine. This is followed by nitrous oxide and oxygen with halothane or enflurane and assisted ventilation.
5. The positional changes necessitate the use of breathing tubes twice the length (190 cm) of the regular tubes (95 cm).
6. During surgery **the patient is rotated to the prone position,** which unfolds the retinal flap. Great care must be taken to do this slowly. A headrest is placed on the patient's forehead to maintain the position of the head.
7. The patient is placed high enough to enable **the ophthalmologist to operate under the patient,** facing the patient's head, which remains in the perpendicular position. When the retina has been satisfactorily incarcerated, the patient is returned to the supine position for completion of the operation.

C. Vitrectomy.

Vitrectomy. The vitreous body is a gel that fills the interior of the eye between the lens and the retina. It contains a lacy network of collagen fibers, which insert into the retina.

1. The most common vitreous disease requiring surgery is vitreous bleeding. This is usually due to diabetic retinopathy, but may also be caused by retinal vein occlusions, trauma, sickle cell disease, or other conditions.
2. In many persons, the vitreous body degenerates with age and begins to liquefy, ultimately collapsing on itself. When collapse occurs, residual attachments of the vitreous body to the retina may create traction and retinal hole formation. It is this process that causes most retinal detachments. However, most detachments can be treated by scleral buckling without vitrectomy.
3. In a few patients, vitreous traction on the retina may be so severe that both vitrectomy and scleral buckling are required. Also, vitrectomy may be required in the presence of a retinal detachment with vitreous bleeding when the ophthalmologist cannot adequately visualize the retina. Additional indications for vitrectomy may be diabetic traction retinal detachment, vitreous bleeding, membrane or retinal detachment due to trauma, or other causes of vitreous opacity.
4. The most common technique for vitrectomy is the so-called pars plana vitrectomy, performed with small cutters through the pars plana region of the eye, under microscopic visualization through a corneal contact lens. This operation may be extremely delicate and requires general anesthesia. When the instruments are inside the eye, it is crucial that patient movement or movement of the operating table does not occur; thus local anesthesia is not used.
5. The preoperative evaluation and preparation and the management of general endotracheal anesthesia is similar to that in patients with retinal detachment.

6. Many of the patients who require vitrectomy have long-standing diabetes, which complicates anesthetic management. Renal failure, hypertension, coronary artery disease, and arrhythmias are common in these patients.

7. During vitrectomy, intraocular fiberoptics are used for visualization. The view is improved by extinguishing all lights, and the anesthesiologist may then have to work with flashlights only.

8. In some patients, scleral buckling may be carried out with vitrectomy.

X. Strabismus (squint)

A. **Surgery on the extraocular muscles** for correction of strabismus is the most common eye procedure in **children.** It is performed in children under general endotracheal anesthesia and in adults under local or general anesthesia.

B. **During surgery,** pinching of the conjunctiva or traction and manipulation of the extraocular muscles, particularly the medial rectus, frequently activates the **oculocardiac reflex.** This is detected by the electrocardioscope. Bradycardia and other cardiac irregularities due to this reflex can be treated with IV atropine and/or retrobulbar injection of a local anesthetic solution. The oculocardiac reflex is explained anatomically through the interaction between the trigeminal nerve and the vagus nerve.

XI. Trauma and tumors

A. **A foreign body** on the cornea or conjunctiva is removed under topical anesthesia with a cotton applicator moistened with saline. The cornea is anesthetized by instilling into the conjunctival sac 2–3 drops of 0.5% proparacaine. Instillation of 1–2 drops of sterile **2% fluorescein** into the conjunctival sac helps to localize a foreign body on the cornea and also indicates the extent of the injury, since any corneal abnormality is stained by the fluorescein and thus can be easily visualized.

B. **Penetrating foreign bodies** are removed as soon as feasible under local or general endotracheal anesthesia.

C. **Lacerations and penetrating eye injuries**

1. **Sealing a leaking wound** and releasing tissues incarcerated in it are urgent tasks. Uveal tissue incarcerated in the wound carries a risk of infection and sympathetic ophthalmia.

2. **A ruptured globe** is sutured immediately to prevent loss of the eye. Prompt surgery is best performed in adults and in children under general endotracheal anesthesia.

3. **A lacerated eye** presents few anesthesia problems. However, the patient may be under the influence of alcohol or may have a full stomach, and any delay in surgery increases the problems of the ophthalmologist. If possible, it is advisable to wait until the stomach empties itself spontaneously.

4. **During induction of anesthesia,** the face mask is placed carefully to avoid any pressure on the injured eye. In the presence of a **penetrating wound,** tubocurarine or pancuronium is used as a muscle relaxant. **Succinylcholine increases the intraocular pressure and so is contraindicated.**

5. **Repair of a lacerated cornea in a child** is considered an **emergency** and is carried out under general endotracheal anesthesia.

D. **Orbital injuries.** Application of a blunt force to the eye may result in fragmentation of the thin bone forming the orbital floor and the roof of the maxillary antrum (blowout fracture) without fracture of the orbital rim, and the contents of the orbit herniate downward into the maxillary antrum. Surgery lasts 3–4 hr and is done under general endotracheal anesthesia.

E. **Orbital tumors** are removed under local or general endotracheal anesthesia. **Exenteration** of the orbital contents may be indicated in the presence of a malignant tumor. A skin graft from the abdomen or inner thigh is used to line the orbit. Later the orbit is fitted with a prosthesis.

F. **The Kronlein operation** consists of resection of the lateral wall of the orbit for the excision of orbital tumors, especially those occupying the retrobulbar space. Surgery is performed under general endotracheal anesthesia. If bleeding is excessive, replacement by transfusion is required.

G. **Enucleation, evisceration, and exenteration**

1. **Enucleation** is excision of the eyeball.
2. **Evisceration** consists of removing the contents of the eye, with only the scleral shell remaining. Both operations are carried out under local or general endotracheal anesthesia.
3. **Orbital exenteration** is the removal of the orbital contents (eyeball, extraocular muscles, and connective tissue). It is a long operation, lasting 2–4 hr, and is done under general endotracheal anesthesia. If blood loss is significant, a replacement transfusion is indicated.

Bibliography

Ausinsch, B., Graves, S. A., Munson, E. S., et al. Intraocular pressures in children during isoflurane and halothane anesthesia. *Anesthesiology* 42:167, 1975.

Ausinsch, B., Rayburn, R. L., Munson, E. S., et al. Ketamine and intraocular pressure in children. *Anesth. Analg.* (Cleve.) 55:773, 1976.

Backer, C. L., Tinker, J. H., Robertson, D. M., et al. Myocardial reinfarction following local anesthesia for ophthalmic surgery. *Anesth. Analg.* (Cleve.) 59:257, 1980.

Balamoutsos, N. G., Droussou, F., Alevizou, F., et al. Pupil size during reversal of muscle relaxants. *Anesth. Analg.* (Cleve.) 59:615, 1980.

Batra, K. Y., and Bali, M. I. Corneal abrasions during general anesthesia. *Anesth. Analg.* (Cleve.) 56:363, 1977.

Cook, J. H. The effect of suxamethonium on intraocular pressure. *Anesthesia* 36:359, 1981.

Cross, D. A., and Krupin, T. Implications of the effects of general anesthesia on basal tear production. *Anesth. Analg.* (Cleve.) 56:35, 1977.

Cunningham, E. E., and Venkataraman, B. Cardiac arrest following fluorescein angiography. *J.A.M.A.* 242:2431. 1979.

Deglin, S. M., Deglin, E. A., and Chung, E. K. Acute myocardial infarction following fluorescein angiography. *Heart Lung* 6:505, 1977.

Duncalf, D., Goldman, K. S., McNeil, J. M., et al. Symposium on ocular care of the hospitalized patient. *Anesth. Rev.* 7:51 (July), 1980.

Fabian, L. W. What are your prime considerations in providing anesthesia for eye surgery? *Surv. Anesth.* 18:488, 1974.

Hess, J. B., and Pacurariu, R. I. Acute pulmonary edema following intravenous fluorescein angiography. *Am. J. Ophthalmol.* 82:567, 1976.

Joshi, C., and Bruce, D. L. Thiopental and succinylcholine. Action on intraocular pressure. *Anesth. Analg.* (Cleve.) 54:471, 1975.

Katz, H., Machida, R. C., Wooth, D. G., et al. A technic of general anesthesia for blepharoplasty and rhytidectomy. *Anesth. Analg.* (Cleve.) 55:165, 1976.

Litwiller, R. W., Difazio, C. A., and Rushia, E. L. Pancuronium and intraocular pressure. *Anesthesiology* 42:750, 1975.

Meyers, E. F., Krupin, T., Johnson, M., et al. Failure of nondepolarizing neuromuscular blockers to inhibit succinylcholine-induced increased intraocular pressure. A controlled study. *Anesthesiology* 48:149, 1978.

Meyers, E. F., Singer, P., and Otto, A. A controlled study of the effect of succinylcholine self-taming on intraocular pressure. *Anesthesiology* 53:72, 1980.

Meyers, E. F., and Wilson, S. Vitrectomy. A new challenge for the anesthesiologist. *Anesth. Analg.* (Cleve.) 54:58, 1975.

Peuler, M., Glass, D. D., and Arens, J. F. Ketamine and intraocular pressure. *Anesthesiology* 43:575, 1975.

Presbitero, J. V., Ruiz, R. S., Rigor, B. M., et al. Intraocular pressure during enflurane and neurolept anesthesia in adult patients undergoing ophthalmic surgery. *Anesth. Analg.* (Cleve.) 59:50, 1980.

Rieser, J. C., and Snow, J. C. Atropine and glaucoma. *Anesth. Analg.* (Cleve.) 55:460, 1976.

Runciman, J. C., Bowen-Wright, R. M., Welsh, N. H., et al. Intra-ocular pressure changes during halothane and enflurane anesthesia. *Br. J. Anaesth.* 50:371, 1978.

Snow, J. C. *Anesthesia in Otolaryngology and Ophthalmology* (2nd ed.). New York: Appleton-Crofts-Century, 1982.

Snow, J. C., Kripke, B. J., Norton, M. L., et al. Corneal injuries during general anesthesia. *Anesth. Analg.* (Cleve.) 54:465, 1975.

40 Anesthesia in Otolaryngology

I. General considerations

A. **Surgery in the ear, nose, oral cavity, pharynx, and larynx** has certain characteristics:

1. **The majority of the patients** are good anesthetic and surgical risks; many are young and free of degenerative, metabolic, or cardiovascular diseases.
2. **Many operations include the larynx or structures around the larynx,** with accompanying hazards of respiratory obstruction.
3. **Very little muscle relaxation** is required. Muscle relaxants are administered to facilitate endotracheal intubation, maintenance of light anesthesia, and/or endoscopic procedures. When the **facial nerve** is tested during mastoidectomy, tympanoplasty, facial nerve decompression, parotidectomy, or excision of acoustic neuroma, the use of muscle relaxants is contraindicated.
4. **The presence of electrocautery** and other electrical instruments precludes the use of flammable anesthetics.
5. **Epinephrine** 1:100,000 or 1:200,000 solution is often used for hemostasis or to increase the duration of effect of local anesthetic drugs. The use of **halothane** is not precluded by the use of minimal amounts of epinephrine. **Enflurane** (Ethrane) has documented compatibility with epinephrine; up to 10 ml of epinephrine 1:100,000 or 1:200,000 containing solution alone or in conjunction with local anesthetics may be injected subcutaneously at a rate of not more than 10 ml/min and no more than 30 ml/hr. More dilute solutions and reduced doses should be used in highly vascular areas.
6. **The anesthesiologist** and the anesthesia machine are placed at a distance from the patient's head to secure a sterile surgical field.

B. **Airway**

1. **It is very important that the airway be protected** from obstruction by blood, secretions, or instruments. Under general anesthesia, this can be achieved by insertion of an endotracheal tube with an inflatable cuff or by efficient pharyngeal packing. The presence of a flexible, nonkinkable tube is a great help. Recently, the technique of Venturi ventilation has been added to our armamentarium.
2. **General endotracheal anesthesia** is indicated for the majority of ear, nose, and throat operations. The use of an endotracheal tube ensures an unobstructed upper airway, reduces dead space, and prevents aspiration of the contents of the mouth and stomach.
3. **The presence of an endotracheal tube** is particularly useful for procedures in which the otolaryngologist and anesthesiologist compete for the patient's airway.

C. **Local and/or general anesthesia**

1. **Excessive bleeding** is the otolaryngologist's main reason for preferring local anesthesia.

2. Local anesthetic drugs

a. For infiltration and nerve block anesthesia

(1) Procaine 2–4% with or without epinephrine 1:200,000.

(2) Lidocaine 1–2% with or without epinephrine 1:200,000.

b. For surface (topical) anesthesia

(1) Cocaine 4%.

(2) Lidocaine 4%.

(3) Tetracaine 2%.

3. General anesthetic drugs used are:

a. Nitrous oxide, oxygen, and halothane or enflurane with spontaneous or assisted ventilation.

b. Nitrous oxide, oxygen, narcotics, and muscle relaxant drugs with controlled ventilation.

II. Anesthesia management

A. Preanesthetic preparation. See Chapter 1.

B. Preanesthesia medication. See Chapter 3.

C. Monitoring. See Chapter 6.

III. Operations on the ear

A. Otoplasty

1. Abnormally protruding auricles (lop ears) are the most common deformity of the external ears; **in children** the surgery is performed under general anesthesia and **in adults** under local anesthesia.

2. Correction of other external abnormalities (macrotia, microtia) is performed under general endotracheal anesthesia.

B. Foreign body in the ear. Removal of a foreign body from the external auditory canal can be done **in adults** under local anesthesia and **in children** with general anesthesia. Ordinarily this procedure is performed on an outpatient basis.

C. Myringotomy (paracentesis tympani)

1. Incision of the tympanic membrane is brief; the great majority of patients are children.

2. Most myringotomies, with or without insertion of middle ear ventilation tubes (using the Zeiss operating microscope), are performed electively. However, in acute purulent otitis media, **emergency paracentesis tympani** may be indicated. These operations can be carried out under general anesthesia on an outpatient basis, provided that intake of food has been restricted for at least 4–6 hr.

3. General anesthesia with nitrous oxide, oxygen, and halothane, enflurane, or ketamine is preferable because myringotomy is painful.

D. Mastoidectomy and tympanoplasty

1. Microsurgery of the ear is carried out **in children** under general anesthesia and **in adults** with either local or general anesthesia.

2. Local anesthesia is satisfactory for operations lasting less than 1–1½ hr, because relatively little congestion and bleeding occur in the patient's field. However, the technique is limited by the patient's anxiety, discomfort, and nausea, which may lead to restlessness, straining, and increased bleeding.

3. **General endotracheal anesthesia** provides satisfactory operative conditions and is preferred in the majority of middle ear operations because adequate time for surgery is provided.

4. **Problems and difficulties** due to general anesthesia arise in the following areas:

   a. **Bleeding** is increased because most of the general anesthetic drugs are vasodilators, and venous pressure is elevated during general anesthesia. The elevated peripheral venous pressure is accompanied by engorgement of superficial veins in anesthetized patients. In addition, whenever controlled ventilation with intermittent positive pressure is used, the intrathoracic pressure is increased, and the venous return to the heart may be decreased with further engorgement of peripheral veins. Thus **spontaneous respiration** with minimal respiratory assistance for maintenance of good gas exchange is preferable.

      (1) **Bleeding can be minimized** during general endotracheal anesthesia by establishment of a satisfactory depth of anesthesia; by achievement of spontaneous respiration without expiratory or inspiratory obstruction; by proper positioning of the patient; and by controlling hypotension at 95 torr systolic BP. The preferred anesthetic mixture includes nitrous oxide, oxygen, and halothane or enflurane (0.1% trimethaphan or nitroprusside may be added). Controlling bleeding is very important in operations requiring use of the operating microscope, because even small amounts of blood obliterate the surgical field.

      (2) **The degree of induced hypotension** is controlled by the depth of anesthesia with halothane or enflurane, positioning, and, if required, titration with trimethaphan or nitroprusside.

   b. **Formation of nitrous oxide bubbles under the flap.** Nitrous oxide is not a desirable anesthetic for use during the closing phases of surgery for mastoid-tympanoplasty. In concentrations ordinarily administered in middle ear surgery, it causes an elevated closed-space pressure. During tympanoplasty the otolaryngologist often observes a bulging of the tissue graft, which increases until it is so pronounced that bubbles of gas escape from under the edge of the graft. Although the graft collapses, the bulging soon recurs. This phenomenon, caused by nitrous oxide, occurs because of the difference between the partition coefficient of nitrous oxide and that of nitrogen in the tissues.

      (1) **Changes occur in air-filled body cavities** because nitrous oxide is 35 times more soluble in the blood than nitrogen. During induction of anesthesia, nitrous oxide invades a closed, air-filled space 35 times more rapidly than nitrogen leaves the cavity, increasing the enclosed pressure or volume. On discontinuation of the anesthetic, the reverse occurs, and a negative pressure is produced.

      (2) **It is recommended** that nitrous oxide be discontinued during the placement of the tissue graft.

   c. **Serious ventricular arrhythmias,** including ventricular fibrillation, may occur secondary to an excessive quantity of epinephrine solution.

   d. **Epinephrine 1:100,000 in minimal dose** is administered subcutaneously and topically for the control of bleeding during mastoid-tympanoplasty surgery, which is carried out under general endotracheal anesthesia with halothane or enflurane. Epinephrine 1:100,000 for local infiltration and/or topical use, not exceeding 5–7 ml in a single injection or application, may be administered safely during halothane or enflurane endotracheal anesthesia for mastoid-tympanoplasty surgery.

E. **Stapes surgery for otosclerosis.** Surgery for removal of the stapes and replacement with a prosthesis is often carried out under local anesthesia. If general anesthesia is required, every effort must be made to ensure that **bleeding is minimal,** because during the critical stages of the microsurgery even a minute amount of bleeding obscures the surgical field.

F. **Labyrinthectomy** is designed for the relief of Meniere's disease. Surgery is carried out under general endotracheal anesthesia.

G. **Facial nerve exploration** is performed under general endotracheal anesthesia and with the aid of the operating microscope. When the facial nerve must be tested with a nerve stimulator, the use of muscle relaxants is contraindicated.

H. **Acoustic neuroma**

1. **A small acoustic neuroma** with coexisting hearing loss is resected via the translabyrinthine route. This approach offers the best opportunity for preserving the facial nerve function.

2. **Larger tumors** can be removed safely, with preservation of facial function, by the translabyrinthine and suboccipital (craniotomy) routes. **The first stage** lasts 5–7 hr and is done by the otolaryngologist, aided by the operating microscope. **The second stage** is performed within a week of the first; it lasts 6–8 hr and is carried out by the neurosurgeon.

3. **In both stages, surgery** is performed under general endotracheal anesthesia. Blood transfusion with 1000–1500 ml is necessary during each stage.

4. **Complications**

a. Bleeding.

b. Thrombosis of a cerebellar artery.

c. Cerebral edema.

d. Cerebrospinal fluid leakage.

IV. **Surgery on the nose and paranasal sinuses**

A. Because it permits better **control of bleeding,** the otolaryngologist prefers **local anesthesia** for surgery on the nose. When this is not practical or feasible, general anesthesia is maintained through an endotracheal tube with an inflatable cuff.

B. **Reduction of nasal fractures**

1. **Fractures of the nasal bones** can be reduced under either local or general anesthesia.

2. **Local anesthesia** can be obtained through bilateral application to the nasal mucosa of pledgets of cotton saturated with 4% cocaine. **Regional nerve blocks** are obtained by injection of 2% lidocaine with epinephrine 1:100,000.

3. **In adults and in children** who may have in their stomachs undigested food or an unknown quantity of swallowed blood, general anesthesia should be delayed for at least 4–6 hr.

C. **Submucous resection of the nasal septum** is ordinarily carried out under local anesthesia.

D. **Nasal polypectomy.** Local anesthesia can be achieved by application of 4% cocaine to the nasal mucosa. If general anesthesia is required, it is performed under endotracheal anesthesia.

E. **Rhinoplasty.** Plastic surgery of the external or internal nasal contours is best performed under local anesthesia because there is much less bleeding than with general anesthesia. A satisfactory nerve block and hemostasis may be produced by injecting 6–12 ml of 1% lidocaine with epinephrine 1:100,000, on both sides of the nose, between the skin and mucosa and between the nasal bony and cartilaginous framework of the nose.

F. Lateral rhinotomy. By means of a lateral rhinotomy, the external nose can be opened and hinged on one side for direct visualization. Surgery is carried out for a complete eradication of malignant tumors of the paranasal sinuses; it is performed under general endotracheal anesthesia. It may last 2–3 hr, during which a considerable blood loss is to be expected. Blood, 500–1500 ml, should be available before induction of anesthesia.

G. Nasopharyngeal angiofibroma, a highly vascular tumor, occurs in young males between the ages of 10 and 20 years. It does not metastasize or infiltrate; the tumor destroys by pressure. During surgery performed under general endotracheal anesthesia, there may be brisk bleeding. This can be minimized by selecting arterial ligation (internal maxillary artery), but 2–3 L of blood should be available before induction of anesthesia.

H. Surgery on the paranasal sinuses

1. The paranasal sinuses include the maxillary, ethmoid, frontal, and sphenoid sinuses.
2. **The airway** is very close to the surgical field. Bleeding may be considerable, and **epinephrine** 1:100,000 is used to control it. **Infection** is generally present, and adequate visualization for surgery is difficult to obtain without destroying structures of cosmetic or physiologic importance.
3. Surgery is done under general endotracheal anesthesia with an inflatable cuff.

V. Surgery in the mouth, pharynx, and salivary glands

A. Tonsillectomy and adenoidectomy

1. Tonsillectomy and adenoidectomy should not be considered minor surgery; the mortality is 1:16,000 cases, of which the main preventable causes are anoxia due to **airway obstruction** and **bleeding**.
2. **In children,** surgery is performed under general endotracheal anesthesia.
   a. **Induction of anesthesia** is carried out with nitrous oxide, oxygen, and increasing concentrations of halothane or enflurane. An endotracheal tube is inserted under a deep plane of anesthesia or IV succinylcholine. **Maintenance of anesthesia** is accomplished with nitrous oxide, oxygen, and halothane or enflurane with spontaneous or assisted ventilation.
   b. **Another popular technique** is IV administration of a sleeping dose of 50–100 mg of 2.5% thiopental or thiamylal, and 20–40 mg of succinylcholine to facilitate intubation. Anesthesia is maintained by nitrous oxide, oxygen, and halothane or enflurane with spontaneous or assisted ventilation.
   c. **The Crowe-Davis mouth gag** has been modified to accept an endotracheal tube within the groove along the undersurface of the tongue blade. The endotracheal tube remains in the midline between the tongue and the tongue blade of the mouth gag; thus the operative field is free of the endotracheal tube.
   d. Either a **semiclosed carbon dioxide absorption system** or a nonrebreathing technique can be used. The semiclosed absorption system may be used even in infants and small children.
3. **In adults,** tonsillectomy is performed under either local or general endotracheal anesthesia.
4. **Complications**
   a. Injury to the teeth.

b. Corneal abrasions.

c. Postoperative bleeding.

(1) Following control of bleeding, a large **gastric tube** should be inserted to decompress the stomach and evacuate blood clots.

(2) If general anesthesia is required, the patient is assumed to have a full stomach of blood clots, so attempts must be made for **awake intubation.** Although the amount of external bleeding may be small, there may be large quantities of blood in the stomach that can produce regurgitation and aspiration. The endotracheal tube must remain in place until bleeding is controlled and the patient is fully reactive and awake.

(3) Occasionally the otolaryngologist inserts a **postnasal pack** to control oozing and/or bleeding in the adenoid area. This presents a difficult problem in airway management and deserves close attention.

B. Peritonsillar abscess. There may be a sudden release of a great amount of purulent material, which may flood the pharynx, larynx, and trachea. Local anesthesia is the method of choice for incision and drainage. A well-functioning suction tube should be readily available at all times. **In many centers, emergency tonsillectomy** is being used for the primary treatment of peritonsillar abscess. After the induction of general anesthesia, succinylcholine can be relied on to relax trismus (muscle spasm) and allow intubation.

C. Salivary glands. Operations on the parotid, submaxillary, and sublingual salivary glands require general endotracheal anesthesia. During **parotidectomy,** the presence of the facial nerve in the surgical area of the parotid gland makes surgery tedious, and it may last up to 3 hr. Blood, 500–1000 ml, for transfusion may be required.

VI. Surgery on the larynx, trachea, esophagus, and neck

A. Laryngoscopy for examination and/or microsurgery on the larynx is done by:

1. Indirect laryngoscopy with a laryngeal mirror inserted into the mouth.

2. Microscopic laryngoscopy with suspension. The management of anesthesia presents many problems because the surgeon and anesthesiologist are in competition for control of the patient's airway. Several anesthesia techniques have been used for microscopic laryngoscopy and endoscopic surgery of the larynx.

a. Surface (topical) anesthesia

(1) Topical anesthesia is indicated in cooperative adults, but in children and uncooperative adults one must resort to general anesthesia.

(2) Cocaine 4% is used.

(3) Lidocaine 4% is less toxic and gives adequate results, but in the practice of otolaryngology, the use of cocaine persists because it is most effective and provides an adequate margin of safety.

(4) Cetacaine, a mixture of topical anesthetics, can be used with ease. It is furnished in a 50-ml aerosol bottle and contains 14% benzocaine, 2% butyl aminobenzoate, and **2% tetracaine.** A 1-sec spray releases 0.1 ml of solution, and only 3–4 sec of spraying are needed to anesthetize the mouth, pharynx, and larynx. Because of the presence of 2% tetracaine, it must be used with great caution.

b. General endotracheal anesthesia with muscle relaxants

(1) In children, nitrous oxide, oxygen, halothane or enflurane, and succinylcholine are used in a continuous slow drip. Respiration is manually controlled through an uncuffed endotracheal tube. The size of the tube varies with the patient's age.

(2) **In adults,** thiopental, nitrous oxide, oxygen, enflurane or fentanyl, and succinycholine are used in a continuous slow drip. Respiration is controlled manually through a cuffed endotracheal tube.

(3) **Venturi or jet ventilation**

(a) **The great advantage** of jet ventilation is that it permits the apneic patient to be ventilated by intermittent injection of oxygen through the suspension laryngoscope or bronchoscope and without an endotracheal tube. It affords unparalleled access to the laryngotracheobronchial tree for both diagnosis and microsurgery.

(b) **A stream of oxygen** is directed, through various-sized needles, within the open lumen of the laryngoscope or bronchoscope. The jet stream of oxygen, at high velocity, is directed via the instrument and (by a suction effect) entrains room air with it, with the result that a large volume of oxygen-rich air is transmitted to the respiratory tree under pressures that are readily adjustable for adequate ventilation of the patient.

(c) **The needle sizes** used are: an 18-gauge jet needle for children under 2 years old, a 16-gauge needle for children over 2 years old, and a 14-gauge needle for adults.

(d) **Pressure gauge settings** are not to exceed 9 kg for children and 13.5 kg for adults. These pressures are based on a two-stage reducing valve.

(e) **A combination** of tracheal intubation and jet ventilation may be alternately used with ease, so that the advantages of the one overcome the disadvantages of the other.

3. **Other techniques**

a. Translaryngeal topical anesthesia.

b. Apneic technique.

c. Emerson chest respirator.

d. Neuroleptanalgesia.

4. **Direct laryngoscopy in a patient with a tracheostomy** does not present problems because there is no competition between the otolaryngologist and the anesthesiologist for control of the airway.

5. **Complications**

a. The occurrence of **cardiac arrhythmias** is common during suspension laryngoscopy, especially in high-risk patients. Continuous cardiac monitoring is a necessity. Sustained arrhythmias, such as premature ventricular contractions, require removal of the laryngoscope from the suspension apparatus.

b. Recurrence of the arrhythmia after resuspending the laryngoscope may require blocking of the mechanism with intravenous lidocaine or a superior laryngeal nerve block with local anesthesia.

B. **Laryngectomy with or without neck dissection**

1. **Carcinoma of the larynx**

a. **Symptoms and signs** include hoarseness, pain, difficulty in swallowing, and bleeding. Respiratory obstruction and dyspnea may be present if the tumor is large.

b. Following **microscopic diagnosis,** treatment of **early** carcinoma of the true vocal cords is usually by x-ray radiation or laser surgery. **Total laryngectomy** is carried out when the laryngeal musculature, perichondrium, or cricoarytenoid joint is invaded by cancer. When there is an extension from the primary lesion to the subglottic or supraglottic areas, **neck dissection** is combined with total laryngectomy.

c. Cancer and edema distort the normal anatomy and may **render intubation difficult.** In addition, there are **two critical periods:** (1) during induction of anesthesia and insertion of the endotracheal tube through the mouth and (2) during the transfer of the endotracheal tube from the mouth to the transected trachea.

2. Anesthesia management

a. **Induction of anesthesia and intubation** are achieved with IV thiopental and succinylcholine. In the presence of a large tumor or possible difficult intubation, **awake intubation** with topical anesthesia is indicated.

b. **Maintenance of anesthesia** is accomplished with (1) nitrous oxide, oxygen, and halothane or enflurane with spontaneous or assisted ventilation or (2) nitrous oxide, oxygen, narcotics, and muscle relaxants with controlled ventilation.

3. Complications

a. Hypotension and/or bradycardia may occur due to carotid sinus reflex.

b. Pneumothorax.

c. Venous air embolism.

d. Hemorrhage.

C. Arytenoidectomy

1. Indications

a. **During thyroidectomy,** when peripheral injury of the recurrent laryngeal nerves paralyzes the vocal cords.

b. Fixation of the arytenoid cartilage in a patient with **cricoarytenoid arthritis**.

2. Under local anesthesia, a preliminary **tracheotomy** is followed by arytenoidectomy. **General anesthesia** is carried out through a flexible, cuffed endotracheal tube inserted through the tracheal opening. Anesthesia is maintained with nitrous oxide, oxygen, narcotics, muscle relaxants, and controlled ventilation.

D. Bronchoscopy. An outline of anesthesia management can be found in Chapter 31, section **III.J.**

E. Tracheotomy

1. Indications

a. To bypass upper airway obstruction.

b. To permit aspiration of secretions from the trachea and lungs.

c. To permit long-term ventilatory support.

2. **Elective tracheotomy** may be performed under local anesthesia. **Emergency tracheotomy** is best performed after awake intubation under topical anesthesia and light general anesthesia.

3. Complications

a. Bleeding.

b. Emphysema (subcutaneous and/or mediastinal).

c. Tube displacement or occlusion.

d. Pneumothorax.

e. Aspiration.

f. Death (2%).

F. **Esophagoscopy** for diagnostic and therapeutic purposes is performed under general endotracheal anesthesia with nitrous oxide, oxygen, enflurane or narcotics, muscle relaxants, and controlled ventilation.

G. **Hemimandibulectomy**

1. **Hemimandibulectomy with radical neck dissection** (commando or composite resection of oropharyngeal cancer) includes excision of part of the tongue, mandible, and lymph nodes of the neck.

2. **Problems** that the anesthesiologist is likely to meet are (a) the local results of preoperative radiotherapy, (b) intraoral and pharyngeal suppuration, (c) low blood volume, (d) malnutrition, and (e) respiratory or cardiovascular disease.

3. **General endotracheal anesthesia** is induced with thiopental and succinylcholine. Anesthesia is maintained with nitrous oxide, oxygen, narcotics, muscle relaxants, and controlled ventilation.

4. **Elective tracheotomy** is done at the completion of surgery.

VII. Hypophysectomy

A. A hypophysectomy is performed for excision of pituitary tumors, pituitary adenomas, or as palliative therapy for **advanced carcinoma of the breast,** diabetic retinopathy, and advanced prostatic carcinoma.

B. **The approach to the pituitary gland** is by way of a frontal **craniotomy** or via the **sphenoid sinus** through a right external ethmoid excision or sublabial incision.

C. With the perfection of the Zeiss operating microscope, the **transsphenoidal route** has become increasingly competitive with the intracranial subfrontal approach employed by the neurosurgeon.

D. **Transsphenoidal hypophysectomy.** The transsphenoidal approach to the sella turcica for hypophysectomy is more direct and has the advantages of lower morbidity and mortality, as well as a shorter convalescent period. The patient can be discharged from the hospital on the sixth to seventh postoperative day. **Intraoperative and postoperative complications,** such as injury to the optic chiasm, seizures, extradural hematoma, brain damage, and cerebral edema, are rare.

1. **Anesthesia management**

a. **Anesthesia is induced** with thiopental and succinylcholine, and a cuffed endotracheal tube is inserted. Tracheal intubation of a patient with **acromegaly** can be very difficult because of **macroglossia;** awake intubation with topical anesthesia is indicated.

b. **Maintenance of anesthesia** is accomplished with nitrous oxide, oxygen, enflurane or halothane, and spontaneous or assisted ventilation.

c. The careful use of **epinephrine** 1:100,000 solution for hemostasis does not preclude the use of halothane.

2. **Corticosteroids** are given during the preoperative, intraoperative, and postoperative periods. Other effects of excision of the pituitary gland on the

general glandular metabolism are not noted for several days (diabetes insipidus or hypothyroidism).

VIII. The laser in otolaryngology. The laser has become accepted as a clinical tool in a variety of therapeutic and surgical applications. It has been used extensively in ophthalmology for the treatment of retinal disorders; in otolaryngology for therapy of tumors of the larynx and trachea; in dermatology for treatment of lesions of the skin; in surgery for hemostasis; and in gynecology for therapy of erosions of the cervix.

A. The laser beam

1. Atom and electrons

a. Each atom has a nucleus, and around this nucleus circulate a number of **electrons.**

b. The distance between an electron and the nucleus can be changed, but only if the electron jumps to another, predetermined level.

c. The electron has the tendency to return to its lowest energy level **(ground state).**

2. Electrons and photons

a. If energy (light, heat, or electricity) strikes an atom, and if this energy is absorbed by that atom, the electron will jump to a higher level. This electron is in the **excited state**. As the electron returns spontaneously to its normal energy level, it releases energy in the form of a **photon**, which is the smallest quantity of light.

b. When a photon bombards another atom that is in the excited state, that atom's electron will fall back to its **ground state,** releasing another photon. This photon has the same frequency as the incoming photon, so it is in step with it and moving in the same direction. This process is called **stimulated emission.**

c. If there are other atoms in the excited state, these photons will continue to multiply in a chain reaction.

B. Production of a laser beam

1. Ruby crystal

a. In a ruby crystal, a great number of atoms are in the ground state. If energy in the form of light from a xenon flash tube strikes the ruby crystal, a great portion of the atoms will go to the excited state. A few atoms will then release **photons** moving in random directions. But a few other photons will travel along the axis of the crystal and stimulate other atoms to release photons.

b. If two special parallel and reflective mirrors are located at each end of the ruby crystal, **released photons will move back and forth between these two mirrors,** stimulating other atoms to emit photons with the same phase, frequency, and direction.

c. If one of the mirrors is partially transparent, part of this radiant energy will escape through it in the form of a powerful beam.

2. Carbon dioxide

a. When energy in the form of an electrical discharge strikes carbon dioxide molecules, the **electrons** move from lower to higher energy levels and thus are in an **excited state**.

b. As the electrons shift back to lower levels, the acquired energy is released, creating spontaneous emission of **photons.**

c. These photons bombard other excited carbon dioxide molecules and produce release of additional photons **(stimulated emission).**

d. **The laser beam,** reflected by mirrors in the surgical arm of the instrument, is then concentrated and focused on the target field.

C. Nature of laser

1. **The laser beam** is light of a specific frequency, which is generated by a special process called Light Amplification by Stimulated Emission of Radiation (LASER).

   a. The laser light is **parallel, monochromatic,** and **coherent.**

   b. It is an extremely intense beam of light that may be focused on a minute area, aimed, concentrated, and controlled like a surgical instrument.

   c. A variety of materials can stimulate laser emissions. The most common materials used in **medicine** are:

   (1) **Solid lasers:** Ruby, neodymium, and neodymium yttrium aluminum garnet (NdYAG).

   (2) **Gas lasers:** Helium, neon, argon, and carbon dioxide.

   d. **Two types of lasers** are used: pulsed (ruby) and continuous wave (argon and carbon dioxide).

D. Carbon dioxide laser

1. **Nature of the carbon dioxide surgical laser**

   a. The carbon dioxide surgical laser is a form of nonionizing, **invisible** electromagnetic radiation.

   b. The wavelength of the laser beam is in the **infrared range (10.6 microns)** of the electromagnetic spectrum. The tissue-destructive capacity of the beam is a **thermal effect.**

   c. This energy is **absorbed** by all biologic tissues, irrespective of pigmentation.

   d. Destruction is in part proportional to the tissue's water content.

   e. It can be used to **vaporize** predetermined volumes of tissue in a precise fashion that is controlled by using the appropriate amount of energy.

   f. The laser beam can be focused to a fine point with the aid of a lens. This concentrated energy can be used to vaporize soft tissues in a **linear fashion.**

   g. **A blue cloud** of vaporized plasma and tissue is emitted.

   h. **The incision is clean and straight.** There is **minimal bleeding,** because the small vessels are cauterized simultaneously. There is very little visible postoperative edema, and the wounds heal with very little postoperative scarring.

   i. In the presence of a carbon dioxide laser beam, **trichloroethylene** breaks down to halides; **halothane** and **enflurane** do not.

2. **The carbon dioxide surgical laser instrument**

   a. The instrument is contained in a standard electronic relay rack and includes: handpieces containing **lenses** of varying focal lengths, the laser **endoscope,** and the **stereomicroscope** laser attachment.

   b. The laser beam is **focused on the target** by an articulated arm that is attached to the surgical **microscope** or **bronchoscope.**

c. **A rheostat** controls the power of the beam, and a footswitch-controlled shutter allows the beam to fall on the target area for an appropriate period.

d. A footswitch activates the laser during surgery.

e. The laser tube draws 15 amp of electrical power from the ordinary 110-V outlet.

3. Advantages

a. The carbon dioxide laser beam offers improved hemostasis and visual control of the lesion.

b. It causes minimal damage to surrounding tissues.

c. There is very little postoperative edema and pain.

d. Healing is rapid, and there is minimal scarring.

4. Disadvantages

a. **Flammable** anesthetic agents cannot be used.

b. The laser beam may cause breakdown of anesthetic drugs.

c. **A fire** starts instantly when latex, rubber, silk, silicone, or plastic endotracheal tubes are exposed to the laser beam.

d. Fire, with released fumes and black smoke, is accelerated by the presence of **oxygen** and **nitrous oxide.**

5. Precautions

a. Fewer safety precautions are necessary during the use of the carbon dioxide laser than with the ruby, argon, or other lasers.

(1) The operating room personnel need only wear **ordinary eyeglasses** to protect the corneas from injury should the laser beam be reflected accidentally from a metal surface.

(2) For the same reason, the **patient's eyes** must be protected.

(3) If an area of tissue close to the target area needs to be protected, it can be shielded adequately by covering it with **moist gauze**, since water dissipates the energy effectively.

(4) There is no harm or injury to a **pregnant patient** or to pregnant personnel in the operating roon. The carbon dioxide laser beam is not like an x-ray; its effect is limited to the areas where it is aimed.

b. **All nonflammable anesthetic drugs** can be administered to patients undergoing laser surgery. For **general anesthesia,** drugs used for high-frequency electrosurgery also can be used for laser surgery.

c. If an **endotracheal tube** is located close to the surgical area, special care should be taken to prevent its being damaged by the laser beam, which could cause it to burn in the presence of oxygen. A thin metal coating, such as self-adhesive aluminum foil, should be wrapped around the distal portion of a red rubber tube (except the cuff) to protect the tube from accidental impact by the laser beam. There is no protection available for the cuff other than covering it with wet cottonoids. The cottonoids must be kept moist at all times. If a cuff is not required, the all-metal (Norton) tube is ideal.

d. In a patient with a **tracheostomy**, a steel or silver tracheostomy tube without further protection, or a red rubber tube wrapped with an aluminum sheath, can be used for the administration of the anesthetics. All currently available endotracheal tubes are flammable except for the Norton steel tubes. Red rubber tubes can be penetrated with the laser only with great difficulty and are much slower to ignite than plastic tubes. Red rubber tubes are therefore preferred at the present time.

e. For protection, all personnel should do the following:

(1) Be aware of possible damage to the cornea.

(2) Place wet gauzes on metal instruments and reflecting surfaces.

(3) Avoid placing objects in the path of the laser beam, to prevent reflection or fire.

Bibliography

Abou-Madi, M. N., Trop, D., and Barnes, J. Etiology and control of cardiovascular reactions during trans-sphenoidal resection of pituitary microadenomas. *Can. Anaesth. Soc. J.* 27:491, 1980.

Barron, W. D. Anesthetic management of microsurgical operations on the ear. *J. Laryngol. Otol.* 90:401, 1976.

Borg, U., Eriksson, I., and Sjostrand, U. High-frequency positive-pressure ventilation (HFPPV). A review based upon its use during bronchoscopy and for laryngoscopy and microlaryngeal surgery under general anesthesia. Anesth. Analg. (Cleve.) 59:594, 1980.

Carden, E., and Vest, H. R. Further advances in anesthetic technics for microlaryngeal surgery. Anesth. Analg. (Cleve.) 53:584, 1974.

Cole, W. H. J. Choice of anesthetic technique for microsurgery of the larynx. *Anesth. Intensive Care* 3:62, 1975.

El-Naggar, M., Keh, E., Stemmers, A., et al. Jet ventilation for microlaryngoscopic procedures. *Anesth. Analg.* (Cleve.) 53:797, 1974.

Eriksson, I., and Sjostrand, U. Effects of high-frequency positive-pressure ventilation (HFPPD) and general anesthesia on intrapulmonary gas distribution in patients undergoing diagnostic bronchoscopy. *Anesth. Analg.* (Cleve.) 59:585, 1980.

Johnston, R. R., Eger, E. I., and Wilson, C. A comparative interaction of epinephrine with enflurane, isoflurane, and halothane in man. *Anesth. Analg.* (Cleve.) 55:709, 1976.

Konchigeri, H. N., Shaker, M. H., and Winnie, A. P. Effect of epinephrine during enflurane anesthesia. *Anesth. Analg.* (Cleve.) 53:894, 1974.

Lindholm, C. E., Ollman, B., Snyder, J. V., et al. Cardiorespiratory effects of flexible fiberoptic bronchoscopy in critically ill patients. *Chest* 74:362, 1978.

Messick, J. M., Laws, E. R., and Abboud, C. F. Anesthesia for transsphenoidal surgery of the hypophyseal region. *Anesth. Analg.* (Cleve.) 57:206, 1978.

Norton, M. L., and DeVos, P. New endotracheal tube for laser surgery of the larynx. *Ann. Otol. Rhinol. Laryngol.* 87:554, 1978.

Norton, M. L., Strong, M. S., Vaughan, C. W., et al. Endotracheal intubation and Venturi (jet) ventilation for laser microsurgery of the larynx. *Ann. Otol. Rhinol. Laryngol.* 85:656, 1976.

Owens, W. D., Gustave, F., and Sclaroff, A. Tympanic membrane rupture with nitrous oxide anesthesia. Anesth. Analg. (Cleve.) 57:283, 1978.

Patterson, M. E., and Bartlett, P. G. Hearing impairment caused by intratympanic pressure changes during general anesthesia. *Laryngoscope* 86:399, 1976.

Reisner, L. S., and Lippmann, M. Ventricular arrhythmias after epinephrine injection in enflurane and in halothane anesthesia. *Anesth. Analg.* (Cleve.) 54:468, 1975.

Sellers, S. L., and Augoustides, A. Anesthesia for endolaryngeal surgery. *J. Otolaryngol.* 5:203, 1976.

Snow, J. C. *Anesthesia in Otolaryngology and Ophthalmology* (2nd ed.). New York: Appleton-Century-Crofts, 1982.

Snow, J. C., Kripke, B. J., and Strong, M. S. Management of general anesthesia for mastoid-tympanoplasty. Anesthesia and surgical considerations. *Laryngoscope* 83:1786, 1973.

Snow, J. C., Kripke, B. J., Strong, M. S., et al. Anesthesia for carbon dioxide laser microsurgery on the larynx and trachea. *Anesth. Analg.* (Cleve.) 53:507, 1974.

Snow, J. C., Norton, M. L., Saluja, T. S., et al. Fire hazard during CO_2 laser microsurgery on the larynx and trachea. *Anesth. Analg.* (Cleve.) 55:146, 1976.

Snow, J. C., Shamsai, J., and Sakarya, I. Effects of epinephrine during halothane anesthesia in mastoidotympanoplastic surgery. *Anesth. Analg.* (Cleve.) 47:252, 1968.

Vourch, G., Tannieres, M. L., Toty, L., et al. Anaesthetic management of tracheal surgery using the neodymium-yytrium-aluminium-garnet laser. *Br. J. Anaesth.* 52:993, 1980.

Wainwright, A. C., Moody, R. A., and Carruth, J. A. S. Anaesthetic safety with the carbon dioxide laser. *Anaesthesia* 36:411, 1981.

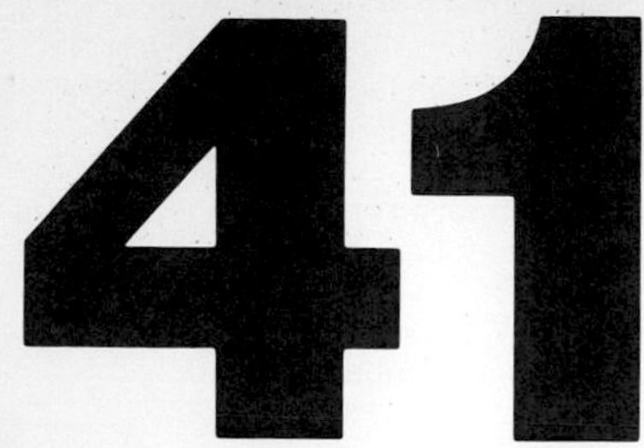

Anesthesia for Urologic Surgery

I. Urologic surgery

A. General considerations

1. Surgery for urologic patients includes endoscopic and open surgery. **Endoscopic surgery** includes cystoscopy and transurethral resection of prostatic obstruction or bladder lesions. **Anesthesia for open surgery** of the external genitalia, bladder, ureters, and kidney has few special problems and is administered as in other abdominal operations. **A diagnostic procedure** requires local, regional, or general anesthesia. The resulting diagnosis may necessitate definitive surgery the following day. Fluids and electrolytes should be replaced adequately, and the patient should be mobilized between procedures.

2. **A great number** of urologic patients are elderly and are suffering from diseases of the kidney or heart or from debilitating malignant lesions. Many of these patients require repeated examinations under anesthesia.

3. **Extensive resection** and reconstruction for cancer or congenital abnormalities exemplify the problem of rising morbidity and mortality as the duration of surgery increases.

4. **The position of the patient** on the operating table for easy surgical approach, particularly in the **nephrectomy** or **perineal prostatectomy** position, can have deleterious effects on respiration and circulation. Pneumothorax after nephrectomy is always possible.

5. **Repeated anesthesia** may create psychological problems in the very young patient undergoing repeated cystoscopies or staged urologic reconstructions.

6. **Electrocautery and x-ray.** Special consideration should be given to the hazards of fire, explosion, electric shock, burns from the electrocautery, and the risk of irradiation during x-ray.

   a. **The use of flammable anesthetics is contraindicated** in the presence of x-ray and electrocautery equipment.

   b. With reasonable precautions and adequate equipment, the **exposure to radiation** during x-ray procedures is minimal. The anesthesiologist or nurse-anesthetist should wear a **lead apron** if it is necessary to stay with the patient during exposures. Stepping back from the patient for 10–20 sec will reduce the radiation dose without increasing the risk to the patient.

7. **The dark room** increases the vision of the urologist but reduces the ability of the anesthesiologist or nurse-anesthetist to maintain visual observation of the patient. Therefore small lights illuminating the anesthesia machine and the patient's head are very important.

8. **Moving the anesthetized patient** through corridors and elevators is a very dangerous practice. The cystoscopy room should be adjacent to the operating room and radiology department.

9. **Outpatient diagnostic and therapeutic procedures** (see Chap. 42). General anesthetics and anesthetic techniques of short duration are available. However, few anesthesiologists are willing to use spinal anesthesia unless they have the opportunity for close observation of their patients for the following 24 hr. Other regional anesthetic techniques may be administered.

B. Anesthesia and the kidney

1. **Regional anesthesia techniques** have the least impact on renal function provided severe hypotension does not ensue.
2. **Alterations in renal hemodynamics** are reversible and can be minimized by adequate preoperative hydration and avoidance of deep anesthesia.
3. **During anesthesia,** the BP is a poor guide to the renal circulation. Renal function is seriously impaired with a BP below 60 torr.
   a. **Methamphetamine** increases renal blood flow; **epinephrine** and **norepinephrine** reduce it. **Isoproterenol** does not have significant effects on renal blood flow or urinary output.
   b. **Cyclopropane, ether, and thiopental** decrease renal flow. The effects of **halothane** are less marked.
   c. The nephrotoxicity of **methoxyflurane** may be produced by a product of its metabolism, inorganic fluoride.
4. **During recovery** from anesthesia, the renal blood flow returns to normal.

C. Instruments

1. **The cystoscope** is used for direct visualization of the urethra and bladder. It consists of a hollow tube or sheath with a light source and a lens system. Water, used as an irrigating solution, distends the area of the lower urinary tract being examined and allows observation. The proper combinations of urologic instruments permit examination of the urethra and bladder and allow the insertion for ureteral catheters. In addition, instruments can be employed for removal of ureteral stones and fulguration of bleeding areas or bladder tumors.
2. **The resectoscope** is an endoscopic instrument utilized for excision of prostatic and bladder tissues through the urethra. It combines a hollow tube or sheath with a light source, cutting loop, and lens system. It locks into the sheath and it has a valve for the irrigating line. The tissues are excised with the movable cutting wire loop by use of a high-frequency current, and bleeding is controlled by fulguration. The irrigating fluid washes blood and cuttings into the bladder until the bladder is filled; then the resectoscope is removed from the sheath and the bladder is emptied.

II. Anesthesia management

A. Preanesthetic preparation. See Chapter 1.

B. Preanesthesia medication. See Chapter 3.

C. Monitoring. See Chapter 6.

D. Anesthesia for pediatric examinations

1. **For diagnostic procedures,** the urologist is in the best position to decide whether general anesthesia is required.
   a. With adequate preparation and **sedative drugs,** many procedures, such as IV pyelography, voiding cystography, and urethral calibration, can be performed without general anesthesia.
   b. **For cystoscopy, urethroscopy,** and repeated diagnostic procedures, general anesthesia is indicated.

2. **Fluid therapy.** It is general practice to restrict oral intake for 12 hr before anesthesia. However, children, especially infants, will become dehydrated during this period. IV administration of appropriate amounts of dextrose and electrolyte solutions will correct this dehydration and reduce the hazards of the postoperative period.

3. **Monitoring.** Heart, respiration, BP, and body temperature should be monitored carefully. In children, body temperature falls because of their larger body surface area in relation to body weight. A short cystoscopy in which cold water is instilled into the bladder and the child is allowed to remain exposed can decrease body temperature significantly.

E. Transurethral resection of prostate and bladder

1. During transurethral resection of prostatic obstruction or bladder lesions, consideration should be given to the following factors:

   a. The patient belongs to an **advanced age group** with a high incidence of degenerative diseases of the respiratory and cardiovascular systems.

   b. He is placed in **the lithotomy position.**

   c. Large amounts of **irrigating solutions** are administered.

   d. **Urethral instruments** are used.

2. **Cardiovascular complications** are the most common causes of operative mortality during transurethal prostatectomy. The cardiovascular and electrolyte status of these patients is changed due to a combination of blood loss, IV fluid administration, and fluid absorption. In the elderly, such hemodynamic changes are not always tolerated.

3. **An irrigating solution** is used during examination of the urethra and bladder. The solution distends the bladder and washes out blood and cuttings to allow clear visualization during cystoscopy.

   a. The irrigating solution is ordinary water, but its absorption into the vascular system may result in hemolysis, bacterial contamination, and water intoxication (dilutional hyponatremia). To avoid hemolysis, **3% sorbitol** is used.

   b. The irrigating solution should be sterile and should be supplied in large quantities, preferably at body temperature.

   c. If an electrolyte solution is used as the irrigating fluid, the electric current will be diffused, and when the loop is activated, there will be no coagulation or cutting.

4. **Venous absorption**

   a. **The venous sinuses** are opened during resection of the prostatic bed and provide direct communication with the cardiovascular system. The larger the prostate, the greater the amount of irrigating solution that is absorbed into the venous system through the opened venous sinuses.

   b. **The pressure** of the irrigating solution within the bladder is greater than the venous pressure. Thus irrigating solution enters the circulation in great volumes, and **three problems** may result:

      (1) **Increased circulating volume.** Because of the absorbed irrigating solution, the weight gain following transurethral resection may be 2–4 kg. However, the average amount absorbed is a few hundred milliliters.

         (a) **Early signs** of increased volume of circulating fluid are increased systolic BP, bradycardia, and bleeding. Development of ventricular failure causes pulmonary edema, leading to cerebral edema.

Asthmatic wheezes, rales, and pink, frothy sputum are present. Cerebral edema causes CNS symptoms of apprehension, disorientation, mental confusion, convulsions, and/or coma.

(b) **Treatment**

i. Endotracheal intubation and administration of oxygen under positive pressure.

ii. Placing tourniquets to the extremities without occlusion of the arterial pulse.

iii. Discontinuation of the bladder-irrigating solution.

iv. Change in body posture to elevate the right atrium and decrease venous return.

v. Administration of diuretics and digitalis.

(2) **Hemolysis of circulating erythrocytes** occurs when large quantities of **irrigating water** are infused from the bladder into the circulation.

(a) **The symptoms** are hypotension, bleeding, tachycardia, and peripheral vasoconstriction with cyanosis.

(b) **The diagnosis** is made by the presence of free hemoglobin in the blood plasma. **Therapy** includes maintenance of renal flow by administration of blood and electrolytes.

(3) **Hyponatremia**

(a) **The serum sodium** is diluted; from a normal level of 131–148 mEq/L, it may be decreased to 120 mEq/L.

(b) **Preexisting conditions predisposing to sodium loss**

i. Heart diseases with sodium restriction and diuretics.

ii. Renal diseases.

iii. Adrenal insufficiency.

iv. Diuresis following complete urinary obstruction.

v. Malnutrition and chronic diseases.

vi. Advanced age.

vii. Preoperative and intraoperative use of water, 5% D/W, or diuretics.

(c) **Under regional anesthesia,** restlessness, confusion, nausea, and vomiting may develop, which may lead to lethargy, coma, or convulsions. Under general anesthesia, changes in BP or convulsions may occur.

(d) **Treatment** consists of IV administration of hypertonic (3%) sodium chloride.

(e) **Prevention.** During transurethral resection, the administration of water or 5% D/W should be restricted. Either can be replaced by 3% sorbitol or 1% glycine irrigating solution.

5. **Hemorrhage.** Estimation of blood loss during transurethral resection of the prostate is very difficult. Because of fluids entering the circulation through the prostate gland, the general signs of hypovolemia are absent.

6. **Hyperfibrinolysis.** Abnormal bleeding is associated with transurethral prostatic surgery because of the release of fibrinolysins, but severe and prolonged bleeding is due to inadequate hemostasis. Abnormal bleeding should be confirmed by examination of a blood specimen in the operating room. Under

normal conditions, a clot should form in 10 min and remain firm. Hyperfibrinolysis is a serious bleeding situation. **Treatment** of suspected systemic hyperfibrinolysis may include the injection of epsilonaminocaproic acid. However, this drug should be administered only on definitive diagnosis or when laboratory findings indicate hyperfibrinolysis.

7. **Disseminated intravascular coagulopathy** with prolonged bleeding may occur during prostatic surgery when tissue materials that induce blood coagulation and platelet aggregation are infused into the blood circulation in great quantities. This complication combines thrombosis and bleeding and activates a secondary fibrinolysis. **Therapy** includes heparin. Epsilonaminocaproic acid is needed for the rare patient with extensive secondary fibrinolysis.

8. **Perforation of the bladder or prostatic capsule** with extravasation of irrigating solution and urine is a serious complication that may lead to death. **The anesthesiologist** may be the first to diagnose this complication, provided he is aware of the symptoms of perforation and extravasation during regional or general anesthesia.

   a. **A perforation** of the bladder or prostatic capsule may occur (1) at the end of an overzealous resection during deep cutting of the prostatic capsule; (2) during fulguration of a bladder tumor; (3) on insertion of the resectoscope into empty, thin-walled trabeculae; or (4) during obturator nerve spasm or obturator nerve stimulation.

   b. With a patient **under regional anesthesia,** a sudden, severe pain may be felt in the lower abdomen. The abdomen becomes tense and tender to palpation. In the less common intraperitoneal extravasation, pain may be felt in the precordium or over the shoulders. Extravasation of **small amounts** of irrigating solution results in hypertension and bradycardia; **larger volumes** tend to cause hypotension and shock.

   c. With a patient **under general anesthesia,** perforation is difficult to diagnose. Changes in respiration and hypotension may lead to the suspicion that perforation with extravasation has occurred. Confirmation of the diagnosis is made by immediate cystoscopy and/or urethrography.

   d. **The therapy** of extravasation is extraordinarily dependent on the presence or absence of urinary tract infection, and it requires immediate termination of the resection and performance of a suprapubic cystotomy with drainage. In the case of a small extravasation, it is necessary to insert an indwelling catheter and administer antibiotics.

9. **Anesthesia for transurethral prostatic surgery**

   a. **Sensory fibers** to the bladder and prostate gland leave the spinal cord at and below the T_{10} segment. Therefore **spinal anesthesia** reaching to the T_{10} dermatome is the first choice, with the following **advantages:**

      (1) The elderly patient tolerates spinal anesthesia very well.

      (2) Satisfactory surgical conditions are obtained from 10–12 mg of tetracaine.

      (3) Inadvertent perforation of the bladder or prostatic capsule is diagnosed by the patient's ability to experience pain.

      (4) Absorption of irrigating solution and fluid overload are recognized by the onset of restlessness.

      (5) Termination of spinal anesthesia is slow and is not associated with emesis, coughing, or restlessness, so the risk of bleeding is considerably reduced.

(6) The incidence of postspinal headache in the elderly also is much reduced.

b. **Continuous lumbar peridural anesthesia** has all the advantages of spinal anesthesia and can be prolonged if necessary.

c. **Spinal, peridural, and caudal anesthesia** are recommended, because the complications associated with transurethral resection are diagnosed easily in the awake patient. However, in a patient with metastasis of **prostatic carcinoma** to the lumbar vertebrae and the concomitant possibility of pain or peripheral neuropathies, the medicolegal implications of the administration of regional anesthesia should be studied carefully.

d. **When general anesthesia** is indicated, surgery requires tranquil respiration and muscle relaxation. The obese, bronchitic, emphysematous, or "bull-necked" patient is best handled by tracheal intubation and controlled ventilation.

F. **For uremic patients, anesthesia** may be necessary for prostatectomy, cystostomy, nephrostomy, renal biopsy, and a few nonurologic emergency procedures. Patients undergoing kidney transplantation have little or no renal function and before surgery are not uremic because they are receiving artificial renal hemodialysis.

1. **In the management of anesthesia** in uremic patients, special consideration must be given to the following:

a. **Renal blood flow and pressure** should be maintained at a level securing glomerular filtration.

b. During fluid therapy, administration of irrigating water may lead to **hyponatremia.** This should not be allowed to occur.

c. Injection of **succinylcholine** may result in **hyperpotassemia** that may in turn lead to cardiovascular collapse and cardiac arrest.

2. **Kidney transplantation**

a. **The kidney donor** is a healthy person. Anesthesia management includes general endotracheal anesthesia and adequate muscle relaxation with pancuronium. The most frequent complication during anesthesia is hypotension, which can occur during positioning of the patient and raising the kidney rest of the operating table.

b. **The recipient** is a chronically ill patient with terminal renal failure, is anemic and hypertensive, and may harbor viral hepatitis. There is a lack of usable veins following repeated hemodialysis and venipunctures for biochemical investigations. The patient may have had multiple procedures, including bilateral nephrectomy, in preparation for renal transplantation.

(1) **The recipient** may receive a kidney from an identical twin, a living donor (usually a relative), or a cadaver.

(2) **Anemia** is the main problem. The patient on chronic hemodialysis has an average hemoglobin level of 6–8 g/100 ml. Due to immunologic problems associated with blood transfusions, every effort should be made to avoid transfusion of lymphocytes. The acceptable blood for these patients consists of **frozen red cells.** Immunosuppressive therapy decreases the patient's ability to combat **infection,** so efforts should be made to protect the patient from this hazard.

(3) **Induction of anesthesia** begins with thiopental, followed (if serum potassium is normal) by succinylcholine to facilitate intubation. **Maintenance** of anesthesia is carried out with nitrous oxide, oxygen, fentanyl, pancuronium, and controlled ventilation.

(a) **The arteriovenous shunt** and/or arteriovenous fistula must be protected from IV use and from the BP cuff.

(b) **Following renal transplantation,** a marked diuresis may develop. Infusion of dextrose and albumin is indicated.

(c) Anesthesia management is similar for the patient scheduled for **removal of a rejected kidney** transplant.

G. Specific urologic procedures

1. **Cystoscopy** and **retrograde pyelography** can be performed on girls, women, and men with topical anesthesia and sedative drugs. Boys require general anesthesia. A few adults may require regional or general anesthesia.

   a. **If bladder distention or electrocautery** to the bladder is needed, general anesthesia or nerve block to T_{10} is required.

   b. Anesthesia may influence the tone of the detrusor and sphincter muscles, so it is best to obtain **cystograms and voiding urethrograms** under local anesthesia.

   c. **Penile erection** is occasionally a problem under local or general anesthesia and can present difficulties during insertion of the cystoscope. Patients with priapism respond to deepening of general anesthesia, amyl nitrite, ketamine, or trimethaphan. This problem does not occur under spinal anesthesia.

2. **Kidney function tests** performed under anesthesia are influenced by the pharmacologic effects of the anesthetic agents. When **cystoscopy** is done under anesthesia, the IV-injected **indigo carmine or methylene blue** in the bladder is delayed. This may be the result of inadequate hydration, depressed circulation, or increased antidiuretic hormone. A similar delay may occur during IV pyelography. These agents may have hypertensive effects.

3. **Circumcision** is perfomed in boys under general anesthesia and in men under local or general anesthesia. If local infiltration is used at the site of the circumcision, vasoconstrictors should be avoided, since skin slough may occur. However, vasoconstrictors can be used with nerve blocks at the base of the penis.

4. **Radical perineal prostatectomy**

   a. **Radical perineal prostatectomy is a long operation,** lasting 5–7 hr and is performed in the most extreme lithotomy position. In this position, there is a great embarrassment of ventilation. General endotracheal anesthesia with controlled ventilation is indicated.

   b. The patient should be **observed carefully** to prevent pressure points and nerve injuries.

   c. The surgical field is highly vascular, and **bleeding** may be excessive. Postural hypotension may develop if the patient is returned to the supine position too rapidly.

5. Anesthesia management for **suprapubic, retropubic, and intraperitoneal surgery** is similar to that for other lower abdominal operations.

   a. **Suprapubic prostatectomy** is associated with abnormal bleeding caused by circulating fibrinolysins, of which the prostate has large amounts (see **E.6**).

   b. **In children,** large abdominal tumors of perirenal origin present anesthetic problems involving the circulation, respiration, and body temperature.

6. **Total cystectomy** is a major procedure that requires good muscle relaxation, decreased bleeding, a collapsed small bowel, controlled body temperature, and adequate urine output.

   a. The major volume of **blood loss** is expected during the actual cystectomy. Following the cystectomy, the urologist's attention is directed toward forming the ileal loop urinary diversion and the ureteric anastomoses.

   b. **Anesthesia** is accomplished by a continuous lumbar **peridural anesthesia,** combined with **general endotracheal anesthesia** and controlled respiration. A moderate degree of hypotension is preferable; this can be achieved by the autonomic anesthesia provided by the peridural anesthesia. At the termination of surgery, the peridural catheter should be left in the peridural space and used for the provision of analgesia in the first postoperative 24 hr.

      (1) Surgery can be performed with a **continuous spinal anesthesia** but with the following **hazards:**

         (a) Postoperative analgesia cannot be provided as safely as usual, because it is not acceptable to leave a spinal catheter in place as long as is allowed for the peridural catheter.

         (b) The incidence of severe postspinal headache is high.

      (2) Surgery can be done under **general endotracheal anesthesia,** but it is difficult to obtain optimal surgical conditions, and the dilated bowel can create difficulties for the urologist.

7. **Renal and perirenal surgery.** Associated problems include the following:

   a. The patient is placed in the **lateral jackknife position.** This extreme situation requires general endotracheal anesthesia with controlled ventilation. Spinal anesthesia is not a good choice.

   b. There is a strong possibility of serious and uncontrolled **hemorrhage** from the renal pedicle or inferior vena cava. Adequate means of rapid transfusion should be kept ready during renal or perirenal surgery.

   c. **Pneumothorax** may result from rib resection or technical difficulties. It can be managed with water-seal drainage.

   d. **Thrombosis** may occur in the dependent extremity due to obstruction of venous flow. **Preventive measures** include (1) use of elastic bandages on both legs, (2) moderation in the flexion of the operating table for the lateral position, and (3) early ambulation of the patient.

   e. **The abdominal approach** to large renal tumors or a giant polycystic kidney presents the problems of severe hemorrhage, need for maximal relaxation, and prolonged surgery.

8. **Adrenalectomy.** See Chapter 34, section **IV.**

9. **Spinal cord lesions**

   a. **Loss of bladder control** due to spinal cord injury causes many urologic difficulties. Repeated cystoscopies and urologic procedures are performed on these patients, most often under local anesthesia. However, general anesthesia is occasionally required for endoscopic diagnosis and surgery to control reflexive contraction of the lower body muscles and extremities.

   b. **Autonomic hyperreflexia in urologic patients**

      (1) During cystoscopy and transurethral surgery, **distention of the bladder** with irrigating fluid in a patient with a high spinal cord lesion (above the T_7 segment) may increase autonomic responses to sensory stimulation that are harmless in a normal person. **Symptoms** are

sudden hypertension, bradycardia, facial flushing, sweating, and throbbing headache.

(2) **The sensory stimulation** due to a distended bladder produces a reflex vasoconstriction below the level of spinal cord injury, with an immediate increase of BP.

(3) **Aortic arch and carotid sinus baroreceptors** are stimulated, producing vagal stimulation and vasomotor center inhibition with resulting bradycardia. However, because the sympathetic pathways are interrupted, vasodilation cannot occur below the level of the spinal cord injury.

(4) The bradycardia, vasoconstriction, and high BP may result in heart failure and retinal or intracranial bleeding.

(5) **For therapy** during local or general anesthesia, trimethaphan is indicated. Spinal anesthesia prevents this phenomenon but for obvious reasons is not recommended in a paraplegic or quadriplegic patient.

c. Succinylcholine. Cardiovascular collapse and **cardiac arrest** may follow IV injection of succinylcholine in patients with spinal cord injury, because these patients release significant amounts of potassium following injection of succinylcholine. The susceptible period begins 1–2 days after injury of the spinal cord and extends at least up to 6 months.

d. Penile erection is seen under local or general anesthesia in a few spastic patients undergoing resection of the bladder neck. In such patients, it can be very resistant to treatment (see **II.G.1.c**).

Bibliography

Desmond, J. Complications of transurethral prostatic surgery. *Can. Anaesth. Soc. J.* 17:25, 1970.

Charlton, A. J. Cardiac arrest during transurethral prostatectomy after absorption of 1.5% glycine. A case report and review of the literature. *Anaesthesia* 35:804, 1980.

Hirshman, C. A., and Edelstein, G. Intraoperative hyperkalemia and cardiac arrest during renal transplantation in an insulin-dependent diabetic patient. *Anesthesiology* 51:161, 1979.

Hurlbert, B. J., and Wingard, D. W. Water intoxication after 15 minutes of transurethral resection of the prostate. *Anesthesiology* 50:355, 1979.

Lindahl-Nilsson, C., Lundh, R., and Groth, G. G. Neurolept anesthesia in the renal transplant operation. *Acta Anaesthesiol. Scand.* 24:451, 1980.

McGowan, S. W., and Smith, G. F. N. Anesthesia for transurethral prostatectomy. A comparison of spinal intradural analgesia with two methods of general anesthesia. *Anaesthesia* 35:847, 1980.

Patak, R. V., Lifschitz, M. D., and Stein, J. H. Acute renal failure: Clinical aspects and pathophysiology. *Cardiovasc. Med.* 4:19-38, 1979.

Snow, J. C., Sideropoulos, H. P., Kripke, B. J., et al. Autonomic hyperreflexia during cystoscopy in patients with high spinal cord injuries. *Paraplegia* 15:327, 1977.

Soulillou, J. P., Fillaudeau, F., Keribin, J. B., et al. Acute hyperkalemia risks in recipients of kidney grafts cooled with Collins' solution. *Nephron* 19:301, 1977.

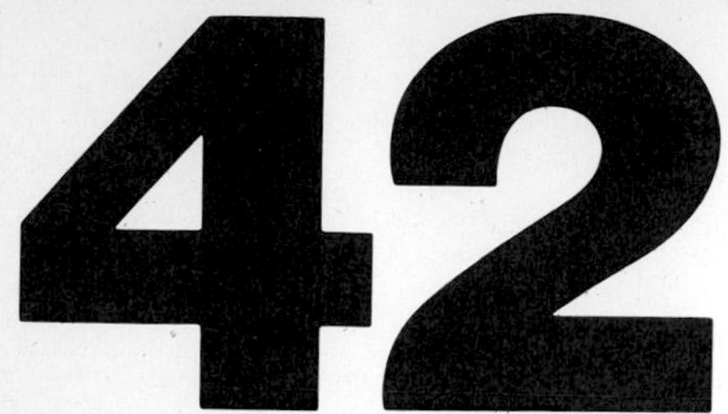

Anesthesia for Outpatient Surgery

I. General considerations

A. Selection of patients

1. **The high cost of hospitalization,** bed shortages, and recognition of the risk of hospital cross-infections have led to the development of hospital ambulatory surgery services, where surgery is performed on a 1-day basis.
2. **Individual cases** are selected for outpatient anesthesia and surgery mainly on the basis of the type of surgery to be performed.
   - a. **Selected operations** are minor, of short duration, and expected to produce minimal bleeding and only minor physiologic derangements.
   - b. **Factors influencing the selection** of patients are the simplicity of the operation, low incidence of postoperative complications, good general health of the patient, psychological acceptance of the procedure by the patient, and cooperation of the surgeon and anesthesiologist or nurse-anesthetist.
3. **Local anesthesia** is indicated in many operations if the patient is cooperative. However, **in children,** general anesthesia is often necessary.

B. The operating room

B. The operating room for outpatient surgery should contain all the equipment found in the inpatient operating room. This includes anesthesia machine, drugs, laryngoscopes and endotracheal tubes, electrocardioscope, suction apparatus, and equipment for bronchoscopy, tracheotomy, and cardiopulmonary resuscitation. A postanesthesia recovery room must be available.

C. Preoperative evaluation and instructions

1. **The preoperative evaluation** of the patient is ordinarily carried out before admission. Much of this can be done in the surgeon's office. The history and physical examination should be done 1–3 days in advance of surgery. If necessary, additional medical or pediatric consultations are requested.
2. **The basic laboratory data** (ECG, chest x-ray, blood tests, and urine tests) are performed within 2 days prior to admission for surgery. Additional tests are done as indicated.
3. **Written instructions** are given to all patients scheduled for outpatient surgery, regardless of whether regional or general anesthesia is to be used. The following points should be included:
   - a. The patient must report to the hospital at least 1 hr before the scheduled time for surgery.
   - b. **Children** and **adults** should have nothing to eat or drink after midnight on the day of surgery; this prohibition includes water, coffee, and orange juice.
   - c. **An informed consent form** will be signed and witnessed before anesthesia, and the patient will be examined by the physician in attendance and by the anesthesiologist.

d. A parent or guardian must accompany a child after discharge from the hospital. An adult patient is not allowed to drive a car and must be accompanied home by a relative or friend.

e. If the patient has a cold, persistent cough, fever, nausea or is vomiting or has not fully recovered from a recent illness, the physician should be notified.

f. If there is any question relating to the patient's health, a medical summary from the family physician or pediatrician should accompany the patient.

II. Anesthetic management

A. Preanesthetic preparation. See Chapter 1.

B. Monitoring. See Chapter 6.

C. Outpatient anesthesia

1. **On arrival in the surgical outpatient** or dental clinic, the patient signs the written informed consent form for administration of anesthesia, and all his or her records are studied and completed in the same manner as are inpatient records.

2. Anesthesia for outpatient surgery is as **hazardous a procedure** as anesthesia for inpatients. Therefore **the same precautions** should be taken, as follows:

   a. Careful check of the record.

   b. Examination of the patient.

   c. Questioning in regard to oral intake, particularly milk if the patient is a child.

   d. Application of monitors.

   e. Securing an IV line for injection of emergency drugs.

   f. Provision of cardiopulmonary resuscitation equipment.

   g. Arrangements to provide an emergency telephone number to be used when the 1-day surgery unit is closed.

3. **Anesthetic methods**

   a. **Local anesthesia,** the most frequent technique for outpatient surgery, is performed by the surgeon in the form of infiltration or field block. Such surgery is similar to procedures carried out in the physician's office.

   b. **Nerve blocks. Brachial plexus block** (see Chap. 17, sec. **III**) is satisfactory for surgery on the shoulder and upper extremity. An interscalene or axillary approach to block the brachial plexus is recommended. The drug used is lidocaine or mepivacaine.

   c. **IV regional anesthesia** (see Chap. 17, sec. **VII**) is an adequate method for outpatient surgery of the upper or lower extremities. The drug used is 0.5% lidocaine without epinephrine. Caution is urged on release of the tourniquet because of systemic absorption of lidocaine.

   d. Spinal, epidural lumbar, and caudal anesthesia are **not satisfactory methods** for outpatient surgery because of postural hypotension (secondary to prolonged sympathetic block) and possible post-lumbar-puncture headache.

   e. **General anesthesia**

      (1) **Minimal medication** is advisable. Premedication may include IM or IV administration of atropine and either a sedative (pentobarbital,

hydroxyzine, or diazepam) or a narcotic (meperidine, alphaprodine, or fentanyl).

(2) **Management of anesthesia**

(a) **In adults,** induction of anesthesia is carried out by IV injection of methohexital, thiopental, or thiamylal, and maintenance is achieved using nitrous oxide and oxygen with halothane, enflurane, isoflurane, or fentanyl. **In children,** induction and maintenance of anesthesia are accomplished by inhalation of nitrous oxide, oxygen, and halothane, enflurane, or isoflurane.

(b) **Respirations** are assisted or controlled. If indicated, tracheal intubation is performed.

(3) Every effort is made to keep the **recovery period** short, so that the patient is able to leave the hospital within a few hours. If necessary, the patient stays longer in the recovery room and may even stay overnight.

Bibliography

Booker, P. D., and Chapman, D. H. Premedication in children undergoing day-care surgery. *Br. J. Anaesth.* 51:1083, 1979.

Frost, E. A. M. Outpatient evaluation. *Anesth. Analg.* (Cleve.) 55:307, 1976.

Riddell, P. L., and Robertson, G. S. Use of doxapram as an arousal agent in outpatient general anesthesia. *Br. J. Anaesth.* 50:921, 1978.

Wright, D. J., and Pandya, A. Smoking and gastric juice volume in outpatients. *Can. Anaesth. Soc. J.* 26:328, 1979.

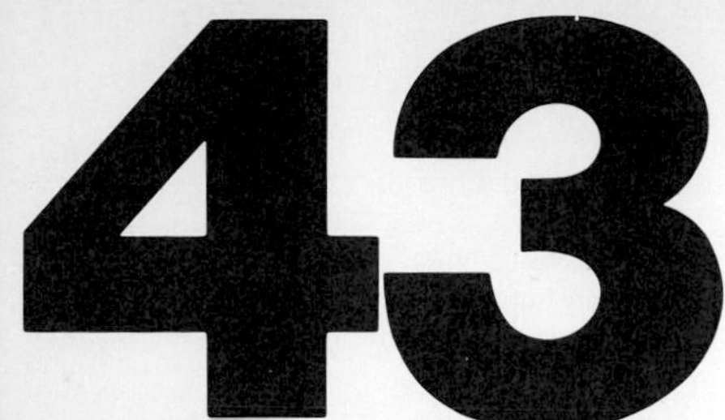

43 Anesthesia for Emergency Surgery

I. General principles

A. The term **emergency** implies that time is important in the successful outcome of the planned surgical procedure. Adequate preparation of equipment and supplies will save valuable time, which is best spent by the anesthesiologist in evaluation of the patient and development of a plan of care.

B. Anesthesia equipment must be kept in working order, and adequate supplies for all possible emergency procedures must be at hand. Although many hospitals employ technicians to maintain equipment and supplies, it is the anesthesiologist's responsibility to ensure that his equipment is kept in proper order.

II. The full stomach

A. Aspiration of stomach contents during induction of anesthesia or emergence is usually a preventable complication.

B. Factors affecting stomach emptying. A careful history of the time and nature of the last solids and liquids ingested and of the interval between the time of the ingestion and the onset of the acute illness or injury are important considerations.

1. **Nature of the materials ingested.** Foods with high fat content prolong emptying time: often 8–10 hr will elapse before emptying is complete. Foods with high glucose content produce an acidic gastric juice.
2. **Emotional distress** will delay emptying.
3. **Medications** such as narcotics delay emptying of the stomach and small bowel.
4. **The time interval between ingestion and the onset** of acute illness, injury, or pain is important. Although many hours may have elapsed since the last oral intake, if the injury or illness occurred within a short time after the oral intake, stomach emptying may have ceased at the time of onset of injury or illness. It is safest to assume that the emergency patient has a full stomach.

C. Hyperventilation or respiratory distress may be associated with air swallowing, creating acute gastric distention, which in turn facilitates regurgitation or vomiting.

D. Patients with nasogastric tubes should be treated as if they have full stomachs, because complete emptying via the tube is never certain. In addition, the tube renders the cardiogastric sphincter incompetent.

E. All women in active labor should be treated as if they have full stomachs irrespective of the time since the last ingestion and the need for anesthesia.

1. Labor delays emptying of the stomach.
2. Pain and fear may cause the patient to swallow air.
3. A long labor will cause a large amount of gastric juice to accumulate.

4. Abdominal contents are pushed cephalad, putting stress on the cardiogastric sphincter and encouraging regurgitation or vomiting.

F. **Patients in coma or semiconsciousness,** regardless of the cause, are prime candidates for aspiration pneumonia. If lavage or gavage is contemplated, the airway should be secured by a cuffed endotracheal tube, or, if cough reflexes are present, the fluid should be instilled after suctioning. The patient should be in a semisitting position, with the larynx at least 40 cm above the cardiogastric sphincter.

1. Usually the force of regurgitation is less than 40 cm H_2O. Therefore the column of regurgitated material should not reach the larynx.
2. Vomiting can occur, but active vomiting is usually associated with a cough reflex.
3. Even with a cough reflex, there is no guarantee that aspiration will not take place.

G. **Techniques for intubating** the patient suspected of having a full stomach include:

1. **Awake intubation.** See Chapter 13, section **V.**
2. **Crash induction,** which may be done in one of two ways:
   a. **Trendelenburg position**
      (1) The patient is placed in a steep Trendelenburg position, so that gastric contents will gravitate to the pharynx instead of the lungs.
      (2) Tubocurarine 3 mg or pancuronium 1 mg is given IV to prevent fasciculations, which would enhance intragastric pressure and aid regurgitation.
      (3) Preoxygenation is done for 5 min.
      (4) The drug of choice for induction of anesthesia is administered rapidly, followed quickly by a suitable dose of succinylcholine (when there is no contraindication to its use).
      (5) There should be no attempt to ventilate; an assistant should compress the trachea firmly against the esophagus as soon as the patient loses consciousness.
      (6) As soon as the masseter muscles are relaxed, the endotracheal tube should be inserted and the cuff inflated immediately.
      (7) It is essential that suction be at hand at all times.
   b. **Reverse Trendelenburg position**
      (1) The patient is put in the steep reverse Trendelenburg position, with the larynx 40 cm above the cardiogastric sphincter. The reason for this position is that the intragastric pressure of fluid during regurgitation seldom, if ever, exceeds 40 cm H_2O. Therefore fluid cannot rise to the level of the larynx, and aspiration cannot occur.
      (2) Follow the steps as in **G.2.a(2)–(6).**
      (3) Failure to abolish fasciculations or permitting the patient to strain during intubation will cause an increase in intraabdominal pressure, and the force of the gastric fluid will be sufficient to permit regurgitation.

H. **Treatment of aspiration**

1. The severity of the effect of aspiration is determined by the pH of the fluid aspirated (the more acidic the fluid, the more severe the pneumonia), by the volume aspirated, and by the particles present in the aspirate.

2. **Treatment of choice**

   a. Immediate intubation, suctioning, and ventilation.

   b. Bronchial lavage with aliquots of 3–5 ml of sterile saline solution and ventilation, followed by additional suctioning.

   c. Repeat the suction-ventilation-lavage-ventilation-suction routine until no more particles are suctioned or there is a clear return fluid.

   d. Start a broad-spectrum antibiotic.

   e. If bronchial spasm is present, 1 g of hydrocortisone is injected IV, and 250 mg of aminophylline diluted in 250 ml of 5% D/W is administered IV slowly but discontinued if arrhythmias or hypotension develops.

3. Measure **the pH of the gastric fluid.** A pH of less than 2 may cause the manifestations of aspiration pneumonia: pulmonary hemorrhage, atelectasis, decrease in the function of surfactant, and severe bronchospasm. Other manifestations may include cardiovascular collapse, hypoxia, tachypnea, dyspnea, and cyanosis.

I. A chest x-ray should be taken as soon as is practical after a suspected aspiration. A repeat film should be taken 6–8 hr later if the initial film was negative for aspiration pneumonia, since there may be a delay between the aspiration and the development of pneumonia.

III. **Hypotension** may be defined as a reduction of 30–35% in the patient's normal systolic BP.

A. **Causes of hypotension**

1. Hypovolemia.
2. Cardiogenic shock.
3. Neurogenic shock.
4. Sepsis.
5. Adrenal hypofunction or failure.
6. Metabolic derangement (i.e., diabetic coma).

B. **Laboratory tests**

1. Blood tests should include a CBC and electrolyte and blood sugar determinations.
2. Additional tests, such as blood culture and blood for toxicology studies, should be ordered when toxic or septic causation is strongly suspected.
3. A blood sample should be taken for blood typing and crossmatching.
4. Arterial blood gases are measured.

C. **To follow the progress of treatment,** the following monitoring system can be employed:

1. **BP,** either by cuff or—more accurate in the presence of severe hypotension—by arterial line with direct reading from a transducer.
2. **Central venous pressure** (CVP), which is more useful in diagnosing right heart overload than the adequacy of fluid replacement. A CVP line offers an additional line through which fluids can be administered.
3. **ECG.**
4. **Temperature probe.** Both hypothermia and hyperthermia can cause serious intraoperative management problems.

   a. **Probes** are designed for tympanic-membrane, esophageal, and rectal placement.

(1) **The tympanic probe** closely monitors brain temperature. It should not be used in a patient with a perforated tympanic membrane or with bleeding from the canal. Care must be used in placement, to avoid damaging the eardrum.

(2) **The esophageal probe** should be positioned at the level of the heart to measure cardiac temperature. If it is placed cephalad to the heart, the cool anesthetic gases entering the trachea will give a false reading, indicating a lower cardiac temperature than actually exists. On the other hand, rapid infusions of cool fluids or exposure of large areas of body surface in a cold operating room will cause the heart temperature to drop. When the heart temperature is near or below 33° C, serious ventricular arrhythmias may occur.

(3) **The rectal probe** has the disadvantage of not indicating the true core temperature, because stool in the rectum acts as an insulating material. The difference can be greater than 1° C.

b. In addition to the direct effect of cold on the myocardium, there can be intense peripheral vasoconstriction that will dampen Korotkoff's sounds and make it difficult to determine BP by cuff.

5. Urinary bladder catheter

a. Urine output indicates both the state of hydration and the rate of blood flow through the kidney. Maintaining a urine flow of 40–60 ml/hr will minimize the possibility of acute renal failure in the immediate postoperative period. The kidney needs a minimum of 80 torr pressure to maintain this flow rate.

b. When urine output is low in the presence of an adequate BP, an osmotic diuretic such as mannitol is a preferred challenge drug. There is little response if the decreased urine output is secondary to hypovolemia.

c. Besides monitoring kidney function, the urinary catheter permits careful monitoring of fluid intake and output in the acutely ill patient.

6. Swan-Ganz catheter

a. When a patient is critically ill and has cardiopulmonary problems, this monitoring system provides valuable information about both right heart and left heart function.

b. The Swan-Ganz catheter measures CVP, pulmonary artery pressure, pulmonary wedge pressure (a measure of left heart function), and, with modifications, cardiac output.

c. Its placement requires skill.

7. Arterial line

a. An indwelling arterial line is useful in continuous measuring of BP and in sampling arterial gases for evaluation of pulmonary status.

b. The radial and brachial arteries are easily accessible.

(1) Before cannulation of the radial (or ulnar) artery, the Allen test should be done to ensure that the radial-ulnar artery arch is intact. A terminal vessel, i.e., one with no collateral circulation, should never be used, since, if it becomes occluded, the tissue it supplies distal to the occlusion will lose its blood supply.

(2) **Allen test**

(a) Occlude both the ulnar and radial arteries by compressing the vessels with your fingers.

(b) Instruct the patient to open and close the hand rapidly several times.

(c) The hand should then appear blanched.

(d) Release the ulnar artery. The hand should become pink again within 5–10 sec.

(e) Failure of the hand to regain its pink color indicates that the ulnar artery is a terminal artery.

(f) Repeat the steps in **(a)** and **(b)**.

(g) Release the radial artery instead of the ulnar artery. Look for pinkening of the hand. If it does not occur, the radial and ulnar arteries in that hand should not be used.

c. **The brachial artery** may be cannulated if the radial and ulnar arteries are unsatisfactory. However, it is a terminal vessel in some patients, and its occlusion, if not diagnosed and treated in time, can require amputation of the hand.

d. The arterial line can be kept patent by a heparin lock or a solution of 1 unit of heparin per milliliter of IV solution flushed through it from time to time.

8. In a major emergency, a **thermal blanket** should be on the operating room table, so that the patient's temperature can be kept within reasonable deviations from normal.

D. **When uncertainty** as to the cause of hypotension or the possibility of adrenal failure exists, or in the presence of septic shock, giving IV corticosteroids equivalent to 1 g of hydrocortisone has been advised.

E. **Support measures,** such as volume replacement and cardiovascular stimulant drugs, should not be withheld while establishing monitoring systems in patients who exhibit signs of shock other than a decrease in BP.

IV. Respiratory distress

A. Mechanical causes of respiratory problems

1. Upper airway

a. **Injuries** involving the soft tissue and bony structures of the face can produce mechanical obstruction of respiration. **Careful inspection of the mouth and pharynx** for foreign bodies, broken teeth, and blood clots should be done before administering any drugs that would obtund the patient's respiratory efforts.

(1) **Swelling of the soft tissues** presents a hazard by displacing the tongue against the soft palate and by occluding the hypopharynx. Anesthesia in such patients may convert a partial obstruction into a complete obstruction, with the risk of anoxic damage. If any doubt exists about the ability to maintain a patent airway during induction of anesthesia, the patient should be **intubated awake.**

(2) A fracture of the middle third of the face introduces the hazard of ethmoid fractures, and nasal intubation should be avoided unless this is the only route to secure an airway. The passage of a nasal tube can track infection to the brain; it is possible to pass a nasogastric tube through a fractured ethmoid plate into the brain.

b. **Effective suction apparatus** is essential, especially in preparing to intubate a patient with facial or intraoral injuries. Care must be exercised not to push debris into the trachea during the preparation for intubation.

c. **Facial injuries** may be associated with trauma to the **larynx.** If the patient has difficulty with vocalization and the voice is similar to that of a patient with bulbar weakness, suspect a fractured larynx. In such a patient, it may be possible to pass only a small endotracheal tube. A **tracheotomy** may be indicated before the emergency surgery is begun.

d. **Aspiration of foreign bodies** is a common emergency.

(1) With a cooperative adult, **topical anesthesia** may be best, since it permits better inspection of the airway, gives ample time for bronchoscopy, and decreases the risk of forcing the foreign body farther down the tracheobronchial tree.

(2) **When general anesthesia is required,** a range of endotracheal tubes must be prepared. A much smaller tube may be needed than is routinely used. To ensure adequate oxygenation, a high inspired concentration of oxygen may be needed if the foreign material is obstructing a main bronchial division.

2. **The thorax and its contents**

a. **Tears in the trachea,** contusion of the lung, and pneumothorax are life-threatening problems that may be associated with blunt trauma to the thorax or penetrating wounds.

(1) The endotracheal tube must be passed beyond the tear in the trachea, and the balloon inflated, to secure the airway.

(2) If the contusion is severe, a tube, such as a Robert-Shaw or Carlens, is indicated for isolation of the affected lung to prevent or minimize spillage into it or to collapse a lung to facilitate repair.

b. **Pneumothorax**

(1) **Preoperative diagnosis** can be made by auscultation, chest x-ray, inspection of respiratory movements and the development of subcutaneous emphysema, complaints of air deprivation, and ashen color of the patient.

(2) **Intraoperatively,** unexplained narrowing of the pulse pressure, tachyarrhythmias, hypoxia, decreased compliance, and then the development of subcutaneous emphysema may be indications of a pneumothorax.

(3) In a patient with a history of adult respiratory distress syndrome or chest injury, taping a chest stethoscope to each side of the thorax and frequent auscultations during the operative procedure will detect the development of pneumothorax before serious problems occur.

(4) **Emergency treatment** of a pneumothorax consists of insertion through the chest wall of a large-bore needle or plastic intravenous catheter attached to a three-way stopcock and a syringe. It will permit rapid and efficient evacuation of the air until a proper chest tube can be inserted.

V. Cardiac tamponade

A. **Cardiac tamponade may be caused** by either trauma or disease. If it is severe, the pericardial sac should be tapped before an anesthetic is administered.

1. In the presence of tamponade, great care should be used in administering any agent that would reduce myocardial contractility.

2. Decreased contractility will limit cardiac output; cardiac arrest may follow, with little chance of resuscitation.

B. **A sleep dose of ketamine** or, in extreme cases, nitrous oxide amnesia or no anesthesia may be used for intubation in association with a muscle relaxant drug. Tubocurarine should be used with caution because of its tendency to induce hypotension.

VI. The central nervous system

A. Spinal cord

1. **The patient with acutely developing lesions,** causing cord compression of the cervical spine, requires careful positioning. A collar for support can prevent transection of the cord and permanent paralysis.

   a. If the patient is cooperative, he or she should be asked to move the head and neck to the point of beginning discomfort. This will give the anesthesiologist knowledge of permissible movement once the patient is anesthetized.

   b. Any positioning of the patient with possible cord injury should be done slowly and with ample personnel to make each movement smooth, preventing any unnecessary stress on the spinal column.

2. **Succinylcholine** should be avoided, since its use may cause hyperkalemia.

3. In the presence of increased intracranial pressure, the depolarizing drug succinylcholine may be used only if a small dose of a nondepolarizing drug (tubocurarine or pancuronium) is used before administering the succinylcholine. The fasciculations caused by succinylcholine increase the intracranial pressure and may compress the medulla.

B. Intracranial disease and injury. The major problem facing the anesthesiologist in dealing with patients with intracranial problems is to avoid increasing the intracranial pressure.

1. **The intracranial pressure may be increased** by:

   a. Improper positioning of the patient. Obstruction of venous return by careless positioning will elevate cerebrospinal fluid pressure.

   b. Fasciculations secondary to depolarizing muscle relaxants.

   c. Hypercapnia from cerebral vasodilation.

   d. The use of **nitrous oxide** if there is free air within the cranial vault. Air used in pneumoencephalography may remain for longer than 36 hr. Because of nitrous oxide's solubility, it will diffuse into air-filled ventricles, creating increased cerebrospinal fluid pressure.

   e. Permitting the patient to strain or buck before the cranial vault is open.

   f. Excessive hydration.

2. **In posterior fossa exploration,** some surgeons want the patient to breathe spontaneously, because respiration characteristics may be altered before cardiovascular changes occur when the surgeon is working near the medullary structures.

3. **Air embolism**

   a. If the patient is in **the sitting position** and ventilating spontaneously, during the inhalation phase of the respiratory cycle, the negative force of inspiration is sufficient to permit air to be sucked into any venous channels that may be open in the neck or above that level, causing air to enter the heart.

   b. **To recognize and treat** air embolism, the following are useful: a precordial or esophageal stethoscope, ECG monitor, and CVP catheter in the right atrium.

      (1) Air entering the heart may produce a mill-wheel murmur that is characteristic of air embolism. Hypotension and irregular respiration

may precede the murmur. (A smaller amount of air may cause only a change in the heart sounds.)

(2) **Rapid treatment** is indicated because the foaming effect will block cardiac output.

(3) With a CVP catheter in the right atrium, the air can be sucked out via the catheter. If practical, the patient's position can be changed from the sitting position to the left lateral position with the head down.

VII. Orthopedic emergencies

A. These emergencies usually are limited to **acute fractures and infection.** If no other injury or disease demands immediate anesthesia, such operations can be delayed until there is an opportunity to obtain an adequate medical workup and correction of underlying problems.

B. Blood loss in closed fractures has been estimated as follows:

1. Fracture of the foot with moderate swelling, 250–500 ml.
2. Fracture of the lower part of the leg with moderate swelling, 500–1000 ml.
3. Fracture of the femoral shaft, 500–2000 ml.
4. Fracture of the knee joint, up to 2000 ml.
5. Fracture of the forearm, 500–750 ml.
6. Fracture of the humerus and shoulder, up to 2000 ml.

C. Estimating blood loss **in the presence of soft tissue damage.** Using the standard volume of a man's clenched fist to represent a volume of damaged tissue, the following is a guide for estimating blood loss:

1. Less than one hand, 10–20% of blood volume.
2. One to three hands, 20–40%.
3. Three to five hands, up to 40%.

VIII. Burns

A. The freshly burned patient may require:

1. Tracheotomy.
2. Fasciotomy.
3. Debridement.

B. Special problems presented by burn patients include:

1. Loss of thermal control because of large areas of skin lost.
2. Massive shifts in fluids, which create a reduced blood volume.
3. Toxins liberated by the damaged tissue, which enhance the hypotension and can damage kidney function.
4. **Hyperkalemia.** Burn patients should not be given succinylcholine. Fatal arrhythmias can develop from the rapid transient rise in potassium during the depolarization of the muscle by succinylcholine.

C. A commonly used formula **for estimating fluid replacement** in burn therapy is the Brook Army Hospital formula.

1. Formula components:
   - **a.** Weight of the patient.
   - **b.** Estimation of the percentage of burn, based on the **rule of nines** (see Chap. 20, sec. **VI.C.3**).

2. To estimate 24-hr replacement:
   a. Body weight in kg × % burn × 0.5 ml colloid.
   b. Body weight in kg × % burn × 1.5 ml isotonic electrolyte solution.
3. Give half of calculated doses in the first 8 hr, the remainder over the next 16 hr.
4. In addition to these calculated requirements, give 0.9% or 0.45% saline in a volume equal to that lost by nasogastric suction.

D. **In severe burns,** additional monitoring should include:
1. Temperature.
2. CVP.
3. Arterial blood gases.
4. Urine volume output and content analysis.
5. Serial blood electrolytes and serum osmolarity.
6. Serial hematocrits.

E. **Acute adult respiratory distress syndrome** may develop because of inhaled toxins, pulmonary burns, oxygen toxicity, or septicemia. Positive end-expiratory pressure has proved of great value in this complication.

IX. Anesthesia techniques for emergency surgery

A. The best technique is the one in which the anesthesiologist is most skilled. An emergency is no time to attempt a new method.
1. There are no absolute contraindications to **general anesthesia.**
2. **Conduction anesthesia** lends itself well to surgical procedures on the forearm, hand, and leg. **Contraindications** to regional or spinal anesthesia are:
   a. **Infection** in the area that the needle must traverse.
   b. **Bleeding disorders.**
   c. **Hypovolemia** with >20% blood volume loss if spinal or epidural anesthesia is indicated, unless it is corrected before administering the anesthetic. This is not an absolute contraindication; judgment should be tempered by consideration of the patient's general health and age. If the spinal or epidural route is selected, replacement of the volume should be accomplished with reasonable speed, with BP supported by vasopressors as indicated.
3. In a patient with a **full stomach,** after all factors have been weighed, **regional anesthesia** should be strongly considered. Spinal or epidural anesthesia gives no absolute protection against aspiration. Regurgitation is possible and, in the absence of abdominal muscle tone, effective coughing to protect the larynx may not be possible.

B. **Patients in shock** require much-reduced doses of any anesthetic agent used because perfusion changes shunt blood preferentially to the heart, brain, kidney, and liver. As the circulatory dynamics improve, additional drugs may be required to maintain a given level of anesthesia.
1. Medications should not be given IM or SQ to a hypotensive patient because of unpredictable absorption rates.
2. The IV route is the route of choice, with dosage alterations as indicated by the manufacturer, by the patient's assessed condition, and by the pharmacology of the agent.

3. Because intrapulmonary shunting is often present during shock, it is advisable to give at least a 50% inspired oxygen concentration to ensure adequate oxygenation.

Bibliography

Ancker, K., Halldin, M., and Gothe, C. J. Nitrous oxide analgesia during ambulance transportation. Airborne levels of nitrous oxide. *Acta Anaesthesiol. Scand.* 24:497, 1980.

Snow, J. C., Kripke, B. J., Sessions, G. P., et al. Cardiovascular collapse following succinylcholine in a paraplegic patient. *Paraplegia* 11:199, 1973.

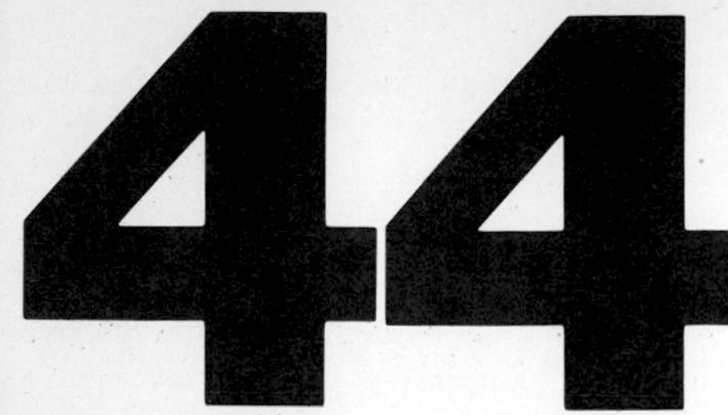

Invasive Hemodynamic Monitoring

I. Indications

A. Patients with preexisting cardiovascular disease compromising normal physical activity.

1. A history of **unstable angina** or **angina at rest** with any of the following:
   a. A history of **recent heart failure** or failure present at the time of the proposed surgery.
   b. A recent history of **ischemia or infarction.**
   c. Symptomatic **mitral or aortic valvular disease.**
2. Severe, uncontrolled **hypertension.**
3. Unstable **arrhythmias.**

B. Patients with preexisting symptomatic **pulmonary disease.**

C. Patients in shock or whose state of hydration is uncertain.

D. Planned surgical interventions that will cause **large shifts in fluids.**

E. One-lung anesthesia.

F. When noninvasive monitoring techniques will not provide adequate information for planning therapeutic interventions, or the information provided would not be accurate.

G. Controlled **hypotension.**

H. Operations done with the patient in the **sitting position.**

II. Problems associated with invasive methods

A. Discomfort to the patient during instrumentation.

B. Potential source of infections if aseptic techniques are not used during the instrumentation and for the care of the sites and equipment used for monitoring.

C. Potential source for thrombi or emboli and cellulitis.

D. Instrumentation can damage adjacent anatomic structures, e.g., hemothorax, pneumothorax, laceration of vessels or nerves.

III. Monitoring equipment

A. Electronic equipment has **three basic components** that must be appropriate for the physiologic event to be measured.

B. The physiologic event being measured is **pressure change.**

C. The **transducer** must be responsive within the range of the pressure being measured.

1. **Pressure waves** are complex events consisting of:

a. Frequency.

b. Amplitude

c. Oscillation and resonance.

d. Phase.

2. **Impedance** and dampening affect transducer response.

D. The **amplifier** must be capable of filtering appropriate signals and transmitting the desired signals to a recording device.

E. The **recording device** must be capable of displaying information in a meaningful way.

F. A difference in a value obtained from an electronic device and one obtained by mechanical means is not unusual. The **best example** is the occlusion method of obtaining blood pressures versus the electronic measurement of the pressure wave.

G. An **error in transducing** can be minimized by the selection of the correct tubing and filters and attention to the details of caring for the cannulas.

IV. Arterial cannulation

A. Indications

1. **Critically ill patients** requiring multiple blood gases and beat-by-beat BP monitoring.

2. Controlled hypotension.

3. One-lung anesthesia.

4. Hypothermic patients in whom mechanical methods of monitoring pressure would be grossly inaccurate.

5. Massively obese patients in whom monitoring by mechanical means would be difficult.

6. Patients with severe aortic stenosis or severe coronary artery disease.

B. Selection of the artery to be cannulated

1. Any readily palpable artery may be chosen.

a. Arteries that are not end-arteries are preferred. If thrombosis occurs in an end-artery because of the cannulation, the patient may experience gangrene in the area served by the artery.

b. If the patient has an injury to the hand in which part of the hand may be lost, it is best not to use the uninjured arm as a site.

2. The **radial or ulnar arteries are the most commonly used** for cannulation. **Allen's test** is done to determine if the palmar arterial arc is intact. If it is, it is usually safe to use an 18-gauge or smaller plastic needle for a cannula for either the ulnar or radial artery.

a. Have the patient extend the arm, palm side up.

b. Palpate the radial and ulnar arteries at the wrist.

c. Manually occlude both arteries.

d. Have the patient elevate the arm to drain the venous blood. The hand will have a pale, ischemic color.

e. Release the pressure on the ulnar artery. The hand should completely return to its normal color within a few seconds.

f. Repeat as above, but release the pressure on the radial artery instead of the ulnar artery.

g. If the flush returns after each release, either artery may be used. If it does not, select other arteries.

3. **The dorsalis pedis** is another convenient artery.

C. Cannulation procedure

1. Prepare a solution of heparin, 1 unit/ml of normal saline.
2. Fill a 10-ml syringe with this solution. Put a stopcock and an extension connector on the syringe, ensuring that the heparinized saline fills the connector.
3. **Secure the forearm and hand** on an arm board. The hand should be palm side up, and a small roll should be placed under the wrist, so that it is comfortably hyperextended.
4. Prepare the skin over the wrist with an iodine solution.
5. **Using a 25-gauge needle,** infiltrate the skin over the selected artery with a local anesthetic. Be careful not to use a large amount since it may obscure the pulsation.
6. **Pierce the skin with a 15-gauge needle.** This will facilitate the passage of the 18-gauge or smaller needle and prevent a skin plug in the needle tip.
7. Partially fill a 3-ml syringe with the heparinized saline, and attach it to the needle selected for cannulating the artery.
8. With your nondominant hand, **palpate the artery,** placing your index and middle fingers over the artery gently. Too much pressure by the exploring fingers may occlude the pulsations.
9. **Insert the needle** through the puncture site. Gently create negative pressure in the syringe as you move the needle toward the artery. Once the bevel of the needle enters the artery, blood should readily enter the syringe. Advance the needle slowly to avoid going through or past the artery.
10. Once the artery has been entered, slip the sheath off the needle and withdraw the stylet.
11. With your nondominant hand, occlude the tip of the catheter in the artery to prevent unnecessary blood loss. Attach the 10-ml syringe with the stopcock and extension to the needle. **Flush heparinized saline** through the system, and turn the stopcock "off" to patient. Secure the line with adhesive tape after applying antibiotic ointment to the puncture site.
12. **A flush solution** of heparinized saline may be attached to a pressurized system that can be opened from time to time to flush the cannula, preventing a thrombus from partially or completely occluding the cannula.
13. The arterial line now may be used to draw samples for blood gas analysis or blood pressure monitoring.

V. Central venous pressure monitoring

A. Indications

1. A **history of heart failure** or suspected heart failure.
2. Expected large intraoperative and perioperative fluid requirements.
3. Direct administration of drugs.
4. Need for parenteral nutrition.

B. Selection of a vessel

1. Any vein large enough to receive an 18- or larger-gauge bore long-line catheter and through which the catheter may be threaded into the right heart.

2. The most accessible veins are the **right basilic vein,** the **subclavian veins,** and the **external or internal jugular veins.**

C. **Preparation**

1. The vessel is selected and prepared in the same manner as for arterial cannulation. Local anesthetic is infiltrated SQ.

2. **If the basilic vein** is selected, a tourniquet is applied to the upper part of the brachium to encourage venous filling. Once the needle is in the vein and the long-line catheter is advanced, the tourniquet is removed.

3. Resistance may be met at the shoulder. Have the patient place the arm at right angles to the body and turn the head in the opposite direction. This may aid in slipping the catheter into the subclavian vein. The line cannot be forced; it may perforate the vein or knot on itself.

4. Once it is presumed that the catheter is in the superior vena cava or right heart, the needle is withdrawn from the vein, and the plastic guard is placed over the needle. The catheter is connected to an IV administering set containing a small amount of methylene blue or Berocca-c and heparin, 1 unit/ml of IV solution. The central venous pressure (CVP) may be monitored by using manometry or a transducer.

5. Placement should be checked by chest x-ray.

6. **The external or internal jugular veins** may also be used. The method of cannulation will be discussed in section **VI.**

D. **When transducing equipment is available,** it is the preferred method of monitoring CVP. In addition to obtaining beat-by-beat CVP values, the waves generated can be evaluated for information about the heart's performance.

VI. **Pulmonary artery pressure monitoring (Swan-Ganz Catheterization)**

A. **Indications**

1. Severe coronary artery disease.

2. Recent evidence of myocardial ischemia or infarction.

3. Existing heart failure.

4. Severe valvular heart disease.

5. Septic shock.

B. **Selection of a vessel**

1. The **cephalic** vein, **subclavian** vein, or **external or internal jugular** veins may be used.

2. **Complications associated with cannulation**

a. **Cephalic vein**

(1) A cutdown may be required.

(2) It may be impossible to float the catheter into the subclavian vein.

(3) Fluoroscopy may be needed for accurate placement.

b. **Subclavian vein**

(1) Inadvertent laceration of the subclavian artery, with subsequent difficulty in controlling hemorrhage.

(2) Potential risk of hemothorax and pneumothorax.

c. **External jugular vein**

(1) The anatomy is variable as to location and size.

(2) There may be difficulty in entering the subclavian vein.

d. Internal jugular vein

(1) Inadvertent laceration of the carotid artery may occur, but the hemorrhage is easier to control than that of the subclavian artery. If the patient has preexisting carotid stenosis, a hematoma may cause a stroke or a transient ischemic attack.

(2) Injury to the brachial plexus.

(3) Pneumothorax.

C. Internal jugular vein. This vein can be used for placement of a flow-directed catheter for monitoring pulmonary artery pressure, cardiac output, CVP, and core temperature.

1. The vessel is relatively easy to cannulate. Using the Seldinger technique there is little risk of injury to adjoining structures.

2. Seldinger technique

a. The patient is supine, with the operating room table in a 20- to 30-degree Trendelenberg position if the patient can tolerate it. This causes distention of the internal jugular vein and prevents air embolism.

b. An **oxygen mask** is placed over the patient's face.

c. Pillows are removed from under the patient's head and he or she is asked to turn the head to a 45-degree angle from the midline. If the head is sharply turned away from the side to be cannulated, the internal jugular vein is brought over the carotid artery, making it more likely that the artery will be entered.

d. **The right internal jugular vein** is the vein of choice because there is almost a straight line from it into the subclavian vein and then into the superior vena cava.

e. The **patient's neck** is prepared from the tip of the mastoid process to below the clavicle and from the midline anteriorly to the anterior border of the trapezius.

f. **The operator scrubs** and puts on gloves and gown using aseptic technique after checking the calibration of the transducer, ensuring that the patient's arterial pressure tracing, ECG, and the channel tracing for the Swan-Ganz catheter will be in view. The heparinized solutions for the catheter flush are prepared as described in section **IV.C**.

g. **The patient is draped using aseptic technique,** with the sterile area extending at least over the entire chest.

h. Kits are available from several manufacturers that will provide all the equipment necessary for introducing a Swan-Ganz catheter. The kit is aseptically handed to the operator, who places it on the patient's chest or a sterile Mayo stand.

i. The operator's left hand identifies the **carotid artery. The heads of the sternocleidomastoid muscle** are identified. The apex formed by the diverging heads of the muscle is found; it is approximately at the level of the cricoid ring, slightly below the external jugular vein, and approximately midway between the tip of the mastoid process and the clavicle, or about 5 cm above the clavicle.

j. **A line may be drawn from the cricoid ring** parallel to the clavicle and another line may be drawn from the tip of the mastoid process perpendicular to the clavicle. The lines' intersection should be slightly above the apex of the triangle formed by the heads of the sternocleidomastoid muscle and the clavicle.

k. A skin wheel of local anesthetics is made at that point. The left hand remains over the carotid artery. A 1.5-inch, 22-gauge needle with a 5-ml syringe filled with local anesthetic is advanced through the skin with the needle directed toward the medial border of the clavicular insertion of the sternocleidomastoid muscle. In the average adult, the **vein** should be encountered before the needle is inserted more than an inch. The direction and depth of the needle are noted, and the needle is withdrawn.

l. **A 16-gauge needle with a plastic sheath** is inserted in the same manner as before. When blood enters the syringe, the plastic sheath is advanced, the needle introducer is withdrawn, and a wire guide is passed through the sheath. A length of the guide wire remaining above the skin should be at least an inch longer than the introducer to be used. If too little remains above the skin, there is a danger that the guide wire may be sucked into the right heart. The tip of the wire should always be readily visible and of sufficient length to be grasped by the operator.

m. The sheath is removed, and an incision about 0.25 inch in length is made completely through the skin at the site of the wire.

n. **The introducer** is threaded over the guide wire and into the vein. Blood should freely return through the introducer after the wire is removed. Heparinized saline is flushed through the introducer.

o. **The Swan-Ganz ports are tested for patency,** and the catheter is threaded through the introducer sheath. The tip port pilot tube is attached to the transducer with appropriate tubing, the balloon-tip pilot tube is inflated, and the catheter is slowly advanced. The pressure tracing waves will inform the operator of the location of the tip. The waveform changes as it passes from the right atrium into the right ventricle and the pulmonary artery, and then when it is in wedge position.

p. **When the catheter is in wedge position,** note the distance the catheter is inserted, secure the introducer sheath by suturing it in place, place antiseptic ointment over the insertion site, and apply a sterile occlusive dressing. Secure the Swan-Ganz catheter so that it will not move in or out of the sheath. The catheter may be withdrawn if needed but may not be advanced once the exterior portions of the catheter are no longer sterile.

3. **If you are uncertain** that the catheter is in a vein or an artery, draw a sample from the arterial cannula and one from the cannula in the questionable vessel. If the blood appears darker from the vessel in question, it is venous. If the color is the same, the vessel is an artery.

D. Normal values

CVP	5–10 torr
RV	22/0 torr
PA	20/10 torr
Wedge	12–15 torr
C.T.	2.5–4 L/min/m^2
C. O.	4–8 L/min
B.P.	140–100/90–60 torr

Bibliography

Bedford, R. F. Radial arterial function following percutaneous cannulation with 18- and 20-gauge catheters. *Anesthesiology* 47:37, 1977.

Bedford, R. F. Long-term radial artery cannulation. Effects on subsequent vessel function. *Crit. Care Med.* 6:64, 1978.

Borja, A. R. Current status of infraclavicular subclavian catheterization. *Ann. Thorac. Surg.* 13:615, 1972.

Brodsky, J. B. A simple method to determine patency of the ulnar artery intraoperatively prior to radial artery cannulation. *Anesthesiology* 42:626, 1975.

Buchbinder, N., and Ganz, W. Hemodynamic monitoring. Invasive techniques. *Anesthesiology* 45:146, 1976.

Ganz, W., et al. A new technique for measurement of cardiac output by thermodilution in man. *Am. J. Cardiol.* 27:392, 1971.

Ganz, W., and Swan, H. J. C. Measurement of blood flow by thermodilution. *Am. J. Cardiol.* 29:241, 1972.

Katz, A. M., Birnbaum, M., Moylan, J., et al. Gangrene of the hand and forearm. A complication of radial artery cannulation. *Crit. Care Med.* 2:270, 1974.

Kim, J. M., Arakawa, K., and Bliss, J. Arterial cannulation. Factors in the development of occlusion. *Anesth. Analg.* (Cleve.) 54:836, 1975.

Kuramoto, T., and Sakabe, T. Comparison of success in jugular vs. basilic vein techniques for central venous pressure catheter positioning. *Anesth. Analg.* (Cleve.) 54:696, 1975.

Mangano, D. T., and Hickey, R. F. Ischemic injury following uncomplicated radial artery catheterization. *Anesth. Analg.* (Cleve.) 58:55, 1979.

Miyasaka, K., Edmonds, J. F., and Conn, A. W. Complications of radial artery lines in the pediatric patients. *Can. Anaesth. Soc. J.* 23:9, 1976.

Ramanathan, S., Chalon, J., and Turndorf, H. Determining patency of palmar arches by retrograde radial pulsation. *Anesthesiology* 42:756, 1975.

Stoelting, R. K. Evaluation of external jugular venous pressure as a reflection of right atrial pressure. *Anesthesiology* 38:291, 1973.

Stamm, W. E., Colella, J. J., Anderson, R. L., et al. Indwelling arterial catheters as a source of nosocomial bacteremia. *N. Engl. J. Med.* 292:1099, 1975.

Johnson, R. W. A complication of radial artery cannulation. *Anesthesiology* 40:598, 1974.

Swan, H. J. C., and Ganz, W. Use of balloon flotation catheters in critically ill patients. *Surg. Clin. North Am.* 55:501, 1975.

Talbot, L., and Berger, S. A. Fluid-mechanical aspects of the human circulation. *Am. Sci.* 62:671, 1974.

Zinner, S. H., Denny-Brown, B. C., Braun, P., et al. Risk of infection with intravenous indwelling catheters. Effect of application of antibiotic ointment. *J. Infect. Dis.* 120:616, 1979.

Index

The Little, Brown SPIRAL™ Manual Series

Little, Brown SPIRAL™ manuals are available at all medical bookstores throughout the United States and abroad. You may also order copies directly from Little, Brown and Company, by tearing out, filling in, and mailing this postage-paid card.

☐ MANUAL OF **MEDICAL THERAPEUTICS**, 23rd Edition—Washington University Department of Medicine; Freitag & Miller, Editors (#924032) **$15.95**

☐ MANUAL OF **CLINICAL PROBLEMS IN INTERNAL MEDICINE:** ANNOTATED WITH KEY REFERENCES, 2nd Edition—Spivak & Barnes (#807141) **$15.95**

☐ PROBLEM-ORIENTED **MEDICAL DIAGNOSIS**, 2nd Edition—Friedman, Editor(#293563) **$14.95**

☐ MANUAL OF **CLINICAL PROBLEMS IN INFECTIOUS DISEASE:** WITH ANNOTATED KEY REFERENCES—Gantz & Gleckman (#303518) **$14.95**

☐ MANUAL OF **ACUTE BACTERIAL INFECTIONS:** EARLY DIAGNOSIS AND TREATMENT—Gardner & Provine (#303275) **$14.95**

☐ MANUAL OF **CORONARY CARE**, 2nd Edition—Alpert & Francis (#035033) **$12.95**

☐ MANUAL OF **CARDIOVASCULAR DIAGNOSIS AND THERAPY**—Alpert & Rippe (#035025) **$14.95**

☐ MANUAL OF **CLINICAL PROBLEMS IN CARDIOLOGY:** WITH ANNOTATED KEY REFERENCES—Hillis, Ormand & Willerson (#364002) **$13.95**

☐ MANUAL OF **ELECTROCARDIOGRAPHY**—Mudge (#589179) **$12.95**

☐ MANUAL OF **CLINICAL PROBLEMS IN PULMONARY MEDICINE:** WITH ANNOTATED KEY REFERENCES—Bordow, Stool & Moser (#102644) **$15.95**

☐ MANUAL OF **SURGICAL THERAPEUTICS**, 5th Edition—Condon & Nyhus, Editors (#152692) **$15.95**

☐ MANUAL OF **MEDICAL CARE OF THE SURGICAL PATIENT**, 2nd Edition—Papper & Williams (#690481) **$13.95**

☐ MANUAL OF **EMERGENCY AND OUTPATIENT TECHNIQUES**—Washington University Department of Surgery; Klippel & Anderson, Editors (#498688) **$14.95**

☐ MANUAL OF **ACUTE ORTHOPAEDIC THERAPEUTICS**, 2nd Edition—Iversen & Clawson (#434310) **$14.95**

☐ MANUAL OF **PEDIATRIC THERAPEUTICS**, 2nd Edition—Children's Hospital Medical Center, Boston; Graef & Cone, Editors (#139114) **$15.95**

☐ MANUAL OF **CLINICAL PROBLEMS IN PEDIATRICS:** WITH ANNOTATED KEY REFERENCES—Roberts, Editor (#749842) **$15.95**

☐ MANUAL OF **NEONATAL CARE**—Cloherty & Stark (#147494) **$15.95**

☐ MANUAL OF **OBSTETRICS:** DIAGNOSIS AND THERAPY—Niswander (#611468) **$14.95**

☐ MANUAL OF **ANESTHESIA**—Snow (#802204) **$15.95**

☐ MANUAL OF **NEUROLOGIC THERAPEUTICS:** WITH ESSENTIALS OF DIAGNOSIS—Samuels, Editor (#769908) **$14.95**

☐ MANUAL OF **PSYCHIATRIC THERAPEUTICS:** PRACTICAL PHARMACOLOGY AND PSYCHIATRY—Shader, Editor (#782203) **$14.95**

☐ PATIENT CARE IN **NEUROSURGERY**—Howe (#375640) **$13.95**

☐ MANUAL OF **RHEUMATOLOGY AND OUTPATIENT ORTHOPEDIC DISORDERS:** DIAGNOSIS AND THERAPY—Beary, Christian, & Sculco (#085758) **$14.95**

☐ MANUAL OF **ALLERGY AND IMMUNOLOGY:** DIAGNOSIS AND THERAPY—Lawlor & Fischer (#516651) **$15.95**

☐ MANUAL OF **DERMATOLOGIC THERAPEUTICS:** WITH ESSENTIALS OF DIAGNOSIS, 2nd Edition—Arndt (#052809) **$14.95**

☐ MANUAL OF **OCULAR DIAGNOSIS AND THERAPY**—Pavan-Langston (#695378) **$15.95**

☐ MANUAL OF **CLINICAL PROBLEMS IN ONCOLOGY:** WITH ANNOTATED KEY REFERENCES—Portlock & Goffinet (#714240) **$13.95**

☐ MANUAL OF **NEPHROLOGY:** DIAGNOSIS AND THERAPY—Schrier (#774774) **$13.95**

☐ PATIENT CARE IN **CARDIAC SURGERY**, 3rd Edition—Behrendt & Austen (#087564) **$13.95**

☐ MANUAL OF **ACUTE RESPIRATORY CARE**—Zagelbaum & Pare, Editors (#984671) **$13.95**

☐ MANUAL OF **CLINICAL PROBLEMS IN OBSTETRICS AND GYNECOLOGY:** WITH ANNOTATED KEY REFERENCES—Rivlin, Morrison & Bates (#747645) **$15.95**

NAME ____________________

ADDRESS ____________________

CITY ____________________

STATE & ZIP ____________________

☐ **My check for $** __________ **is enclosed.** Publisher pays postage. MA, CA, NY residents please add state sales tax. All orders–please add handling charge.

☐ **Please bill me for book(s) plus postage and handling.** (Outside continental U.S.A., payment *must* accompany order.)

HANDLING CHARGE: on all orders, please add 50¢ per book, not to exceed $2.50 per total order.

T denotes a tentative price. Prices listed are Little, Brown prices, current as of April, 1982, and do not reflect the prices at which books will be sold to you by suppliers other than Little, Brown. All prices subject to change.

NO POSTAGE
NECESSARY
IF MAILED IN THE
UNITED STATES

BUSINESS REPLY MAIL
FIRST CLASS PERMIT NO. 2117 BOSTON, MA.

POSTAGE WILL BE PAID BY ADDRESSEE

LITTLE, BROWN AND COMPANY
MEDICAL DIVISION
200 WEST STREET
WALTHAM, MASSACHUSETTS 02154